PROMOTING EMOTIONAL RESILIENCE

PROMOTING EMOTIONAL RESILIENCE

Cognitive–Affective
Stress Management Training

RONALD E. SMITH
JAMES C. ASCOUGH

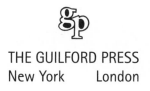

THE GUILFORD PRESS
New York   London

The authors have checked with sources believed to be reliable in their efforts
to provide information that is complete and generally in accord with the
standards of practice that are accepted at the time of publication. However,
in view of the possibility of human error or changes in behavioral, mental
health, or medical sciences, neither the authors, nor the editor and publisher,
nor any other party who has been involved in the preparation or publication
of this work warrants that the information contained herein is in every
respect accurate or complete, and they are not responsible for any errors or
omissions or the results obtained from the use of such information. Readers
are encouraged to confirm the information contained in this book with other
sources.

Library of Congress Cataloging-in-Publication Data

Names: Smith, Ronald Edward, 1940– , author. | Ascough, James C.
    (Psychologist), author.
Title: Promoting emotional resilience : cognitive–affective stress management
    training / Ronald E. Smith and James C. Ascough.
Description: New York, NY : Guilford Press, [2016] | Includes bibliographical
    references and index.
Identifiers: LCCN 2016006015 | ISBN 9781462526314 (hardcover : alk. paper)
Subjects: | MESH: Stress, Psychological—therapy | Resilience,
Psychological | Cognitive Therapy—methods
Classification: LCC RC489.C63 | NLM WM 172.4 | DDC 616.89/1425—dc23
LC record available at *http://lccn.loc.gov/2016006015*

About the Authors

Ronald E. Smith, PhD, is Professor of Psychology and Director of Clinical Training at the University of Washington, where he also has served as head of the Social Psychology and Personality Program. His major professional interests are psychological stress and coping, therapeutic assessment, and performance enhancement research and intervention. A past president of the Association for Applied Sport Psychology, Dr. Smith's publications include numerous books and more than 200 articles and book chapters, over 60 of which are in the areas of anxiety, stress, and coping.

James C. Ascough, PhD, is semi-retired and in part-time private practice at Mascouten Associates in West Lafayette, Indiana. He served on the faculties of the University of Georgia and Purdue University, and was Director of Child and Adolescent Services at Wabash Valley Hospital in West Lafayette, Indiana. Dr. Ascough's research focused on autonomic nervous system arousal, measures of affect, and models of cognitive imagery and behavior change. He is a recipient of the Sagamore of the Wabash Award, Indiana's highest state honor, for his contributions to youth mental health.

Contents

Introduction and Overview

The concept of resilience has played an increasingly prominent role in scientific and clinical discourse over the past three decades. *Resilience* first received widespread attention in the developmental psychopathology literature on longitudinal studies of children who defied the odds not only by surviving, but also by thriving—despite growing up in deprived and abusive environments where they were subjected to unremitting stress. Borne in part on the wave of positive psychology, resilience became a topic of increasing interest. Today, the concept of resilience is studied and applied across the entire lifespan. It also encompasses the ability to adapt not only to chronic stressors, but also to acute stressors of varying levels of intensity and duration.

Resilience has been operationalized in a variety of ways. Sometimes it is defined purely by the absence of negative physical or psychological consequences in the face of exposure to stressors, with little or no attention paid to factors that mediated the successful outcome. Others regard resilience as a trait that is assumed to have transituational applicability, not taking into account that people can show resilience in some situations, but not in others. Both of these definitions have their shortcomings. We favor instead an interactional process perspective. That is, we prefer to define resilience in terms of reciprocal causal links among features of the environment, individual and environmental resources that facilitate adaptation, and the types of functioning that are preserved (or even enhanced, as in the case of posttraumatic growth). This perspective takes into account the fact that resilience is likely to vary as a function of the nature of the stressor, the demands it imposes on the individual, the kinds of adaptive resources needed to cope successfully with it, and the domain of functioning that is involved, be it cognitive, emotional, or behavioral in nature. It also reflects the recognition that people are likely to be resilient to some stressors and not to others, depending on their developmental histories, idiosyncratic coping resources, and environmental supports. The intrapersonal variation seen in the process of coping and its outcomes is at odds with a conception of resilience as a stable trait, and it invites individual-level analyses to assess idiographic patterns. It also requires an assessment of the "active ingredients" of situations that are linked to successful or unsuccessful adaptations and the ability to "bounce back" in the face of adversity. Across the lifespan, new developmental tasks and life situations may create challenges that test or exceed the person's resources, resulting in differing individual trajectories of adaptation.

A substantial body of literature has now emerged on resilience and the factors that enhance or negatively impact responses to stressors. Among these factors are external influences such as a history of close relationships and a supportive social network; educational opportunities; connectedness to social institutions; an intimate relationship with a mentor, spouse or partner; and a fulfilling work environment. Personal resources include social, intellectual, and vocational skills; problem-solving ability; positive self-regard; self-efficacy and feelings of personal control; a sense of meaningfulness in life; positive affect; commitment to one's work and to others; and the ability to select and successfully apply coping skills relevant to the demands of the stressful situation. As noted above, resilience may be reflected in specific areas of cognitive, emotional, or behavioral functioning. When manifested in the emotional domain, the term *emotional resilience* may be applied.

"Emotional resilience" is defined as the ability to engage in overt and/or covert emotion self-regulation behaviors that allow the person to minimize negative affect in the face of stressful life events. Negative affect and ineffective attempts to cope with it are central underlying mechanisms of many psychological disorders and many physical ones as well. There is abundant evidence (reviewed in Chapter 1) that deficits in emotion regulation skills render people susceptible to psychological disorders in the wake of both routine stressors and extreme or traumatic events. Moreover, emotional dysregulation has a negative impact on many forms of cognitive, behavioral, and physiological functioning. From this perspective, increasing emotional resilience is a key to enhancing physical, social, and psychological well-being in a world where nobody can avoid stressful life events.

The focus of this book is on promoting emotional resilience by helping people acquire emotion-focused coping skills that enhance affective self-regulation. To this end, we put forth a brief, empirically supported coping skills program called *cognitive–affective stress management training* (CASMT). This program can be applied in either an individual or group format, to clinical populations as a treatment regimen or to nonclinical ones as a prevention program designed to enhance stress resilience and reduce the potential for future psychological disorder. Utilizing a variety of empirically supported techniques, including relaxation training, cognitive restructuring, self-instructional training, mindfulness meditation, and defusion, the program is designed to help clients develop a range of cognitive and arousal-control skills that increase emotion regulation capabilities.

Much evidence indicates that skill acquisition proceeds most effectively when people are able to practice a skill in situations that are similar to the *future* settings in which the skill will be applied. One important aspect of future encounters with stressors is the high affective arousal they are likely to elicit. As the relaxation and cognitive coping skills are being developed in CASMT, a learning-based procedure known as induced affect (IA) is used to elicit high levels of emotional arousal, and the client uses relaxation and self-selected stress-reducing self-statements to practice reducing the arousal. The program helps clients develop a combined relaxation and cognitive-based "integrated coping response" tied into the breathing cycle that can be applied to control arousal in stressful situations. The high level of arousal elicited by IA is designed to create high levels of coping self-efficacy. In addition to its skill acquisition benefits, this procedure also helps counter emotional avoidance, and it is consistent with a proposition endorsed by therapists of all persuasions that the active experiencing of emotion within the therapy room is a key component in successful outcome.

CASMT is conducted within a collaborative assessment framework in which therapists and clients work as a team, utilizing a Stress and Coping Diary to discover relations among stressful situations in clients' lives, their appraisals of those situations and of themselves, their emotional reactions, and their use of coping strategies. In the daily diary, clients report descriptions of stressful events, the feature(s) of the situation that made it stressful, and the automatic thoughts that may have led to their emotional reaction. They also generate alternative thoughts that could have changed their emotional reaction, and they report their use of various coping behaviors (e.g., relaxation techniques, rethinking the situation, practicing acceptance, seeking social support) in response to stressful situations, as well as the effectiveness of those behaviors. This diary can be done in either a paper-and-pencil format or electronically.

The procedures used in CASMT are grounded in a social–cognitive theoretical framework and in empirically supported principles and research results. Chapters 1 through 3 provide the conceptual and empirical bases of both CASMT and IA. Chapter 1 reviews research on stress, coping, and emotion regulation. Chapter 2 discusses the pivotal role of emotional experiencing in psychotherapy and describes the IA technique, which is not only an integral part of CASMT, but also a stand-alone treatment that could be applied in other forms of therapy. Empirical evidence for the applicability and efficacy of IA is also presented. Chapter 3 provides an overview of CASMT and the evidence underlying its status as an empirically supported intervention.

Chapters 4 through 9 present a detailed guide for the administration of CASMT. Designed as both a training manual and as a potential research protocol, one chapter is devoted to each of the six sessions (or phases) of the intervention. Each chapter presents the rationale and step-by-step instructions for how to administer the session, using extensive therapist–client transcripts to illustrate the procedures (and to standardize the administration for research purposes). However, the intervention can be extended beyond six sessions when needed to optimize clinical outcomes or to incorporate additional treatment components.

Appendices A and B provide practical tools needed to administer CASMT. Appendix A contains all session-related training resources for clients, including the Stress and Coping Diary and the instructional handouts for each skill, together with forms for clients' homework assignments. Appendix B contains resources for therapists' and trainers' presentations, including conceptual models of stress and the CASMT elements, a Subjective Units of Distress Scale (SUDS), and tables illustrating dysfunctional core beliefs and sample hierarchies for self-desensitization. These can be given to clients in hard-copy form during sessions or used as presentation overheads or PowerPoints. For your convenience, we have also made the reproducible forms and worksheets available online, so individual book purchasers can download and print them as needed in a convenient 8½" × 11" size. Also available is an audio recording of the muscle relaxation training exercise (in Handout A-2), which can be streamed directly from the Internet or downloaded in MP3 format. This audio track is available in two different locations: (1) on the clinician's webpage, together with the reproducible forms and worksheets (*www.guilford.com/smith8-materials*), and (2) on a webpage developed specifically for clients (*www.guilford.com/smith8-audio*). You can direct your clients to this second website to access the recordings on their own. Alternately, you may wish to download the audio track yourself and burn it onto a CD or copy it to a USB flash drive to distribute to each client. See the copyright page for the terms of use of these items.

We use the terms "therapists" and "trainers" to recognize that CASMT can be administered not only by clinicians, but also by other professionals working with clients who are dealing with stress-related issues, as well as by researchers who wish to study or evaluate the intervention. In addition to addressing the goal of contributing to the training of clinicians at all levels of professional development, from graduate students to seasoned professionals, we are also interested in encouraging more research on the treatment package and on the IA procedure. The explicit step-by-step procedures and transcripts in Chapters 3 through 9 should ensure high treatment fidelity in administering the CASMT protocol. We hope this book will achieve both the clinical and scientific goals that inspired us to write it.

CHAPTER 1

Emotion, Stress, and Coping
Implications for Intervention

Life without emotions would be bland and empty. Our subjective experiences of love, anger, fear, joy, and other emotions energize and add color to our lives. Modern psychology's focus on the study of emotion echoes a timeless fascination expressed in songs, paintings, stories, poems, and scholarly treatises. However, emotions are a two-edged sword; they can foster happiness and well-being, or they can contribute to psychological and physical dysfunction.

NEGATIVE EMOTION AND STRESS

Negative emotions such as anxiety, depression, and anger are core components in psychological stress; are involved in many physical and psychological disorders; and are the most pervasive targets of psychological interventions (Barlow, Sauer-Zavala, Carl, Bullis, & Ellard, 2014; Mennin & Fresco, 2010). Anxiety is the most prevalent form of stress response (Narrow, Rae, Robins, & Regier, 2002). Epidemiological studies reveal that nearly one in five Americans suffer from a diagnosable anxiety disorder in any given year. In more than 70% of cases, anxiety-based disorders interfere significantly with life functions or cause the person to seek medical or psychological treatment (Kessler, Chiu, Demler, & Walters, 2005). A survey of 340,000 college students who sought treatment at campus counseling centers revealed that 86.2% of them presented with anxiety or depression as their primary complaint. The survey also showed that anxiety self-referrals had increased from 39.3 to 46.9% since a similar survey in 2007. In a national survey of 150,000 entering college students, 34.6% reported feeling "overwhelmed" by schoolwork and other commitments (Higher Education Research Institute, 2015). Many other people who do not meet criteria for a mental disorder experience high levels of stress that interfere with their functioning and reduce life satisfaction.

Failure to cope successfully with stressful life events takes a significant toll on people's physical, social, and psychological well-being. Stressful life events, negative emotional responses to them, and failures to cope effectively are prime components or causal factors in a wide range of illnesses and psychological disorders (Folkman, 2011; Taylor, 2014; Zautra, 2006). In *Stress in America: Missing the Health Care Connection*, a nationwide survey of adults and teens, commissioned by the American Psychological Association (2013), the average level of life stress reported by adult respondents was 4.9 on a 10-point scale, but 20% of the adults reported stress levels of 8, 9, or 10, frequently accompanied by physical and psychological symptoms. Sixty-five percent said managing their stress is very or extremely important, but just 38% reported doing an excellent or very good job managing stressful situations and their responses to them. A sizeable proportion of respondents said that their stress level had increased in the past year, and only 17% of the high-stress respondents reported doing a good job of managing their stress. Teens reported even higher average stress levels at 5.8, and they reported similar levels of emotional and physical symptoms as the adult sample.

Nearly half (47%) in the Stress in America survey thought psychologists and other mental health providers could help with stress management, but more than half reported that they did not receive needed support from their health care provider. In a discussion of emerging public health needs, Kazdin and Blase (2011) cited the need for brief, effective stress management treatments that can be widely administered to individuals and groups for both preventive and treatment purposes as a key element in "rebooting psychotherapy" to respond to current mental health needs. It is widely accepted that helping people cope more successfully with stress would make a positive contribution to the nation's levels of physical and psychological well-being (American Psychological Association, 2013).

"Affect" is a general term that subsumes emotions (both positive and negative), moods, and stress responses (e.g., Gross, 2014b; Scherer, Schorr, & Johnstone, 2001). Contemporary developments in affective science and psychotherapy research provide a useful integrative framework for understanding and treating a wide range of psychological disorders that involve negative emotional states (e.g., Barlow et al., 2014; Mennin & Fresco, 2014).

There are seven empirically supported postulates about emotion that are acknowledged by therapists across a variety of therapeutic orientations (e.g., Barlow et al., 2014; Goldfried, 2013; Linehan, 2014; Messer, 2013; Renninger, 2013; Paivio, 2013).

1. Negative affect and ineffective attempts to cope with it are central underlying mechanisms of many (though not all) psychological disorders, and many physical ones as well.
2. Deficits in emotion regulation capabilities render people susceptible to psychological disorders in the wake of both routine stressors and extreme or traumatic events.
3. Regardless of type of therapy, clients' avoidance of emotional engagement can create an impediment to successful treatment.
4. Success in treating emotional disorders depends in part on the ability of the therapist and the treatment technique to counter emotional avoidance.
5. Active experiencing of emotion within the therapy room is a key component in successful outcome.
6. Emotional engagement often facilitates the emergence of related thoughts, memories, and action tendencies that are important aspects of the client's personality functioning.
7. Techniques are needed that can effectively activate the cognitive–affective networks, emphasized in current emotion science, which are the targets for therapeutic change.

Evidence-based interventions for developing client emotion regulation and stress management skills should be a part of every clinician's skill set. In this book, we provide just such a skill set in the form of cognitive-affective stress management training (CASMT), which addresses each of the postulates listed above. This brief six-session (or six-phase, if expanded) stress management program helps clients to access and control negative affect (particularly anxiety and anger) by applying empirically supported cognitive and somatic coping skills. In CASMT, experiencing and controlling high levels of affect are accomplished using a procedure known as "induced affect" (IA). Though developed within a behavioral framework and used in CASMT, the IA procedure can also be used in any therapeutic modality to elicit affect, or it can be used as a stand-alone treatment. We use the technique not only to achieve insights into cognitive–affective–motivational relations specific to the individual, but also to provide clients with an opportunity to rehearse previously acquired coping skills, such as somatic relaxation, adaptive cognitions, and mindfulness strategies to respond to and control affective arousal.

WHAT IS CASMT?

CASMT was initially developed as a clinical intervention of indeterminate length for the treatment of individuals presenting with high levels of anxiety and distress (Smith, 1980; Smith & Ascough, 1985). It constitutes a coping skills alternative to deconditioning treatments (i.e., systematic desensitization and extinction-based treatments such as exposure), which have exhibited little evidence of generalizing to new stressors. CASMT has also been adapted to a brief six-session group format that is described in this book. The intervention is applicable to both nonclinical and clinical populations. In addition to clinical applications, the brief manualized program has been applied successfully in a group format to a variety of nonclinical populations, including test-anxious college students (Smith & Nye, 1989), heavy college-age drinkers (Rohsenow, Smith, & Johnson, 1985), stress-ridden medical and graduate students (Chen et al., in press; Holtzworth-Munroe, Munroe, & Smith, 1985; Shoda, Wilson, Chen, Gilmore, & Smith, 2013), military officer candidates undergoing stressful training (Jacobs, Smith, Fiedler, & Link, 2012), and athletes and coaches whose performances were negatively affected by stress (Crocker, Alderman, & Smith, 1988; Smith, 1984; Watson, 1998; Ziegler, Klinzing, & Williamson, 1982).

Although CASMT differs in some important respects from other coping skills programs, such as self-control desensitization (Goldfried, 1971), stress inoculation training (Meichenbaum, 1977, 1985) and anxiety management training (Suinn & Richardson, 1971), and the self-guided multimedia Stress Management and Resilience Training for Optimal Performance (SMART-OP) program (Rose et al., 2013), it also has some notable similarities. Like these interventions, the CASMT program combines a number of empirically supported clinical techniques into an emotion self-regulation intervention. The current version of CASMT is also informed by recent theoretical and empirical developments in the burgeoning area of emotion regulation discussed later in this chapter; the result is the recent addition of several empirically supported training elements and client resource materials.

Although the conceptual and treatment models for CASMT predate Mischel and Shoda's (1995) cognitive–affective processing system (CAPS) model (described below), the CAPS metamodel is highly compatible with the CASMT program and has served to guide recent developments in collaborative assessment as well as our current research agenda (Chen et al., in press; Shoda et al., 2013; Smith et al., 2011). The CASMT program focuses on associative links among appraisals, affects, and self-regulatory competencies. Specifically, the program is designed to help people discover and modify dysfunctional appraisals that cause needless distress, acquire empirically supported cognitive and somatic coping skills, and thereby gain increased control over their affective responses. The process is designed to enhance stress-resilience by altering the demands-to-resources stress equation and by increasing the client's "learned resourcefulness." In essence, CASMT combines the principles derived from stress and coping research with the affect regulation methods described later in this chapter. It therefore addresses the goal of the current dissemination-implementation movement to "synthesize existing knowledge about evidence-based practices into modular components and tailor them to the implementation context" (Shoham et al., 2014, p. 10).

Though clearly not as comprehensive as some recently developed treatment packages, the CASMT protocol is more narrowly focused and, at six sessions, is appreciably shorter than the 15–25 sessions required by other empirically supported interventions, such as Barlow et al.'s (2014) unified protocol; Leahy, Tirch, & Napolitano's (2011) emotional schema therapy; Berking and Schwarz's (2014) affect regulation training; Mennin and Fresco's (2014) emotion regulation therapy; and other stress management programs that average 10 or more sessions (van Dixhoorn & White, 2005). Nonetheless, given its empirical support (summarized in Chapter 2), CASMT can help address the widely articulated need for brief interventions that provide economical treatment and prevention programs to the many people with stress-related problems who receive no assistance from the current health care system (American Psychological Association, 2013). To respond to today's mental health needs, brief, effective treatments that can be widely disseminated are needed for both treatment and prevention of stress-related disorders (Kazdin & Blase, 2011). Such interventions are consistent with current National Institute of Mental Health priorities that emphasize "reach"—that is, that address specific mechanisms of psychological disorders in a highly focused fashion, that can be disseminated at a population level as part of a stepped-care approach, and that can be administered in either a clinical context or in an educational or group format (Insel, 2012; Insel & Cuthbert, 2013; Onken, Carroll, Shoham, Cuthbert, & Riddle, 2014).

CASMT occupies a niche with several other brief and efficacious interventions focused on specific disorders, such as a one-session extended exposure treatment for specific phobias (Ollendick & Davis, 2013; Öst, 1989), a five-session treatment for panic disorder (Otto et al., 2012), and brief motivational interviewing treatment for addictive disorders (Miller & Rollnick, 2002). As Kazdin and Blase (2011) point out, brief interventions, whether they are stand-alone treatments or techniques that augment existing empirically supported therapies, can have a positive impact by addressing the mental health needs that threaten to overwhelm the traditional treatment delivery system. If a cost-effective intervention can be disseminated to enough people, even small outcome effect sizes can translate into large societal benefits.

As noted earlier, there exists a large untreated stress-ridden population that is on its way to developing clinical disorders in the absence of preventive intervention (Lahey, 2009; Kendler, Gatz, Gardner, & Pederse, 2006). In nonclinical populations, high negative affective reactivity to daily stressors predicts the development of clinically significant anxiety and depressive disorders in future years (Charles, Piazza, Mogle, Sliwinski, & Almeida, 2013). The lower rungs of a stepped-care approach using brief interventions can help reduce this trajectory toward psychological disorders.

In the remainder of this chapter, we review literature that is relevant to the emotion regulation interventions discussed in the remainder of the book. We review key concepts of emotion, the relation of emotion to other psychological phenomena, and the role of emotion in psychopathology. We then survey current knowledge about stress, coping, and emotion regulation and the relevance of this body of theory and research to clinical practice. In Chapter 2, we provide an overview of CASMT intervention strategies and the empirical support for the program. In Chapter 3, we address the topic of affect elicitation in therapy and review theoretical principles and techniques that have been employed in the service of affect elicitation and emotional processing. We focus in particular on the IA procedure, how it is employed in psychotherapy and coping skills training to elicit and control affective arousal, and how it has been successfully applied in a variety of clinical and nonclinical populations. Chapters 4 through 9 present session-by-session guidelines for conducting CASMT with either a group or an individual. End-of-book appendices provide all of the assessment and training materials used in the intervention.

EMOTION: COMPONENTS AND PROCESSES

As noted above, emotion is one type of affective response, distinct from moods in being more transitory and from stress in being either positive or negative in nature, rather than primarily negative. Psychologist James Averill (1980) found more than 550 words in the English language that refer to various positive and negative emotional states. We surely do not have 550 different emotions, but the emotions we do have share four common features.

1. Emotions are responses to external or internal stimuli that become the focus of attention (Gross, 2014b). Attentional processes

are biased toward the detection of stimuli that have survival implications or are relevant to a currently salient goal or motivational state or to an already-existing emotional response (Joorman & Siemer, 2014). Attentional biases have been found in a variety of emotional disorders (Mathews & MacLeod, 2005).

2. Stimulus input triggers *appraisal* of these stimuli, which gives the situation its perceived meaning and significance (Arnold, 1960; Gross, 2014b; Lazarus, 1991a). These appraisals need not be linguistic in nature; they can be represented within a number of subcortical and cortical brain structures that permit varying levels of conscious awareness (Kihlstrom, 2008; LeDoux, 2000).

3. Our bodies respond physiologically to our appraisal of the stimuli. The *physiological response* can involve an array of biological systems both within and outside of the brain (Ochsner & Gross, 2014). We may become physically aroused as in fear, joy, or anger, or we may experience decreased arousal, as in contentment or dysphoria. Situational features help define the meaning of the arousal (Lazarus, 1991a). As arousal occurs, it acquires stimulus properties and feeds back into the ongoing appraisal process. For example, internal cues from an intense arousal response may result in a more negative reappraisal of the situation or of one's capacity to deal with it. Behavioral signs of intense arousal may also serve as social stimuli that affect the behavior of others, thus changing the eliciting situation.

4. Emotions include *action tendencies*. Some are expressive behaviors (e.g., exhibiting surprise, smiling with joy, crying) that are innate, but also subject to cultural display rules. Others are instrumental behaviors—that is, ways of doing something about the stimulus that aroused the emotion (e.g., studying for an anxiety-arousing test, fighting back in self-defense, running away). Some theorists (e.g., Frijda, 1986) assume that each of the basic emotions has its own innate action tendency shaped by evolutionary forces (e.g., attack in anger, avoidance or escape in fear, withdrawal from activity in depression).

Emotion is thus a dynamic ongoing process of reciprocal causal relations involving the situation, the person, and the person's behavior (Bandura, 1986; Lazarus, 1991a). Moreover, emotion is not only a biopsychological network unto itself, but it is also embedded in broader networks that involve other important psychological phenomena, including cognitive, motivational, behavioral, and personality factors (Bower, 1981; Mischel & Shoda, 1995; Rumelhart & McClelland, 1986). In this respect, emotions operate both as stimuli that activate other processes and as responses from other psychological processes, such as self-schemas (Baldwin, 1999). They thus comprise a central hub for psychological functioning. Most contemporary emotion theorists acknowledge functional links between motives and emotions (e.g., Gross, 2014b; Lazarus, 1991a, b; Scherer et al., 2001). Lazarus (1991b), for example, insisted that there is *always* a link between motives and emotions, because we react emotionally only when our motives and goals are gratified, threatened, or frustrated. Emotional reactions are especially strong when an experience is pertinent to goals that are very important to us. Each emotion, therefore, has its own "core relational theme," appraisal pattern, and innate action tendency.

Table 1.1 summarizes Lazarus's (1991b, p. 826) proposed relational themes that link specific motives with emotions. These relational themes are central concerns in psychotherapy as therapists and clients work on important client agendas. Successful therapy occurs when clients are empowered to pursue meaningful positive goals and are unshackled by impediments, including fears and self-defeating behavioral tendencies. Moreover, emotional reactions act as a window through which one can gain insights into important motivational factors. This premise is reflected in the importance ascribed to emotional expression in most therapeutic orientations, and it is the underlying theme for this book's focus on affect elicitation in psychological treatments.

Emotion plays an important role in virtually every theory of personality. For example, today's cognitive-behavioral therapy (CBT) movement shares a close kinship with social-cognitive personality theory (Shoda & Smith, 2004). In the CAPS model of personality functioning advanced by Mischel and Shoda (1995), emotions play a prominent role because of their associative links with four other psychological processes: appraisals, expectancies and beliefs, goals and values, and cognitive-behavioral competencies and self-regulatory skills. As in other network models, CAPS units can have either excitatory or inhibitory associations with other units, creating distinctively different personality structures. This dynamically organized personality system interacts continuously with the social world in which it functions, generating distinctive patterns of behavior that can differ markedly across different situations.

Entry into the personality system at the level of affect can be an important means of understanding the person's idiographic system of cognitions, memories, and motives. For example, self-schemas activated by a particular encoding can create specific sensitive areas or emotional vulnerabilities that contribute to psychological disturbances (Leahy et al., 2011). Finally, many forms of therapy are directed at the improvement of self-regulation competencies, including emotion regulation capabilities (e.g., Barlow, Allen, & Choate, 2004; Berking & Schwarz, 2014; Mennin & Fresco, 2014). Because of its heuristic and explanatory value, the CAPS

TABLE 1.1. Core Relational Themes Underlying Basic Emotions, According to R. S. Lazarus

Emotion	Relational theme
Fear	Perceived threat of imminent harm
Anxiety	Facing an uncertain threat
Guilt	Personal violation of a moral standard
Shame	Failure to live up to idealized standards
Sadness	Perception of an irrevocable loss
Depression	Complex themes relating to loss, shame, guilt, hopelessness, self-deprecation
Envy	Desire for what someone else has
Jealousy	Combination of anger and envy themes
Relief	Departure of an imminent threat
Happiness	Perceived progress toward or achievement of a prized goal or object
Pride	Ego enhancement from attaining a prized object or accomplishment
Disgust	Exposure to a revolting object or act by another
Hope	Fearing a negative outcome but yearning for a more positive one
Love	Desiring or experiencing affection for another
Compassion	Vicarious suffering and desire to help

Note. Based on Lazarus (1991b).

metamodel is increasingly being applied to clinical topics (e.g., Cervone, Shadel, Smith, & Fiori, 2006; Freitas & Downey, 1998; Huprich & Bornstein, 2007; Rhadigan & Huprich, 2012; Shoda & Smith, 2004; Shoda et al., 2013).

POSITIVE AND NEGATIVE EMOTIONS: STATES AND DISPOSITIONS

Like other psychological processes, emotions have important adaptive functions, many of which have evolutionary origins (Ochsner & Gross, 2014; Scherer, Schorr, & Johnstone, 2001). Some emotions are part of an emergency arousal system that increases the chances of survival by energizing, directing, and sustaining adaptive behaviors. The most basic of these behavioral tendencies, seen in virtually all species, is fighting, freezing, or fleeing when confronted by threat. The physiological arousal that is so central to the emotions of anger and fear energizes and intensifies such behaviors.

Positive and negative emotions have different adaptive functions (Fredrickson, 1998). Evolutionary survival pressures have sculpted negative emotions to *narrow* attention and action tendencies so that the organism can respond to a threatening situation with a focused set of responses. In contrast, positive emotions usually arise under conditions of safety and goal attainment in which high physiological arousal is not needed. Rather than narrowing attention and behavior tendencies, positive emotions such as interest, joy, contentment, and love broaden our thinking and behavior so that we explore, consider new ideas, try out new ways to achieve goals, play, and savor what we have. In these ways, positive emotions also are highly adaptive for humans.

The distinction between positive and negative emotions has strong empirical support. Factor analytic studies, whether involving affective state measures collected over time or trait measures that ask how one generally feels, consistently reveal statistically independent dimensions that have been labeled "positive affect" (PA), including such feelings as energetic, happy, relaxed, and optimistic, and "negative affect" (NA), which encompasses fear, anger, and sadness (Tellegen, Watson, & Clark, 1999). Unless conflicting emotions are being simultaneously experienced, people's momentary emotions typically fall along a single dimension featuring PA at one end and NA at the other (Russell & Carroll, 1999).

The majority of emotional problems involve inappropriate levels, duration, or modulation of NA such as anxiety, depression, and anger (Barlow et al., 2014). As a disorder of negative affect, anxiety involves experiences of tension, physiological hyperarousal, worry, concentration disruption, and negative self-appraisals. In addition, it is an emotional marker for Gray's (1991) NA-related behavioral avoidance system of retreat from threat. Depression involves not only NA (typically sadness), but also a marked reduction in the capacity to experience PA (Clark & Watson, 1991). Like anxiety and depression, anger loads strongly on the NA dimension, but it also has a unique property lacking in the other two emotions: namely, a disposition toward approaching and engaging the offending object, presumably reflecting the joint operation of Gray's (1991) behavioral approach system (Harmon-Jones, 2003).

Other disorders also represent variations in NA and PA. Emotion dysregulation, including marked affective instability in both NA and PA, is especially pronounced in borderline personality disorder (Linehan, 1993; Neacsiu, Bohus, & Linehan, 2014). Among the many maladaptive behaviors linked to attempts to downregulate negative emotions and/or upregulate positive emotions are substance abuse and eating disorders (Kober, 2014). However, in contrast to disorders that involve high levels of NA, psychopathy is marked by low baseline levels of affect, contributing to a lack of capacity to experience anticipatory anxiety or guilt (or to experience empathic emotion) that would inhibit acting out in most people, thereby resulting in dysfunctional impulsive behaviors (Raine, 2008). Finally, although PA is more generally associated with positive adjustment than is NA, one notable exception exists in manic reactions, where unbridled energy, optimism, and faulty judgments regarding the long-term consequences of impulsive approach behaviors can have dire consequences (Meyer & Baur, 2009).

Neuroticism (Negative Affectivity) as a Target for Intervention

PA and NA have dispositional as well as state properties. The disposition to experience frequent and intense NA states in response to threat, frustration, or loss has been termed "neuroticism" (Eysenck, 1947; McCrae & Costa, 2003). Its psychometric markers include such terms as "anxiety," "worry," "depression," "sadness," "vulnerability," "irritability," "anger," and "negative self-consciousness." In contemporary personality research, neuroticism is regarded as a global, transculturally consistent dispositional construct and is a prominent component (along with extraversion, conscientiousness, agreeableness, and openness to experience) in the five-factor model (FFM) of normal personality functioning (McCrae & Costa, 2003). At the extremes of the dimension, neuroticism also involves the construal of the world as dangerous and threatening and of oneself as incapable of coping with the challenges it presents. Current conceptualizations of emotional disorders view neuroticism as the major dispositional variable underlying the development and maintenance of anxiety, depression, and other NA disorders, as well as the common or core factor in the high levels of comorbidity observed among the emotional disorders (Weinstock & Whisman, 2006). This personality variable figures prominently in the dimensional emphasis in the *Diagnostic and Statistical Manual of Mental Disorders, Fifth Edition* (DSM-5; American Psychiatric Association, 2013), and it has therefore become a prime target for intervention (e.g., Barlow et al., 2014). Successful treatment of neuroticism implies, in part, the ability to gain regulatory control over NA by acquiring effective coping skills.

There are very good reasons to target neuroticism, given that it has been established as an important factor in both mental and physical health. In a meta-analysis involving 33 population-based samples, high effect sizes exceeding 1.0 were found for elevated neuroticism in mood disorders, anxiety disorders, somatoform disorders, eating disorders, and schizophrenia (Malouff, Thorsteinsson, & Schutte, 2006). Medium effect sizes have been found for associations between neuroticism and border-line, avoidant, and dependent personality disorders (Saulsman & Page, 2004). In a prospective study involving more than 20,000 participants with no previous history of major depression, each standard deviation in neuroticism scores was associated with a 31% increase in the likelihood of developing a major depressive disorder over the next 25-year period (Kendler et al., 2006). Highly elevated risk for future suicide attempts (Fergusson, Woodward, & Horwood, 2000) and for developing schizophrenia (van Os & Jones, 2001) has also been found in individuals with high neuroticism scores. Finally, in a daily diary study with a nonclinical sample, levels of daily NA and affective reactivity to daily stressors predicted self-reported anxiety and depressive disorders 10 years later (Charles et al., 2013). The combined estimated 12-month prevalence of psychological disorders shown to be strongly or moderately related to neuroticism may exceed 20% of the U.S. population (Narrow et al., 2002; Lahey, 2009).

High levels of chronic NA are associated with other adverse life outcomes as well, including low marital satisfaction and future separation and divorce, poor occupational success, and low levels of subjective well-being in both clinical and nonclinical populations (Lahey, 2009; Ro & Clark, 2013). Importantly in terms of our previous discussion of life stress, individuals high in neuroticism are more prone to negative psychological, physical, and behavioral outcomes when they encounter stressful life events, and they react more strongly to such events than do low-NA individuals (Vogeltanz & Hecker, 1999).

In addition to its negative relation to psychological well-being, neuroticism is a risk factor for physical health outcomes, including lowered longevity (Sareen, Cox, & Asmundson, 2005; Smith & MacKenzie, 2006). Even in nonclinical populations, neuroticism is associated with increased risk of illness, such as cardiovascular disease (Suls & Bunde, 2005), asthma (Huovinen, Kaprio, & Koskenvuo, 2001), irritable bowel syndrome (Spiller, 2007), and atopic eczema (Buske-Kirschbaum, Geiben, & Hellhammer, 2001). It is also associated with a heightened tendency to engage in health-compromising behaviors, such as smoking, drug and alcohol use (Malouff et al., 2006), and unprotected sex (Hoyle, Fejfar, & Miller, 2000). Given the associations of neuroticism with reduced physical and psychological well-being, together with the personal and societal costs involved in its negative outcomes and their treatment, Lahey (2009) has argued persuasively that neuroticism is a major public health issue that requires attention at both the prevention and intervention levels. Barlow et al. (2014) have targeted their unified protocol to the treatment of emotional disorders and the reduction of neuroticism. In like manner, the techniques presented in this book are designed to decrease negative emotional overreactivity to stressful events through the development of emotion regulation skills.

STRESS AND COPING

As noted above, "emotion" and "stress" are closely related affective concepts. Emotion is a broader construct because it involves both PA and NA states, whereas stress (when discussed as a mind–body response) involves only NA states (Gross, 2014b; Lazarus & Folkman, 1984). According to Lazarus, "The concept of emotion includes that of stress, and both are subject to appraisal and coping theory" (1993, p. 12).

The concept of stress has been a focus of scientific interest and research for many decades in psychology, medicine, psychiatry, and other disciplines, and the term has been used in several different ways. Various theorists have treated stress as a stimulus, as a response, or as a process that involves an interaction between the situation and the individual.

The first (stimulus) usage refers to situations that tax the physical and/or psychological capabilities of the individual. The focus here is on the balance between the demands of the situation and the personal and environmental resources available to the individual. Situations are likely to be labeled as *stressors* when the demands test or exceed the resources of the person. Life event scales (e.g., Holmes & Rahe, 1967; Sarason, Johnson, & Siegel, 1978) are often used to operationally define stress in stimulus terms.

In the second use of the term, stress refers to cognitive, affective, and behavioral responses to a stressor. This conception of stress was popularized in the work of Walter Cannon (1932), Hans Selye (1956), and Harold G. Wolff (1953), all of who treated stress (or in Selye's case, *distress*) as an organized pattern of physiological responses to noxious stimulation. Clearly, these two uses of the term are not synonymous, since people may vary considerably in how "stressful" they find the same situation.

The third and most comprehensive model of stress combines the stimulus and response conceptions into a transactional process model that involves reciprocal, recursive transactions among the person, the person's behavior, and the environment, the latter used broadly to refer to both external and internally generated stimuli (e.g., Lazarus & Folkman, 1984). Stress involves a subset of negative emotional responses to threats to well-being; thus the concept of stress aligns closely with prevailing theories of emotion. Although anxiety, anger, and other emotional states involving physiological arousal are the emotions most often included under the umbrella of stress, the stress response can be broadened to include the entire range of negative or aversive emotional states, including guilt, shame, and depression, which constitute the more global concept of "distress" (Lazarus, 1991a).

A Transactional Model of Stress

Derived from the contributions of several theorists, including Richard S. Lazarus (1966), Stanley Schachter (1966), Magda Arnold (1970), and Albert Ellis (1962), the model of stress shown in Figure 1.1 emphasizes relations among cognition, physiological responses, and behavior. This model has four major elements: (1) the situational demands; (2) the person's cognitive appraisals of the situation, his or her ability to cope with it, its possible consequences, and the personal meaning ascribed to the consequences should they occur; (3) physiological arousal responses; and (4) instrumental and coping behaviors. As in the case of emotion in general, personality and motivational variables are assumed to influence each of the four primary components.

Situational Demands

The stimuli that constitute the situation may be either external or internal in origin. Although one ordinarily thinks of affect as being elicited

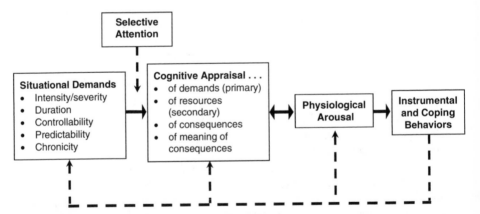

FIGURE 1.1. A mediational and recursive model of stress involving reciprocal relations among (1) the situation; (2) the person's cognitive appraisal of the situation, his or her ability to cope with it, and its possible consequences; (3) physiological arousal responses; and (4) instrumental and coping behaviors. Personality and motivational variables can influence each of the four primary components, and behavioral responses can alter any of the previous components in the model. Adapted with permission of the author from Smith (1993).

by external situations, internal cues in the form of thoughts, images, or memories may also be stimuli that elicit a stress response. Whatever the exact nature of the situation, it involves an imbalance between the demands of it and the resources at hand. This imbalance taxes the coping resources of the person and threatens his or her well-being or goals in some fashion.

As shown in Figure 1.1, stressors can differ in a number of ways that affect their capacity to generate stress responses. One dimension of differentiation is intensity or severity. Intensity or severity of stressors can range from the micro level, such as minor inconveniences and annoyances, to the macro level of major events, such as the death of a loved one or a serious illness. The most severe stressors are catastrophic events that affect large numbers of people. In addition to intensity or severity, several other characteristics of stressors have been identified as important, as shown in Figure 1.1. In general, events over which the person has little or no perceived control, which occur suddenly and unpredictably, and which impact a person over a long period of time seem to take the greatest toll on physical and psychological well-being (Lazarus & Folkman, 1984; Taylor, 2014).

Cognitive Appraisals

Cognitive appraisal processes are of critical importance in the stress response. Although clients (and people in general) typically view their emotions as direct responses to situations, in most instances situations exert their effects through the intervening influence of thoughts and beliefs that create the psychological reality to which they respond. These effects occur in part through selectively attending to particular features of situations—features that then become the "active ingredients" or "hot buttons" to which individuals are particularly reactive (Shoda & Smith, 2004; Shoda et al., 2013). In a social situation, for example, one person may be especially attuned to cues of disapproval, whereas another may be selectively vigilant to indicators of disrespect. Thus, the same "objective" or nominal situation may elicit anxiety in the first person and anger in the second because of attentional biases and differential reactivity to the array of cues that is present to both people. Distinctive feature reactivity profiles or stress signatures have been demonstrated in CAPS-inspired research (Shoda et al., 2013).

As shown in Figure 1.1, the nature and intensity of stress responses are a function of at least four different appraisal elements, all of which are frequent therapeutic targets, particularly in cognitive therapy. The first (termed "primary appraisal" by Lazarus, 1966, 1991a) involves a construal of the demands and their relevance to the person's well-being.

Stress appraisals include judgments of harm or loss, threat, and challenge. *Harm or loss* relates to the consequences of previous transactions, whereas *threat* concerns losses or harms that are anticipated. This appraisal is the cognitive representation of the demands element in the situational component of the model.

The second appraisal element corresponds to Lazarus's (1966; 1991a) process of secondary appraisal in which the person evaluates the extent to which he or she has the resources to cope with the perceived demands. Resources may be capabilities, knowledge, social support, or tangible ones such as money. In a related social-cognitive theoretical model, Bandura (1997) emphasized the role of self-efficacy expectancies in effective behavior.

The third appraisal is the construal of the nature and likelihood of potential consequences if the demands are not met. Obviously, strong negative consequences that are deemed highly likely to occur have the greatest capacity to arouse negative emotional responses. Worrisome rumination about the possibility of threatening outcomes (sometimes specific and sometimes nonspecific) is a significant factor in generating and maintaining anxiety states (Barlow, 2004; Borkovec, Alcaine, & Behar, 2004). Worry has also been shown to be strongly associated with stress responses in nonclinical populations (Szabo, 2011).

The fourth appraisal element relates to the personal meaning of one's success or failure to cope adequately with the demands. Again, this set of appraisals is strongly linked to the person's motivational structure and commitments—that is, to what has personal meaning and importance. The greater the strength of a commitment, the more vulnerable the person is to a perceived threat in that area (Lazarus, 1991a, b). For a person whose self-esteem is strongly tied to successful achievement, anticipated or actual failure can be devastating. Individual differences in the nature and strength of commitments can result in completely different appraisals and emotional responses.

Excessive or inappropriate stress responses can result from errors or distortions in any of these appraisal elements, and such distortions are prime targets for cognitive therapy (A. T. Beck, 1976). Thus, a person with low self-confidence or self-efficacy (but objectively adequate resources) may misappraise the balance between demands and resources as "too much for me to handle" so that negative consequences seem imminent. Misappraisals in the other direction can cause one to underestimate the demands and inhibit the engagement of coping responses. Likewise, appraisal errors may occur in relation to the subjective likelihood and/or valence of the potential consequences, as when a person anticipates that the worst is sure to happen. Finally, personal belief systems and internalized standards influence the ultimate meaning of the situation for the person. For example, an internalized belief that self-worth depends on success will attach a different and more urgent meaning to performance outcomes than will occur for someone who can divorce self-worth from success or failure. Finally, as Ellis (1962), A. T. Beck (1976), and other cognitive theorists have noted, many people are victimized by irrational "should" and "ought" beliefs concerning the meaning and importance of success and social approval, and such beliefs predispose them to inappropriate stress reactions (Strauman et al., 2013).

Physiological Arousal

The third component of the stress model shown in Figure 1.1 is physiological arousal. It is related in a bidirectional or reciprocal fashion to the appraisal processes described above. Physiological responses can differ along a number of dimensions, including frequency, intensity, and duration. Whether and to what extent people react with emotional arousal depends largely on mediational cognitive responses. When appraisal indicates the threat of harm or danger, physiological arousal occurs as part of the mobilization of resources to deal with the situation. Arousal, in turn, provides feedback concerning the intensity of the emotion being experienced, thereby contributing to the process of appraisal and reappraisal (Lazarus & Folkman, 1984). Thus, a person who becomes aware of somatic cues of increasing arousal may appraise the situation as one that is very stressful or upsetting, thereby creating a spiraling acceleration of emotional arousal, as occurs in panic disorders (Barlow, 2004). Conversely, a person who experiences evidence of low physiological arousal in a potentially stressful situation is likely to appraise the situation as less threatening and as one with which he or she can cope successfully, thereby enhancing self-efficacy and reducing anxiety (Bandura, 1997).

Instrumental and Coping Behaviors

The fourth component of the model consists of the behavioral responses to the situation. There are countless ways that people can respond to a stressor. Many different classes of coping strategies, some adaptive and others generally maladaptive, have been described (e.g., Aldao, Nolen-Hoeksema, & Schweizer, 2010; Carver, Scheier, & Weintraub, 1989; Holahan & Moos, 1986; John & Eng, 2014). One popular classification divides coping strategies into three categories: problem-focused coping, emotion-focused coping, and seeking social support. Problem-focused coping strategies involve attempts to confront and directly deal with the demands of the situation, or to change the situation so that it is no longer stressful. Emotion-focused coping strategies are efforts to manage the emotional responses that result from encountering the situation. A third class of coping strategies involves seeking social support, that is, turning to others for assistance and emotional support in times of stress. Social support can come in a variety of forms, including informational support, tangible support, and emotional support. In psychotherapy, a positive client–therapist relationship can be a potent source of emotional support.

Research on Coping Strategies

Although it is widely recognized that coping with stress is situation-specific and that what is effective in one situation may not be effective in another, researchers have nonetheless assessed the general effectiveness of various coping strategies. These studies have also helped to identify some of the stressor and person characteristics that influence coping efficacy.

Using a diary methodology, Holahan and Moos (1986) tracked coping episodes and psychological outcomes in more than 400 adults over a 1-year period, asking respondents to rate the extent to which they used a variety of different coping strategies. Although people typically reported using several coping methods in dealing with a given stressor, problem-focused coping methods and seeking social support were most often associated with favorable outcomes. In contrast, emotion-focused strategies that involved denial, avoiding feelings, denigrating or blaming oneself, or taking things out on other people predicted less satisfactory outcomes.

In children and adults and across many different types of stressors, customary use of emotion-focused strategies that involve avoidance, denial, and wishful thinking are related to poorer outcomes (Aldwin, 2007; Snyder, 2001). Problem-focused coping, positive reappraisal of demands, and infusing ordinary events with positive meaning (e.g., focusing on the enjoyment derived from an interaction with a friend) helps generate positive emotional responses that counter distress created by life stressors (Tugade, 2011). Adaptive emotion-focused strategies, such as identifying and changing irrational negative thinking and learning relaxation skills to control arousal, can reduce stress responses without avoiding or distorting reality, and they can be effective ways of dealing with stress (Gross, 1998; John & Eng, 2014). Physical exercise also has well-established stress-reduction effects (Taylor, 2014).

Despite the evidence generally favoring problem-focused coping, attempts to change the situation are not always the most adaptive way to cope with a stressor. Problem-focused coping works best in situations where there is some prospect of controlling the stressor, given that the coping behaviors are well executed (Lazarus & Folkman, 1984; Park, Armeli, & Tennen, 2004). However, there are other situations where situational control is absent or limited. In those instances, problem-focused coping may be ineffective and may actually worsen the situation. Instead, emotion-focused coping may be the most adaptive approach we can take, for although we cannot master the situation, we may be able to prevent or control maladaptive emotional responses to it (Auerbach, 1989). Likewise, acceptance can be a preferred strategy in such situations (Berking & Schwarz, 2014). Of course, in the long run, total reliance on emotion-focused coping can be counterproductive if it prevents people from acting to change situations in which they actually *do* have control.

Although we have stressed the context-dependent nature of coping and its outcomes, we should expect not only variability but also some degree of transituational consistency in coping strategy use (Lazarus & Folkman, 1984). Although dispositional preference measures (e.g., "How do you generally cope?") are poor predictors of coping in specific situations, distinctive patterns of coping preferences do emerge from single-event reports when aggregated over time (Ptacek, Smith, Raffety, & Lindgren, 2008).

Research with dispositional coping measures that ask people how they *typically* cope with stressful situations they encounter (as opposed to assessing coping strategies within discrete situations) has revealed differential relations of coping strategies with measures of NA and maladjustment. As would be predicted from the laboratory studies described above as well as clinical research, habitual use of strategies such as rumination, suppression, denial, and avoidance has been associated with maladaptive outcomes, whereas problem-focused coping, reappraisal, acceptance, and mindfulness have been linked to generally positive outcomes (e.g., Aldao et al., 2010; Goldin, McRae, Ramel, & Gross, 2007; Hoffman, Heering, Sawyer, & Asnaani, 2009; Kring & Sloan, 2010). However, in both community and clinical populations, positive correlations between putatively maladaptive strategies and psychopathology symptoms such as anxiety and depression have been larger than the negative correlations found for adaptive strategies such as reappraisal and acceptance. Across anxiety, depression, eating disorders, and substance abuse disorders, meta-analytic results revealed stronger effect sizes for rumination, suppression, and avoidance than for reappraisal and acceptance. Of the adaptive strategies, problem solving exhibited a larger positive effect size with adaptive outcomes than did reappraisal and acceptance (Aldao et al., 2010). However, in a community sample, Aldao and Hoeksema (2012) found that adaptive strategies exhibited positive relations with adjustment only in people who also reported high levels of maladaptive strategy use, suggesting that adaptive strategies can serve a compensatory function, helping to blunt or cancel out the negative effects of maladaptive strategies. This finding indicates the importance of teaching people adaptive coping skills, such as those that are the focus of CASMT. Such skills can help counteract the use of previously acquired maladaptive coping strategies, eventually replacing them as the adaptive skills are executed more effectively and are reinforced by positive outcomes.

Approaches to Stress Reduction

We now come to the model's implications for clinical practice. In stress theory and research, the term "coping" includes in part the concept of emotion regulation in emotion research, but it focuses on the downregulation of negative emotional states. Emotion regulation, however, involves upregulation of PA as well as downregulation of NA. Lazarus and Folkman have described the process of coping with stress as "constantly changing cognitive and behavioral efforts to manage specific demands that are appraised as taxing or exceeding the resources of the person" (1984, p. 141).

The process model of stress shown in Figure 1.1 suggests a variety of ways in which stress can be reduced. In a general sense, any of the model's components can be a target for action. Thus, coping and interventions can be directed at the situational, cognitive, physiological, or behavioral components of stress, as well as at the broader level of the personality and motivational variables that are assumed to influence the four basic components. It is important to recognize, however, that measures taken to modify any one of the components will almost certainly affect other components as well.

Problem Solving for Situational Demands

At the situational level, changes in certain features of the environment can dramatically alter its capacity to generate stress. Problem-focused coping may involve attempts to reduce demands, to increase resources, or both. Among clinical interventions, training in problem solving is typically directed at dealing with situational demands by generating alternative solutions, choosing among them, removing obstacles to goal attainment, and acting (D'Zurilla & Nezu, 2007). In work settings, stress reduction interventions can be directed at changing the physical environment (e.g., through noise reduction or greater privacy), the work requirements (e.g., by decreasing workloads), or the interpersonal environment (e.g., through changes in leadership or human relations training of supervisors and coworkers). Interventions for couples can help create a less conflictual setting as new relational skills are learned.

Clearly, the environment influences behavior, but the environment is also influenced and sometimes transformed by behavioral changes.

Problem-focused coping can also involve acquisition of social, problem-solving, or work skills to increase personal resources and reduce demands. Acquiring parenting skills can reduce problematic behaviors in noncompliant children that create family stress. Social skills training can increase the resources that socially anxious people can bring to bear in social situations, reducing social avoidance and the stresses of anxiety and loneliness. Assertiveness training can help create a more benign and less exploitative interpersonal environment. Besides affecting the situational component, behavioral changes affect future situational appraisals and self-efficacy expectancies.

Modifying Cognitions and Controlling Physiological Arousal

Intervention strategies can be directed at modifying cognitive responses. This is a key component in the model, since other model components are ultimately mediated by or exert their effects through the appraisal processes (Lazarus & Folkman, 1984). Even if the situation cannot be changed, people can be trained to discover, challenge, and change the appraisal elements that are, in actuality, generating their stress responses. They can also use covert self-instructional strategies to focus on task-relevant cues and engage in goal-directed behavior.

Second, stress can be reduced at the level of physiological arousal. Arousal-control skills such as muscle relaxation and meditation can be highly effective in reducing affective arousal and preventing it from interfering with performance. These cognitive and arousal-control interventions are the focus of the emotion-focused coping techniques presented in this book. We now turn to a review of the research on emotion regulation strategies and their effects, including cognitive reappraisal and control of physiological arousal. This literature has clear implications for evidence-based practice.

The Evidence on Emotion–Focused Coping Strategies

Although teaching problem-focused coping strategies is an appropriate aim of treatment and can easily be combined with training in adaptive emotion-focused skills, CASMT has a fundamentally emotion-focused treatment orientation. Over the past decade, emotion regulation has been the focus of much research (extensively reviewed in Gross, 2014a) and intervention (e.g., Barlow et al., 2014; Leahy et al., 2011; Mennin & Fresco, 2014). The study of emotion-focused strategies by emotion regulation researchers has produced a wealth of information concerning their range of application and the conditions under which certain strategies are most likely to yield positive or negative outcomes (Webb, Miles, &

Sheeran, 2012). Such information provides an empirical basis for developing coping skills interventions.

Much theoretical and empirical attention has focused on six strategies for the self-regulation of NA: attentional deployment (especially distraction), suppression, reappraisal, acceptance, mindfulness, and somatic relaxation. Derived from both laboratory and treatment research, the findings have clear relevance to clinical interventions and are the focus of the discussion to follow. All are also coping strategies taught in the CASMT program described later in the book. Although some of the strategies have been deemed more generally adaptive than others, we shall see that this is not universally the case and that contextual factors can markedly influence each strategy's degree of adaptiveness. Even rumination, considered to be a generally maladaptive strategy, can be helpful as a defensive strategy in some situations by focusing attention on thoughts and thereby deflecting attention from gut-level affective experience that could have a disorganizing impact (Borkovec et al., 2004). Healthy adaptation therefore requires flexibility in the use of coping strategies, skillfulness in executing them, and discriminative facility in judging their applicability to the stressful situation at hand (Bonanno, Papa, Lalande, & Coifman, 2004).

Attention Deployment (Distraction)

Self-regulation may occur very early in the emotional process. As noted in the CAPS model, every situation contains numerous stimulus features or potential "active ingredients" that can be the focus of attention, and attentional deployment is necessarily selective (Mischel & Shoda, 1995). One relatively simple strategy is to move one's attention away from aversive stimulus elements and to focus on more innocuous ones. This is the essence of distraction strategies, which require few cognitive resources and can be easily learned and widely applied. Distraction has a long history of efficacy as a physical pain tolerance strategy (McCaul & Mallott, 1984). In one medical application, the use of distraction by means of a virtual reality intervention presented during wound cleaning has proven highly effective in reducing subjective pain ratings in burn patients (Hoffman, Patterson, Canougher, & Sharar, 2001).

Successful distraction cuts off emotional processing before it can create a negative primary appraisal that elicits or augments NA. Laboratory studies in which participants were exposed to noxious visual stimuli, such as gory pictures, have shown that distraction manipulations (e.g., instructing participants to subtract numbers by 7's or to focus attention on innocuous aspects of the situation) have resulted in reductions in NA and decreased activation in the amygdala and other affect-generating brain structures (Ochsner & Gross, 2014). Distraction appears more useful (and more preferred by participants) than other cognitive strategies when affect intensity is high and higher-order cognitive processing, such as reappraisal, is thereby impaired. Experimental studies have also shown that training in attentional avoidance of negative information and in focusing instead on positive stimuli can reduce NA arousal in the laboratory as well as in response to real-world stressors. Likewise, distraction that involves generating a pleasant memory or imagining a pleasant situation has positive effects on physiological arousal (MacLeod & Grafton, 2014). Clinically, redirection of attentional focus to external stimuli (e.g., the 5-4-3-2-1 exercise described in Chapter 9) can be a temporary antidote to distressing internal cognitions.

One potential disadvantage of distraction is that, if successful, it can prevent processing of information that could be useful in guiding problem-focused coping or in evaluating the situation from the perspective of personal agendas and goals (Hayes, Strosahl, & Wilson, 2012). Not surprisingly, distraction has been found to be maladaptive when used repetitively over the long term (Kross & Ayduk, 2008). Like other coping strategies, distraction can be a two-edged sword if used indiscriminately.

Suppression and Avoidance

As we shall see in Chapter 3, virtually every school of psychotherapy cites the expression and processing of affective arousal is a primary treatment goal. Moreover, terms such as "defensive avoidance," "affect phobias," and "experiential avoidance" reflect an assumption that suppression and avoidance of emotional arousal and expression are detrimental to treatment effectiveness. Emotion regulation researchers have examined the consequences of emotion-avoidant coping, as have psychopathology and treatment researchers. Emotional suppression occurs as an attempt to modulate expressive and/or experiential emotional responses after they have been elicited. Avoidance, in contrast, involves attempts to prevent or block emotional responses from occurring.

Emotion suppression strategies can be beneficial in situations when intensive emotional displays would be dysfunctional or inappropriate (Bonanno & Keltner, 1997). Suppression of expressive behavior can be appropriate and adaptive in some situations where "maintaining one's cool" helps to facilitate problem solving and goal attainment, or helps defuse a potential confrontation. Used habitually, however, suppression can have an array of negative consequences (John & Eng, 2014), though apparently more so in Western cultures than in Asian ones, where it is more normative (Soto, Perez, Kim, Lee, & Minnick, 2011). In Western samples, scores on measures of habitual suppression are related to higher levels of NA, lower levels of PA and life satisfaction, and less intimate and satisfying relationships (English, John, & Gross, 2013). The cognitive and behavioral demands required for successful suppression of emotional responses can degrade the processing of socially relevant information. Though intended to dampen emotional arousal, suppression can result in increased sympathetic nervous system responses and greater activation in the amygdala and other brain regions that are involved in affect generation (Ochsner & Gross, 2014). Emotional constraint takes a toll on the body and is associated with an array of health problems (Eysenck, 1994; Kring & Sloan, 2010).

The many cues present in any situation can include "active ingredients" that have special significance to an individual, which in turn may trigger suppression or avoidance. In anxiety disorders, according to the hypervigilance–avoidance model (Barlow, 2004), attentional biases increase sensitivity to threat-related stimuli and engage avoidance behaviors, including efforts to deny or escape threatening information, reduced processing of both external and interoceptive emotion-related cues, and overt avoidance behaviors. Worry and rumination can also serve a defensive function by deflecting attention away from emotional experience. With time and repeated instances of negative reinforcement in the form of anxiety reduction, disengagement strategies may generalize from high-intensity situations, where they can be adaptive in the short term, to low-intensity ones that would ordinarily not require disengagement (Campbell-Sills, Ellard, & Barlow, 2014).

Cognitive Reappraisal

As noted in the model of stress presented in Figure 1.1, reappraisals can change the perceived demands-to-resources balance by reevaluating the demands as less threatening or the resources as more numerous or potent. One might also reappraise the seriousness or likelihood of the threatening consequences. At the most complex level of reappraisal, the "personal meaning" of the consequences can influence or reinforce important elements of the self-concept. Such personalized appraisals are often the target of cognitive restructuring and other CBT interventions that are intended to change negative self-construals (e.g., A. T. Beck, 1976; Ellis, 1962; Leahy et al., 2011).

Across a large number of studies, reappraisal has proven to be an effective coping strategy, both for decreasing NA and for increasing PA (Webb et al., 2012). In laboratory studies, perspective-taking reappraisal (e.g., "See it from a third-person perspective, noting that it doesn't affect you") seems easier to do and has stronger effects than stimulus reappraisal (e.g., "It's not really happening right now"). Reappraisal has also proven to be a more effective emotion regulation strategy than expressive and experiential suppression for reducing subjective NA, autonomic arousal, and activation of emotion-related brain regions, such as the amygdala (Gross, 2014b; Webb et al., 2012). Mediational analyses in both laboratory and clinical studies show that reappraisal self-efficacy (i.e., belief in one's capacity to generate stress-reducing self-statements) is a powerful mediator of successful stress management (Goldin et al., 2012).

Reappraisal has also been compared with distraction. Meta-analytic results indicate that, overall, the two strategies have similar overall effects in reducing NA. However, the effects of reappraisal can dissipate at high levels of arousal, and distraction then becomes more effective and more likely to be preferred by participants. Whereas distraction is relatively simple from a cognitive resources perspective, reappraisal requires more complex cognitive processes because the generation of alternative construals is in conflict with the original emotional appraisal and because it occurs later in the stress process (Sheppes, 2014). This is one reason why, in the training of reappraisal skills, a primary goal should be to replace dysfunctional appraisals with more adaptive ones. This relearning should occur in the process of treatment as the prevention or dampening of NA negatively reinforces adaptive self-statements (Smith, 1980). It is this process that is reflected in statements such as "Since I changed my attitude, the situation doesn't bother me anymore." From this perspective, successful cognitive therapy can be seen as a process of changing the appraisal response hierarchy so that, with time, adaptive appraisals become stronger and more likely to occur than dysfunctional ones.

From a clinical practice perspective, these studies provide evidence that relatively simple and easily learned reappraisals can reduce subjective and physiological stress responses to aversive stimuli. As also demonstrated in the pain control literature (Ehde, Dillworth, & Turner, 2014), relatively brief cognitive interventions that help clients to adopt a small number of stress-reducing self-statements as substitutes for catastrophizing appraisals can be effective. As discussed in Chapter 2, this can also be accomplished in our brief stress management intervention.

Acceptance

In his classic treatise on physical pain, Melzack (1973) differentiated between the sensory aspect of aversive stimulation and the emotional component, which turns aversive sensory stimulation into emotion-infused suffering. In one effective pain reduction strategy, patients are told to focus on the stimulus characteristics in an objective, nonemotional fashion rather than on its aversiveness (McCaul & Mallott, 1984; McCracken & Vowles, 2014).

The same principle is applicable to emotional pain, and it is reflected in the recent emphasis on acceptance in third-wave behavior therapies, particularly acceptance and commitment therapy (ACT; Hayes et al., 2012), in which experiential avoidance is viewed as a major contributor to maladjustment and a major target for intervention. The client is encouraged to regard emotional responses in a manner that divests them of their avoidance-eliciting and personalized aversive qualities. In ACT, the goal is to gain a new perspective on emotions as natural responses that are best accepted and not avoided.

To the extent that people can be receptive to whatever inner experiences are occurring and can divest them of their negative implications for personal identity, the experiences can be used to guide and stimulate movement toward fulfilling life values. Decentering and defusion exercises—which sometimes take the form of turning emotions into objects like waves that rise and fall on a sea that will become calm in time, or the image of standing on a sturdy mountain that remains stable and permanent as storms come and go and the angry clouds give way to sunshine—can be useful metaphors for the natural trajectory of emotional experience. This notion is similar to one associated with Gestalt therapy: "Emotions are neither good nor bad; they simply are" (Perls, 1969, p. 27). According to Hayes et al. (2012), acceptance is an important mechanism that not only helps people divest themselves of nonadaptive construals of who they are, but also fosters sustained movement toward intrinsically valued goals.

Experimental studies have shown that instructions to accept emotional experiences are associated with lowered subjective stress and behavioral avoidance (e.g., Wolgast, Lundh, & Viborg, 2011). A meta-analysis of acceptance instructions for confronting negative stimuli yielded a modest but statistically significant effect size of 0.31 over 30 separate experimental comparisons (Webb et al., 2012).

Acceptance has been established as an adaptive coping strategy and has been incorporated into many contemporary CBT protocols. In addition to ACT, these include dialectical behavior therapy (Linehan, 2015), emotion regulation therapy (Mennin & Fresco, 2014), emotion schema therapy (Leahy et al., 2011), and affect regulation therapy (Berking & Schwarz, 2014), all of which have as a treatment goal the reduction of experiential avoidance and enhanced emotional regulatory competence. Berking and Schwarz (2014) regard the ability to feel acceptance and tolerance as a critical skill, particularly whenever affective arousal cannot be handled with other coping skills, such as reappraisal or relaxation.

Mindfulness

Mindfulness is both a specific state of consciousness and a meditation-based procedure that has experiential acceptance as a core objective

(Farb, Anderson, Irving, & Segal, 2014). It is designed to foster present-moment experiential awareness through a focus on interoceptive attention and an attitude of acceptance. One major vehicle is a passive meditation technique derived from Buddhist practices and built upon the Benson meditation technique popularized in the 1970s as a stress management procedure (Benson & Klipper, 1976; Benson & Proctor, 2010).

The Benson technique was designed to promote a hypometabolic state of lowered arousal that is incompatible with the stress response. One of its chief principles is the acceptance of immediate experience without evaluation. Kabat-Zinn (1982) adapted the technique first as a pain reduction treatment, then as a stress management intervention. The prototype meditation technique involves a focused attention on one's breathing, which in itself lowers metabolic activity. Awareness of internal and external stimuli is encouraged, but the stimuli are to be regarded in a nonjudgmental manner. All experiences are to be accepted, even lapses in the meditation process, in which case the person simply returns interoceptive attention to the act of breathing. A goal is to promote new appraisals of experience, thereby allowing the person to approach experiences with a sense of exploration and curiosity. Recent evidence suggests that mindfulness training helps prevent sensory input from activating brain regions (e.g., the midline prefrontal cortex) that are involved in negative self-referential evaluation (Farb, Segal, & Anderson, 2013). Mindfulness training is being successfully applied as a stress reduction technique in both nonclinical and clinical populations (Alidina, 2015; Chiesa & Serretti, 2009), and it is being used efficaciously in the treatment of many medical problems as well (Farb et al., 2014).

Somatic Relaxation

Somatic relaxation has a long history as an emotion regulation strategy. Early on, it was recognized as a physiological response that is incompatible with the emotional arousal produced by the autonomic and endocrine systems (Cannon, 1932; Jacobson, 1938; Wolpe, 1958). Relaxation training has been applied within behavior therapies for more than a half century either to countercondition anxiety (e.g., Wolpe, 1958) or as a voluntarily applied self-control skill (e.g., Goldfried, 1971). It continues to be incorporated in many CBT modalities as an arousal-control coping skill.

WHAT'S AHEAD

Having considered the nature of emotion, stress, and coping, as well as the relative effectiveness of various emotion regulation strategies, and drawing on the evidence regarding the effectiveness of emotion regulation coping strategies, we apply this scientific base to the practical matter of helping clients develop more effective emotion regulation skills. In Chapter 2, we describe CASMT, which assists clients in acquiring and then utilizing relaxation and cognitive coping skills to reduce high levels of affective arousal created by the use of the IA technique. CASMT also incorporates empirically supported stress reduction techniques reviewed above, including acceptance, defusion, and mindfulness training. As we shall see in the research described in Chapter 2, success in controlling such arousal has salutary effects on coping self-efficacy, stress resilience, and performance measures.

CHAPTER 2

An Overview of Cognitive–Affective Stress Management Training

Coping with stress is a complex process, and a variety of coping skills may prove effective in preventing or reducing stress responses. Coping efficacy requires that the appropriate strategy be selected and that it be skillfully executed. Both individual and situational determinants influence how effective a given coping skill will be. It therefore follows that an intervention should teach a variety of generalizable coping skills; it should also provide the opportunity not only for skill acquisition, but also for rehearsal of the coping skills to provide for their optimal use in response to future stressors. Cognitive–affective stress management training (CASMT) is designed to accomplish these goals. The CASMT program is applicable to stress responses involving anger as well as anxiety in both clinical and nonclinical populations because of the cognition–arousal parallels in these emotions. We do not consider CASMT a treatment of choice for depression, and there is no empirical support for its efficacy for that problem. However, in comorbid cases, the training procedures to control anxiety could be applied to the anxiety component of depression within a multimodal treatment plan, with the cognitive restructuring portion of the intervention focusing on both anxiety and depression. In such instances, the duration of the treatment would necessarily extend beyond the protocol described in this book.

INTERVENTION STRATEGIES

Figure 2.1 illustrates the relation of the interventions that are the focus of the CASMT program to the model of stress presented in Chapter 1

(Figure 1.1). The main intervention targets are cognitive appraisals and physiological arousal—the central components of the model of stress. Cognitive restructuring and self-instructional training address appraisals, and relaxation skills target physiological arousal. These interventions are then combined to constitute an *integrated coping response* that is unique to CASMT. The goal is to help the client acquire and rehearse adaptive, emotion-focused, distress reduction skills. We should note that the treatment of an individual could be (and frequently is) expanded to focus on the other two components of the model: situational demands and coping behaviors. At the situational level, a therapist might work with a client to change aspects of the situation that produce or increase demands. For example, a worker might be encouraged to talk with his or her boss about changing a work schedule that is causing stress. Modeling and role playing might be used to refine the skills needed to approach the boss. At the coping behavior level, adoption of a structured time management procedure might help a college student function more efficiently and meet study and assignment demands more effectively, thereby decreasing performance anxiety. Likewise, social skills training might be implemented with a client whose social anxiety is based in part on skill deficits. Relationship-based stressors may be dealt with in similar fashion, while at the same time teaching the client (or a couple) emotion-focused coping skills and problem-focused communication skills. New behavioral competencies can help reduce situational demands that are taking a toll on the client by altering the demands-to-resource equation in the client's favor.

As noted earlier and shown in Figure 2.1, the cognitive and relaxation skills training is a prelude for combining them into a "body–mind" integrated coping response that can be readily applied before or within stressful situations without disrupting ongoing task-related or social behavior. Its development and rehearsal is the defining aspect of CASMT, as well as the explicit goal of treatment.

The CASMT protocol can be divided into four partially overlapping phases: (1) pretraining assessment, (2) presenting the rationale, (3) skill acquisition, and (4) skill rehearsal and generalization enhancement. When administered on a group basis, the preliminary assessment phase is generally less extensive unless research data are being collected or baseline measures are being obtained using our Stress and Coping Diary (Form A-1, p. 295). Table 2.1 shows a schedule of sessions based on the six-session protocol. Following pretraining assessment, CASMT sessions typically occur on a weekly basis over 6 weeks. Each session lasts an hour. The first two sessions and daily homework assignments are devoted to the acquisition of relaxation skills and stress-reducing self-statements. In working with groups and individuals, we have found that 2 weeks of conscientious adherence to the training results in the level of coping skill

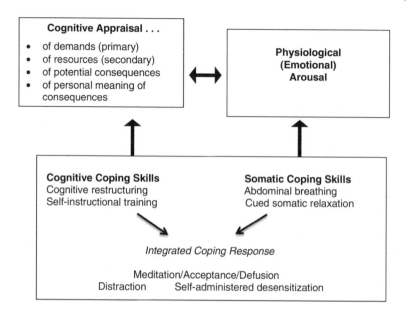

FIGURE 2.1. Cognitive–affective conceptual model of stress and its relation to the CASMT intervention components. The cognitive and somatic relaxation skills are combined into an integrated coping response that is phased into the breathing cycle. Other emotion regulation strategies taught in the program are also shown.

competency needed to move on to the rehearsal phase in the third session. Obviously, we expect skill levels to increase throughout the remaining sessions. However, we should also note that a therapist working with an individual client (or, for that matter, a trainer working with a group) could choose to extend the skill acquisition or rehearsal phase, including more intensive training in some of the skills to ensure a satisfactory level of mastery. Chapters 4 through 9 detail how to conduct each of the six sessions, but we can also conceptualize the treatment protocol in terms of six *phases*, each of which could involve multiple sessions as needed.

Pretraining Assessment

When the program is administered to individuals, several sessions may be devoted to assessing the nature of clients' stress responses, the circumstances under which these responses occur, the manner in which their functioning is affected, and the coping responses they are currently using. This phase is also directed at assessing a client's cognitive and behavioral

TABLE 2.1. Schedule of CASMT Training Sessions

Pretraining assessment

Interview, questionnaires and rating scales, self-monitoring

Training rationale and skill acquisition

Session 1. Orientation and relaxation training. The nature of emotion and stress is discussed, as is the nature of coping with stress. Training is begun in deep muscular relaxation, which serves as a physical coping response.

Session 2. Continuation of relaxation training and discussion of the relations between thoughts and feelings. Implications of these relations for coping with stress are discussed.

Skill rehearsal

Session 3. Practice in the use of relaxation and adaptive self-statements to control emotional responses. The IA technique is used during the session through the imagining of stressful situations. The development of mental coping responses is continued.

Session 4. Practice in using relaxation and stress-reducing mental statements to control emotional reactions induced through imagination and IA. Participants are introduced to the practice of mindfulness meditation.

Session 5. Practice in the use of relaxation and mental coping mechanisms is continued, with emphasis on application to actual life situations. Instruction in mindfulness stress reduction exercises is provided.

Session 6. Coping skills are rehearsed, main principles are summarized, and procedures that can be used to build on the stress management program, including self-administered exercises (e.g., self-administered systematic desensitization), are described.

strengths and deficits so that the program can be tailored to his or her specific needs. For example, the focus of training for a person who already has fairly good relaxation skills but has little control over self-defeating thought processes will tend to be on developing cognitive skills. On the other hand, a primary focus on the development of relaxation and self-instructional skills, as utilized by Meichenbaum (1985), may be the preferred approach for a chronically tense child and for clients who lack the psychological mindedness that would make them good candidates for cognitive restructuring.

A variety of assessment techniques can be employed during this phase, including careful interviewing, administration of questionnaires and rating scales, and self-monitoring by clients. For example, to assess affective states, we frequently employ a 100-point "tension thermometer" or "anger thermometer" that can be completed in seconds to obtain "readings" from the person in various *in vivo* situations. The Perceived Stress Scale (PSS; Cohen, Kamarck, & Mermelstein, 1983) is a measure of the degree to which situations in one's life are appraised as stressful. The PSS developers have published both college student and community norms, and these can be useful in identifying clients who could profit from stress management. We typically do both individual and group work with individuals who fall above the 80th percentile on this measure. We also use the Positive and Negative Affect Scale (PANAS; Watson, 2000) to assess clients' positive-to-negative affective balance. Extensive norms are also available for this measure. These measures can be used to assess current stress level as well as a means of tracking changes as treatment proceeds. Clients can also be asked to monitor the frequency with which certain kinds of thoughts occur before, during, and after problematic situations. The Analyzing Thoughts and Feelings worksheet (in Appendix A, Form A-2) can also be brought forward and used in the initial assessment phase. Measures such as the Irrational Beliefs Test (Jones, 1968) can be useful in targeting chronic self-defeating ideas for cognitive restructuring.

Stress and Coping Diary

We have developed a daily diary instrument based on the stress model to collect information on situations, appraisals, emotional responses, and coping strategies (Shoda et al., 2013; Smith et al., 2011). The Stress and Coping Diary can be administered in paper-and-pencil form (in Appendix A, Form A-1). The latter will eventually be available as a free-access instrument that can be utilized by clinicians. However, its use is strictly regulated by Health Insurance Portability and Accountability Act (HIPAA) statutes, and it is incumbent upon any practitioner or researcher using it to ensure that a secure website is established to protect the confidentiality of data. To utilize the online system, our clients log onto a website using a therapist-generated ID number and a client-generated password and complete the diary on their computer or tablet. The client's responses are transmitted directly to a secure server, where they are immediately accessible to the trainer and from which they can be downloaded to other data-processing systems, such as Excel and SPSS. The diary is useful to help both client and therapist discern patterns among situational characteristics, appraisals, emotional responses, coping strategies, and consequences.

The diary contains both open-ended response windows and rating scales. It can be self-administered in 5–10 minutes by most clients as they report and reflect on the most stressful event of the day. The diary begins with a general rating of situational stressfulness since the last entry, followed by 14 positive and negative affect descriptors. The respondent is next asked to describe the most stressful event experienced, followed by a series of items designed to assess the "active ingredients" of the situation that made it stressful (i.e., the extent to which the client felt incompetent, exhausted, excluded, helpless, irritated, confused, etc.). The client then rates the intensity of his or her emotional response to the event when it occurred and the extent to which the client felt personal control over (1) the situation, and (2) his or her emotional reaction to the situation. The latter item is used to track emotional regulation capability.

Having described key elements of the situation, the next set of items relate to cognitive appraisals that triggered the NA response and the self-statements that might have prevented or reduced it. The first question helps reveal the client's stress-producing appraisals and the second helps the client to reappraise the situation and develop stress-reducing self-statements that will become part of the integrated coping response. In conjunction with the "active ingredients" questions, clients become more aware of their particular situational vulnerabilities, how they typically appraise such situations, and ways to cognitively reappraise and deal with them.

The final portion of the diary assesses the client's coping strategies and their perceived effectiveness. A brief definition of each coping strategy is provided, an approach that has been shown to have strong validity (Smith, Leffingwell, & Ptacek, 1999). Clients are asked to rate the extent to which they applied each of 12 coping responses to the situation and to rate how effective each one they applied was in reducing their stress. The 12 strategies include those discussed in the previous chapter, some shown in research to be more (generally) adaptive than others. The strategies include rethinking the situation (reappraisal), relaxation techniques, seeking social support, direct problem solving (problem-focused coping), distraction, avoidance (behavioral and emotional), counting one's blessings, wishful thinking, physical activity, blaming oneself, blaming others, and acceptance. Clients then rate their stress levels when the event occurred and then after their efforts to cope. Finally, clients rate their general life satisfaction, a single-item measure used extensively in studies of subjective well-being (e.g., Diener & Larson, 1993).

Having shown clients the Stress and Coping Diary, the therapist can introduce the collaborative assessment procedures.

THERAPIST: As we work together, it will be as a team, and you will have a very important role in what happens. One thing we will be doing is monitoring closely what is happening on a day-to-day basis in your life, particularly the situations you confront, your thoughts and feelings, and how you choose to cope with them. I'll ask you to complete some forms, one of which is this Stress and Coping Diary. It's part of your becoming a personal scientist who collects data on yourself and gains greater self-understanding and a sense of personal control. To get this ball rolling, I'm going to ask you to tell me the questions you'd like to have answered as you achieve greater self-understanding.

CLIENT: Well, I'd like to understand why I worry so much about things that don't bother most people. Also, why I tend to get irritated so easily when I'm under stress. Then I feel guilty and like a loser later on. I'd like to get rid of the worry, tension, and irritability.

THERAPIST: Those are very worthwhile goals, and I think you'll find some useful answers to those questions, plus you're going to learn some new skills to counter those tendencies. The information you provide on the diary will also allow us to see changes that occur as we work together.

Having clients complete the measure on a daily basis helps to counteract the inaccuracies that occur when reports of coping skills are done retrospectively (e.g., Smith et al., 1999). By collecting data over time, we can discover patterns of "if–then" relations in the client's response patterns in particular situations and plan treatment in a collaborative fashion with the client. We have found this method to be very valuable in engaging clients in treatment as a collaborative "personal scientist." In a clinical trial on CASMT, a correlation of .52 was found between number of diary entries made by clients and self-reported stress reduction on the PSS over a 6-week period (Chen, 2015). Although the correlation could be a product of a third variable, such as commitment to the program or conscientiousness in carrying out all training assignments, it is also possible that the feedback provided by the diary facilitates the development of stress management skills.

Presenting the Rationale

In any program aiming to facilitate behavior change, initial conceptualization of the problem is of crucial importance in obtaining compliance and commitment to the program. Both client and the clinician should share the same conceptualization, which itself should be understandable, plausible, and have clear intervention implications. At every stage of the program, clients should understand exactly what is being done and why. We sometimes construe the intervention as a relationship between the client and a "stress management coach" whose function it is to guide the client's development of coping skills.

We have found it fairly easy to ensure that clients arrive at our basic conceptual model of stress simply by asking them to describe a recent stressful incident or by examining a Stress and Coping Diary report. This description should contain situational, cognitive, physiological, and behavioral components, which can usually be elicited by follow-up questions if they are not mentioned spontaneously (e.g., "How did you *feel* when that happened?"; "What kinds of *thoughts* went through your mind when he said that?"; "How did you try to *handle* that feeling?"). Labeling these elements and the relations among them provides an introduction to the conceptual model and its intervention components. We then present the client with a printed or written version of Figure B-1 (in Appendix B) and fit the client's reports into the model. Next we provide an overview of the training program and describe the procedures that will be used to intervene at the cognitive and physiological levels. This orientation provides a credible rationale and conceptual framework for clients, who are able to relate it to their own experiences.

THERAPIST: Let's see if we can fit your experience to the model. To recap what you just told me, at the party on Friday your date started paying attention to someone else, who is very attractive, and basically ignored you. That's the situation. You interpreted this behavior as a lack of interest in you, decided that you were no match for your rival, that the relationship you want is going on the rocks, and that you're not attractive enough to keep a relationship going. [Refers to the appraisal portion of the model.] Those thoughts match different kinds of appraisal in our model: what you thought about the situation, about your resources or your ability to cope with the demands, about the consequences of the situation, and about the personal meaning of the consequences should they occur. Your body reacted with a lot of anxiety and anger as well. That's the arousal part of the model, and the more upset you got, the more negatively you interpreted what was going on. Those are the two-way arrows between appraisal and arousal. Finally, you found yourself nearly in tears and you bolted from the party. Is that accurate?

CLIENT: Yes, that's what happened, although I didn't see it in these terms until now.

THERAPIST: So, we can see how this stressful situation and your responses to it fit the model. I think we can also see how the ability to adjust your thinking and to control your body's arousal response could be useful. Those are the kinds of stress management skills you're going to learn. Does that make sense?

CLIENT: Yes, it does.

THERAPIST: Let me be more specific about what we're going to do. (*Shows the client a replica of Figure B-2.*) Here's another version of the stress model, this one with the training elements included. As you can see, we're going to be working on the parts of the model inside the brackets—that is, inside you. You're going to learn some techniques, including relaxation techniques, which will allow you to quiet your body and keep your emotional responses under control. You're also going to learn some ways of programming your thinking to minimize rather than increase your stress response. Finally, you're going to learn to put these coping skills together so you can apply them with each breath, even in highly stressful situations. You'll also learn other coping skills that have scientific support, so that you'll leave the program with a variety of stress management skills. Does this approach make sense to you?

When implementing CASMT with nonclinical populations or as a preventive intervention, a therapist can choose to describe it as an educational program in self-control of emotion (rather than as psychotherapy) to destigmatize participation. With clinical cases, we present it as a therapeutic intervention. In both populations, we emphasize that the components of "mental toughness" or "resilience"—that is, the ability to better handle adversity—are specific skills that can be learned in the same way that other skills are learned, and these concepts are well received. Another term that we use is "learned resourcefulness," applied in this case to the learning of coping skills that become personal stress resistance resources.

The second point we emphasize is that the results of the program will be a function of how much commitment the person makes to the effort involved in acquiring the skills. Our goal here is to place the locus of responsibility on the client so as to maximize compliance with the homework assignments and also to ensure that clients attribute positive changes to themselves, rather than to the therapist. This internal locus should enhance both self-efficacy and the durability of change, and it is consistent with the self-regulation orientation of the program.

Skill Acquisition

The end product of the cognitive–affective program is the development of an "integrated coping response" having musculoskeletal, autonomic, and cognitive components (Figure 2.2, p. 50). The skill acquisition phase thus consists of the learning of somatic and cognitive relaxation skills and the development of cognitive coping responses through cognitive restructuring and/or self-instructional training.

Somatic and Cognitive Relaxation Training

The acquisition of relaxation skills is faster and easier for most clients than are the cognitive modification procedures. For this reason, we begin with training in somatic and cognitive relaxation skills. These skills are useful in controlling the physiological arousal component of the stress response, enabling a client to prevent an increase in arousal beyond the optimal arousal level for performance of the task at hand. They also increase the client's sensitivity to the internal arousal cues associated with anxiety or anger, thereby making it possible for clients to apply coping skills while their affect is more easily controlled.

MUSCLE RELAXATION

We start by teaching abdominal breathing and a self-command during exhalation that is designed to produce a relaxation response during the integrated coping response. Muscle relaxation training is carried out using an abbreviated version of Jacobson's (1938) progressive muscle relaxation technique. Over the years, the relaxation protocol has become increasingly briefer, moving from an initial 16 muscle groups addressed in the 1970s to nine groups, and currently to only three body sections (see Appendix A, Handout A-2), with a special emphasis on the breathing component.

Although some of the skills training is done by the therapist, most of it is accomplished through daily practice in the form of homework assignments. Training is designed to combine three components: the exhalation phase of the breathing cycle, a cue word such as *relax* or *calm*, and self-induced muscle relaxation. Special emphasis is placed on the use of abdominal breathing to facilitate relaxation. The mental command, *relax*, is repeatedly paired with the exhalation phase of the breathing cycle and with voluntary relaxation so that in time, the command becomes an eliciting cue for inducing relaxation and eventually an important component of the integrated coping response. The cue-controlled somatic relaxation skill provides a coping response that can quickly be utilized within stressful situations without interfering with ongoing task-oriented behavior.

COGNITIVE RELAXATION: MEDITATION TECHNIQUES

Davidson and Schwartz (1976) made an important distinction between somatic relaxation of muscular and autonomic processes and cognitive relaxation—that is, quieting of the mind. Anyone who has had difficulty sleeping while somatically relaxed because an active mind churned out intrusive thoughts can appreciate this distinction. We teach cognitive relaxation by means of an updated variant of Benson's (Benson &

Klipper, 1976; Benson & Proctor, 2010) meditation technique and a derivative mindfulness technique described by Kabat-Zinn (1990). The Benson technique has been taught in CASMT since its inception, and empirical support for both this approach and the mindfulness variant has prompted their inclusion in CASMT. Both exercises involve a nonjudgmental and acceptance-based focus on immediate experience and the sensations of breathing. In the Benson technique, intrusive thoughts or sensations are dealt with mentally by saying "Oh, well" and redirecting attention to the focus word, such as *one* or *peace*. Pollak, Pedulla, and Siegel (2014) describe the mindfulness variant as follows: "Rather than thinking about or analyzing these sensations, we allow the mind to be with them, bringing an attitude of interest, curiosity, and acceptance to the experience" (p. 6). We teach both the Benson and mindfulness meditation exercises so that clients can experience and use the one(s) they find most helpful (Appendix A, Handouts A-4 and A-5).

Unlike cue-produced somatic relaxation, meditation as traditionally practiced (for 10–20 minutes) cannot readily be used as a coping skill in stressful situations, though it can be extremely useful as a means of producing a general hypometabolic state of relaxation that yields a sense of tranquility and rejuvenation (Benson & Proctor, 2010). Moreover, the mindfulness perspective produced through meditation creates the ability to be receptive to whatever internal experiences are occurring, to regard them nonjudgmentally as simply experiences that come and go, and thereby to increase stress resilience. These mindfulness skills can be applied within stressful situations (Alidina, 2015; Hayes et al., 2012; Kabat-Zinn, 1990).

Empirical support has increased for the relative efficacy of these mindfulness-based approaches. One meta-analysis of laboratory studies of ACT treatment components reported moderate effect sizes for several components, including acceptance of immediate experience and "defusion," which is the ability to psychologically distance oneself from one's thoughts and to regard them as "simply" thoughts and not truths (Levin, Hildebrandt, Lillis, & Hayes, 2012). Other reviewers have concluded that ACT seems to rival other CBT interventions in efficacy for the treatment of mood-based problems (Powers, Zum Vorde Sive Vording, & Emmelkamp, 2009). Benson and Proctor (2010) review an array of positive outcomes of the relaxation response, including changes in gene expression that favor healthy functioning and reduced stress responses (Dusek et al., 2008).

Cognitive Coping Skills: The Anti-Stress Log

In cognitive coping skills acquisition, we place special emphasis on reducing tendencies to catastrophize about events and their meanings. To "catastrophize" is to exaggerate the demands and aversiveness of situations, to expect highly negative outcomes, and to feel helpless to control the situation and one's emotional reactions to it. Extensive evidence supports the central role of catastrophizing in producing stress reactions in both nonclinical and clinical populations (Boersma, MacDonald, & Linton, 2012; Garnefski, Lagerstee, Kraaij, van den Kommer, & Teerds, 2002). Moreover, component analyses of CBT interventions indicate that decreases in catastrophizing is an especially influential mediator of treatment success (Turner, Holtzman, & Mancl, 2009; Kalisch & Gerlicher, 2014). Our experience in administering the CASMT program, reinforced by single-client process studies using the Stress and Coping Diary (Shoda et al., 2013), suggest a similar conclusion. If one assumes that emotional response intensity is proportionately related to the "awfulnesss" of the situational appraisal (A. T. Beck, 1976; Ellis, 1962; Lazarus & Folkman, 1984), then we should expect reduced catastrophizing to be of crucial importance in stress reduction and to be a fundamental target for intervention.

REAPPRAISALS

Using an abbreviated cognitive restructuring approach, we want clients to uncover some of their more important stress-producing appraisals and then develop and rehearse a set of "anti-stress" reappraisals that will be generally effective in preventing or dampening physiological arousal in their "hot-button" areas of functioning. Using self-instructional training, as in stress inoculation training (Meichenbaum, 1985), we also want to help clients develop a set of adaptive self-directing cognitions that they can employ prior to, during, and following stressful encounters.

In contrast to traditional cognitive therapy, which involves much in-session discussion of cognitive distortions, core beliefs, and their logical analysis, we cover some basics of this approach in this second session, but our in-session efforts are supplemented by bibliotherapeutic materials on cognitive restructuring and self-instructional training that are the most important vehicle for guiding clients' development of the cognitive elements needed for the integrated coping response. Extensive evidence indicates that clients with a variety of affect-based disorders can benefit from such materials, sometimes to a level equivalent to that of therapist-administered live treatment (e.g., Furmark et al., 2009; Gregory, Schwer Canning, Lee, & Wise, 2004; Schelver & Gutsch, 1983). One meta-analysis of 17 outcome studies of cognitive bibliotherapy for depression yielded an overall effect size of 0.77, which compares favorably with some therapist-administered CBT outcomes (Gregory et al., 2004).

Training in cognitive coping skills begins with a didactic description of the manner in which emotional responses are elicited by the *psychological situation* created by ideas, memories, images, and self-statements. Conveying these concepts is easily accomplished by asking clients to analyze a recent stressful event and helping them see how their appraisals gave rise to their emotional response. For example, a client whose high level of life stress often involved encounters with a noncompliant child described a situation in which she became unduly upset with her child:

CLIENT: When Adam defied me again last night, I really got upset and screamed at him. Felt bad about it later.

THERAPIST: Why did you feel bad later?

CLIENT: I totally overreacted. He's just a kid and it wasn't that big a thing.

THERAPIST: What you just said, "He's just a kid and it wasn't that big a thing," must be very different from the thoughts you had when you got upset. Any idea what you told yourself initially in order to get that upset?

CLIENT: That what he was doing was terrible and he had no right to talk to me that way. I thought he was being a real brat.

THERAPIST: It seems as if at two different times you had two different ways of thinking about the situation and about Adam, and they made a big difference in how upset you felt.

CLIENT: Yes, it does make a difference.

THERAPIST: This is a good example of how our thoughts can affect our feelings. What you said initially caused you to overreact emotionally. Another way to look at it is that you may have overreacted initially at the level of thinking, so the feelings followed right along. In contrast, a statement like "It's not that big a thing," or "He's just a kid," which may seem more appropriate to the situation, upon reflection, produced less of a stress response.

Because many cognitive patterns are well practiced and automatized, clients often have limited awareness of the appraisal elements that underlie their dysfunctional emotional responses. To facilitate identification of stress-inducing cognitions and development of adaptive self-statements, clients are given the written materials in Handout A-3 (in Appendix A) to read as well as daily homework forms (see Appendix A, Forms A-2 and A-3) on which they describe a situation that they found upsetting, the emotion they experienced, what they must have told themselves about the situation in order to have upset themselves, and what they might have told themselves instead that would have prevented or minimized their upset. This cognitive restructuring procedure is designed to help clients identify, rationally evaluate, and replace dysfunctional and irrational ideas that underlie their maladaptive emotional responses. Among these is the idea of a "master stressor," identified by Ellis (1962). This is the notion that "It's awful, terrible, and catastrophic when things (me, other people, life circumstances, events in the past) are not the way I demand that they be, and I can't stand it when things are that way." This idea captures the common elements of egocentricity (demandingness), conditions of worth, catastrophizing, and overreacting that characterize many stress-evoking appraisals. Because research shows that catastrophizing cognitions activate brain regions involved in NA (Kalisch & Gerlicher, 2014), they are prime targets in CASMT. Indeed, variations on the master stressor appraisal above underlie most of the irrational ideas that cognitive therapists encounter in their clients.

Handout A-3 and Forms A-2 and A-3 provide cognitive restructuring materials to help clients ferret out and challenge dysfunctional appraisals and develop countering reappraisals. Although we obviously do not provide the depth of training that would occur in formal cognitive therapy, research has shown that adaptive reappraisals (including anticatastrophizing ones) can be learned in a single experimental session with positive results on affective responses (e.g., McRae, Cielielski, & Gross, 2012). Our own process studies have also shown that clients can acquire and utilize adaptive self-statements based on our training materials (e.g., Smith et al., 2011; Shoda et al., 2013).

SELF-INSTRUCTIONAL TRAINING

In self-instructional training, the focus is on helping clients develop and use specific task-relevant self-commands that direct attention, prevent or reduce emotionality, and enhance performance. As Meichenbaum (1985) describes the process, people learn to talk to themselves in an adaptive fashion in their ongoing internal monologues. Stressful situations are broken down into four phases and specific self-instructions are prepared for each phase:

1. *Preparing for a stressor.* "What do I have to do?"; "I can develop a plan to deal with it"; "Don't get shook up—just think about what you have to do"; "I'm feeling stressed—that's natural"; "Worrying won't help anything; instead, make a plan."
2. *Confronting the stressor.* "Take a deep breath and relax"; "What do you need to focus on?"; "As long as I keep my cool, I'm in command of the situation"; "Don't think about my stress, just about what I need to do"; "What's the best way to cope with this situation?"; "Don't make more out of this than I have to."

3. *Coping with feelings of being overwhelmed.* "Don't try to eliminate the stress totally, just make it manageable"; "Relax and slow things down"; "Keep your focus on the present"; "You can handle this"; "Take a long, slow breath."
4. *Poststress.* "It wasn't that bad, and I handled it"; "What can I learn from this? How can I do it better next time?"; "I dealt with it pretty well, and next time I'll do even better"; "I have the skills I need to cope better"; "I did it! Way to go!"

People who are not psychologically minded enough to profit from extensive cognitive restructuring can profit a great deal from self-instructional training alone. In most cases, however, both cognitive restructuring and self-instructional training are employed in CASMT as clients develop an individualized set of anti-stress self-statements that work for them.

Cognitive skills training proceeds via written materials (Handout A-3), in-session discussion, and the use of out-of-session training materials (Forms A-2 and A-3) or the Daily Stress and Coping Diary, Form A-1). The client begins to develop an anti-stress log (Form A-4); clients list their irrational self-statements in one column and one or more adaptive anti-stress substitutes for each in an adjacent column. These self-statements will be utilized during the coping skills rehearsal phase under IA and in stressful situations. The client also creates coping cards (see Handout A-3) containing stress-inducing situations and self-statements on one side and stress-reducing ones on the other (cf. J. S. Beck, 2011). These cards can be carried around by clients and referred to frequently to enhance their internalization of their own stress-reducing self-statements.

The Integrated Coping Response

In the relaxation training, as described earlier, a cue word (e.g., *relax*), voluntary muscle relaxation, and exhalation (which facilitates relaxation) are repeatedly combined so as to enhance voluntary control of relaxation. In the early development of CASMT, we taught clients to use relaxation and cognitive appraisals as separate coping strategies. A major step forward, originally suggested by a client, was to combine relaxation with a reappraisal or self-instructional cognition within the breathing cycle. The result is the *integrated coping response*, a unique feature of CASMT (Smith, 1980).

The exhalation phase of the breathing cycle enhances relaxation, which leaves the inhalation phase of the breathing cycle as an opportune place to insert a stress-reducing cognitive coping response. Thus, as the client inhales, she subvocally says or thinks a stress-reducing or task-oriented self-statement chosen from her Anti-Stress Log. At the peak of inhalation, she says or thinks the words *so* or *and*, and as she exhales, she gives the self-instruction—*relax*—while inducing voluntary muscular relaxation. The integrated coping response can be modified as appropriate and employed repeatedly within the stressful situation without disrupting ongoing behavior. With each breath, a client can potentially use a new stress-reducing self-statement upon inhalation. For example, while inhaling, the client says, "It's not that important. . . . " At the peak of the breath, the client says, "So," and then exhales while saying "relax." A statement based on self-instructional training may also facilitate concentration on task-relevant cues and thus enhance performance. Additional examples of integrated coping responses are shown in Figure 2.2.

Skills Rehearsal

Stress coping skills are no different from any other kind of skill. In order to be most effective, they must be rehearsed and practiced under conditions that approximate the real-life situations in which they will eventually be employed.

In the CASMT program, the IA technique (see Chapter 3) is used to generate high levels of emotional arousal, which are then controlled by

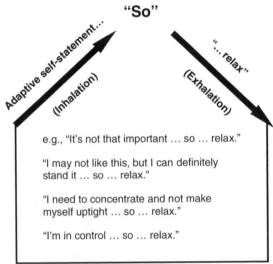

e.g., "It's not that important … so … relax."

"I may not like this, but I can definitely stand it … so … relax."

"I need to concentrate and not make myself uptight … so … relax."

"I'm in control … so … relax."

FIGURE 2.2. The integrated coping response, incorporating relaxation and stress-reducing reappraisals and self-directing cognitions into the breathing cycle. Adapted with permission of the author from Smith (1993).

employing the coping skills learned in the preceding phase of the program. IA is designed to allow rehearsal of coping responses in the presence of two kinds of cues: (1) imaginal representations of external cues that tend to elicit stress, and (2) internal somatic and cognitive cues resulting from emotional arousal. Whereas the external cues are fairly specific to certain situations, the internal cues are probably common to differing emotional responses that may occur across a variety of situations. Practice in dealing with the latter class of cues should help to maximize generalization of the coping skills across a wide variety of stressful situations, as originally suggested by Goldfried (1971) and Suinn and Richardson (1971).

It should be emphasized that CASMT is based on a self-regulation or self-control model designed to develop and provide rehearsal for generalizable emotion regulation skills and overall coping self-efficacy; it is not based on a deconditioning extinction model, as prolonged exposure methods are. Therefore, the IA technique is not employed until the trainer is certain that the client has learned the requisite coping skills well enough to ensure success in controlling the level of arousal that is generated. We want the client to experience a notable reduction in affect level so as to increase his or her sense of coping self-efficacy. During initial use of the technique, arousal is kept at a moderate level. On the initial administration, we typically tell the client to signal us with a "thumbs up" when a level of 50 is reached on a 100-point Subjective Units of Distress Scale (SUDS; see Appendix B, Figure B-4). The scale ranges from no distress, completely "calm, relaxed" to "unbearable, worst imaginable." Clients can establish affect control through relaxation. As the client demonstrates successful control, the level of arousal is allowed to increase to its maximum. In those rare instances in which a client has difficulty controlling a high level of arousal with his or her own application of relaxation or the integrated coping response, the therapist administers relaxation instructions until affective arousal returns to a baseline level. Such occasions can be (1) reframed as a demonstration to clients of how relaxation can reduce arousal and (2) used to encourage clients to further develop the relaxation skills so as to duplicate on their own what the therapist has just accomplished. In decades of experiences of applying the IA technique in CASMT, we (and our students) have never failed to successfully reduce arousal.

The IA Technique

During skill rehearsal, which begins in the third session of the protocol, IA is used to evoke affective arousal. The procedure is described in greater detail in Chapter 3; here we describe its basic elements. The client is asked to imagine, as vividly as possible, a stressful situation that he or she has reported (e.g., a spider-phobic patient may be asked to visualize being trapped in a small room with several large spiders; a basketball player may be asked to imagine getting ready to shoot a free throw in a critical situation; a businessman may be asked to imagine approaching the podium to give an anxiety-arousing presentation). The client is then asked to direct attention inwardly and to focus on the feeling that the situation elicits. It is suggested that as the client focuses on it, the feeling will begin to grow and to become stronger and stronger. The suggestions continue as the client begins to respond with behavioral signs of increased emotional arousal, and indications of arousal are verbally reinforced and encouraged by the therapist, as described in the next chapter. At intervals during the IA phase, the therapist asks the client to label the feeling being experienced, note the kinds of thoughts occurring, and say these thoughts out loud. This information is used to elaborate upon the arousal ("That's it. Focus even more on that feeling of fear about what that person will think of you"). This work also provides information, often previously unreported by the client, concerning the cognitive appraisals that accompany (and, it is hypothesized, mediate) the arousal.

Once an appropriate level of arousal has been elicited, the client is instructed to "turn it off" with his or her coping responses. Two IAs are carried out in the third session. In the first induction of the third session, abdominal breathing and relaxation alone are used as the active coping skill ("Now, focus on your breathing. Each time you exhale, tell yourself to relax, feel your body obey, and watch the feeling begin to drain away"). In the second IA, the client is asked to choose a stress-reducing self-statement from his or her Anti-Stress Log to be paired with the relaxation technique. Self-statements are combined with relaxation in all future IAs to create the integrated coping response that ties the self-statements and the relaxation response into the natural inhalation–exhalation breathing cycle.

IA is used later to rehearse other arousal-relevant skills, such as the mindful acceptance technique (in Appendix A, Handout A-5). This process provides an explicit method of rehearsing defusion under conditions of arousal, but within the safety of the treatment environment. In like manner, we believe that IA could be applied in the unified protocol treatment modules on emotional avoidance and becoming mindfully aware of emotional experience; increasing awareness and identifying the role of physical sensations in emotional experiences; and facilitating exposure to both interoceptive and situational cues associated with emotional experiences (Barlow et al., 2004).

Other empirically supported stress reduction techniques are also taught in CASMT, including self-desensitization, distraction, and covert rehearsal (Clum & Watkins, 2008; Rosen, Glasgow, & Barrera, 1976;

Meichenbaum, 1985). The goal is to provide clients with training in a variety of empirically supported emotion-focused coping techniques that can be flexibly used in response to the particularities of the circumstances that clients encounter. CASMT can also provide a base upon which therapists may introduce other training elements and interventions to suit the needs of their clients. Finally, relapse prevention principles (Marlatt & Gordon, 1985) are presented in the latter portions of treatment to prepare participants to deal with unsuccessful coping episodes and to persist in developing their coping skills.

Additional Skills Taught

Defusion, Mindful Acceptance, and Distraction Techniques

"Defusion" is the process of separating thoughts—verbal events in the mind—from direct experience to help reframe the meaning of subjective experience in a manner that can reduce distress (Hayes et al., 2012). It involves stepping back from negative thoughts or feelings and regarding them nonjudgmentally, as transient events, rather than as inherent aspects of the self or as faithful representations of reality. Defusion is of special interest because it may be a treatment mechanism that is common to both ACT and CBT. In both treatments, clients are encouraged to engage their thoughts, but for different reasons. In ACT, the goal is to develop a nonjudgmental willingness to experience the thoughts, with no active attempt to change them. In contrast, CBT involves increasing metacognitive awareness of one's "automatic thoughts" as a first step to challenging and modifying them (Ingram & Hollon, 1986; Teasdale, Segal, & Williams, 1995). In both treatments, however, the literalness, believability, and "reality basis" of the thoughts is challenged. Given the empirical support for defusion, in recent years we have expanded the range of coping skills in CASMT to include defusion strategies in Session 5. We should note that because of their recent inclusion in CASMT, defusion and distraction were not present in any of the empirical studies on CASMT presented later in this chapter, and we have no evidence at this time that their addition enhances the efficacy of CASMT. We can say, however, that in recent CASMT applications, clients have provided positive feedback about these elements. We have been able to make logical transitions from the cognitive treatment of automatic thoughts by showing clients that both cognitive restructuring and defusion can serve to decrease the believability of dysfunctional thoughts.

In laboratory, clinical, and real-life settings, people often report that reappraisal is difficult to accomplish once a high level of affective arousal has occurred and higher-order cognitive processing is thereby impaired

(John & Eng, 2014). When affect cannot be controlled using cognitive–somatic coping skills, then distraction can be used to help people disengage cognitively from distressing thoughts and emotions. Distraction appears more useful than other cognitive strategies when emotion intensity is high, and it is preferred by participants in laboratory studies. It can be used upon initial exposure to noxious situations to blunt affective arousal and preserve resources for behavioral coping. Successful distraction applied early in an encounter with a stressor can cut off emotional processing before it is represented in working memory and has the opportunity to create a negative primary appraisal that evokes or increases NA. Laboratory studies in which participants were exposed to noxious visual stimuli have shown that distracting manipulations (e.g., instructing participants to subtract numbers from 100 by 7's, or to focus attention on innocuous aspects of the depicted situation) reduce NA and decrease activation in the amygdala and other affect-generating brain regions (Ochsner & Gross, 2014). Training in attentional avoidance of negative information and in focusing instead on positive stimuli that might be present can reduce NA arousal in both the laboratory and in response to real-world stressors. Likewise, distraction that involves generating a positive memory or thinking of a positive situation can dampen physiological arousal (MacLeod & Grafton, 2014). Given evidence of efficacy, we introduce participants to a simple, easily applicable technique in Session 6.

Desensitization and Covert Rehearsal

The learned resourcefulness orientation that is explicit in CASMT implies that acquisition and refinement of coping skills should continue after CASMT ends. Because participants are likely to encounter new life stressors that have not been rehearsed during the stress management program, it is desirable that they have a means at their disposal to enhance their own emotion regulation in those situations. It is unlikely that participants will be able to (or want to) self-administer the IA rehearsal technique. Therefore, we provide training in a modified self-desensitization procedure, using the integrated coping response in place of traditional relaxation.

Considerable empirical evidence indicates that given appropriate guidance, self-administered desensitization and other CBT procedures can be highly efficacious (e.g., Clum & Watkins, 2008; Rosen et al., 1976). Covert rehearsal of coping responses and adaptive behaviors can also be an effective means of preparing for stressful encounters, acquiring new behavioral skills, and increasing self-efficacy (Bandura, 1997; Meichenbaum, 1985). Covert rehearsal has been a successful component in both stress inoculation training and anxiety management training, and we therefore introduce it in conjunction with the modified self-desensitization procedure in

Session 6, providing take-home guidelines (Handout A-6) as well so that participants can learn these supplementary coping techniques.

Finally, a brief relapse prevention element is presented to prepare participants to deal with unsuccessful coping episodes. The goal is to emphasize that no one becomes "stress-proof," no matter what kinds of training they receive. We normalize the fact that clients can expect to be overmatched at times by situations that are either novel or that are especially demanding. The brief relapse prevention element can help ensure that clients do not backslide into a sense of learned helplessness but instead use their unsuccessful coping attempts as information that helps them improve their skills.

A half century after Donald Kiesler (1966) posed the "specificity question" about what type of treatment administered to what type of client in which format and by what kind of therapist leads to what kinds of outcomes, gaps remain in our knowledge, particularly in relation to individual client variables. Therefore, it seems appropriate for multimodal interventions such as CASMT to include a range of empirically supported procedures, even if they derive from seemingly divergent theoretical positions. This policy of inclusion is clearly occurring as acceptance-based concepts and methods are incorporated into a new generation of eclectic CBT approaches (e.g., Leahy et al., 2011; Linehan, 2015; Mennin & Fresco, 2014; Segal, Williams, & Teasdale, 2002)

Although acceptance and self-control models of emotion regulation both have extensive empirical support, we remain proponents of a self-control coping skills approach as a first-line intervention for stress management. If people are able to exert self-regulatory control over NA early in the process through relaxation techniques and adaptive reappraisals, then there is no need to tolerate distress with mindful acceptance. We recognize, however, that different strategies may be effective at different stages of the stress process and in response to different stressors. This complexity also argues for the teaching of diverse coping strategies.

ONGOING COLLABORATIVE ASSESSMENT IN CASMT

CASMT is a collaborative enterprise in which clients and therapists work cooperatively to help the clients become more effective "personal scientists," able to discern and understand the relations between situations, cognitions, emotions, and behaviors as a means of developing more effective self-regulatory competencies. We use intervention-specific measurement data to provide feedback, to monitor client progress, to adjust clinician behavior and, as a result, to improve outcomes (Shoham et al., 2014; Weisz, Ng, & Bearman, 2014).

In collaborative assessment, clients are involved in defining assessment goals, and therapists and clients discuss assessment results. The goal is to use the process as a therapeutic intervention in which clients are invited to explore the meaning of the results and to gain new understandings of the contingencies operating in their lives (Fischer & Finn, 2008). We consider such assessment to be an ongoing activity that extends over the course of treatment. An emerging body of evidence supports the therapeutic effects of collaborative assessment, whether provided during a single feedback session or on multiple occasions (Ackerman, Hilsenroth, Baity, & Blagys, 2000; Pegg et al., 2005; Newman & Greenway, 1997; Poston & Hanson, 2010).

The Stress and Coping Diary is one tool used for ongoing collaborative assessment. Feedback from the daily diary promotes therapeutic progress by helping clients increase their awareness of relevant situation-related coping patterns in their lives. It also allows clients to see the results of their efforts over time, while also allowing the therapist/trainer to monitor the course of training and make adjustments if progress is not occurring or if there is a setback. As an example of tracking the use of adaptive and maladaptive coping strategy over the course of treatment, Figure 2.3 shows daily diary data provided by a client whose stressful working situation led him to seek treatment. His responses showed a clear pattern in which his favored strategy of avoidance seemed to exacerbate his interpersonal distress, causing him to deeply resent a working situation in which he saw himself as being exploited by coworkers who foisted their work on him, even as he avoided expressing his concerns to them. Feedback and discussion of this clearly apparent pattern, together with his training in CASMT coping strategies, resulted in a progressive decrease in his use of avoidance and an accompanying significant increase in a composite measure of adaptive coping strategies, including relaxation, cognitive restructuring, and problem-focused coping (in his case, becoming more assertive in requesting that coworkers do their share of the work). These coping strategies were associated with lowered situational and personal stress. Finally, the collaborative relationship between the client and the therapist enhanced their therapeutic relationship and encouraged the client's compliance with program requirements and his persistence in treatment (Smith et al., 2011).

APPLICATIONS AND EMPIRICAL RESULTS

When CASMT was developed in the mid-1970s, IA as a stand-alone treatment had demonstrated its potential utility as a coping skills rehearsal technique in both outcome and process studies and seemed well suited for this emotion self-regulation intervention. In the intervening years,

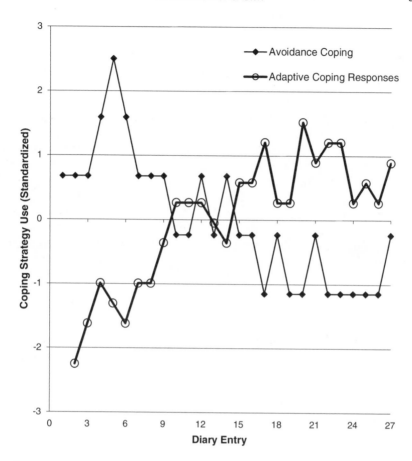

FIGURE 2.3. Changes in group-based standard scores of one client's use of maladaptive (avoidance) and adaptive (relaxation, cognitive restructuring, problem-focused) coping strategies over the course of stress management training. Both the use of avoidance coping and the use of adaptive coping strategies changed significantly ($p < .01$) from baseline (reports 1–9) through treatment (reports 10–27). From Smith et al. (2011). Copyright 2011 by the American Psychological Association. Reprinted by permission of the author.

CASMT has been applied to a wide variety of nonclinical populations as well as to clients suffering from anxiety and anger issues. More recently, we have focused on intensive analyses of single-client data using the Internet-based Stress and Coping Diary, derived from the original cognitive–affective stress and coping model (Smith, 1980; Smith & Ascough, 1985) and from the CAPS model (Shoda et al., 2013). We now summarize the experimental and single-client applications of CASMT to a variety of populations suffering high levels of life stress.

Stress Management Training of Medical Students

Medical school is a highly stressful environment, and the negative effects of stress on medical students and residents have been well documented (Rogers, Creed, & Searle, 2012). Holtzworth-Munroe et al. (1985) assessed the effects of the CASMT program on first- and second-year medical students in a medical school that had experienced a series of suicides, attributed in part to stressful training demands and evaluative pressures. Forty volunteer students who stated that they were experiencing high stress were randomly assigned to either a CASMT treatment group or to a no-treatment control group told that the study was about medical school experiences. To evaluate program efficacy, self-report measures of stress, general anxiety, test anxiety, depression, and self-esteem were administered at pretreatment, posttreatment, and a 10-week follow-up.

Although group differences at posttreatment were in the expected direction for the treatment group and the two groups were beginning to separate on all measures, they did not attain significance at this point. However, at the 10-week follow-up, the CASMT group reported significantly less test anxiety during the stressful period immediately before taking their board exams. Results on a questionnaire administered at posttreatment and at follow-up yielded significant group differences at both times. The trained students reported greater awareness of tension and greater ability to cope with school stress than did students in the control group. The findings suggest that stress management might fruitfully be added to medical school curricula to help decrease student and physician impairment.

Military Officer Candidates

During Officer Candidate School (OCS), prospective military officers are intentionally subjected to highly stressful conditions designed to test their psychological fitness. Because of an inability to function at a satisfactory level under such conditions, up to 70% of officer candidates either withdraw voluntarily or are mustered out of the program. Undoubtedly, the military loses potentially successful officers as a result of stress-coping deficits. It seems possible that coping skills training could be beneficial for both the individuals involved and for the military.

In addition to the attrition issue, previous research has shown a surprisingly low correlation between leader intelligence and leader performance across a variety of leadership contexts, ranging from business settings to the military. One meta-analysis involving 151 samples that included more than 40,000 leaders yielded an average correlation of .17 between intelligence and performance (Judge, Colbert, & Illies, 2004). Fiedler (1995) identified stress as a factor that contributes to the overall low correlation. He provided evidence that under conditions of high inter-personal stress like that created by OCS training officers, intelligent leaders seem unable to utilize their superior cognitive resources, often resulting in a null or negative correlation between intelligence and leader performance in highly stressed leaders.

In a 12-month field experiment that tested propositions derived from Fiedler's (1995) cognitive resource theory, CASMT was adminis-tered to 51 candidates at National Guard OCSs in the states of Oregon and Washington in an attempt to counteract the deleterious effects of situational stress on performance and on the utilization of intellectual abilities (Jacobs et al., 2013). A switching-replications quasi-experimental design was used (Cook & Campbell, 1979). After a baseline assessment, the randomly selected Washington candidates were trained during the first 3 months, and the candidates at the other school (Oregon) served as a no-treatment control. At Time 2, the CASMT program was intro-duced to the Oregon school while the Washington group began a 3-month follow-up period. At Time 3, follow-up measures were collected from the Washington group and posttreatment measures from the Oregon group.

Results of the study regarding performance are shown in Figure 2.4. The two groups of candidates did not differ significantly in baseline performance ratings made by training instructors who were blind to the intervention. Following CASMT, significant differential increases were found on standardized performance ratings of candidates, as indicated by a highly significant conditions × time interaction effect. Particularly notable was a large performance separation between groups beginning at Time 2, when the Washington candidates were presumably applying their already-acquired coping skills to counteract training stressors and training was about to begin for the Oregon group (Cohen's $d = 1.72$). Rate of improvement increased between Time 2 and Time 3, and supe-rior performance to the Oregon group was maintained at Time 3 ($d = 1.20$). Significant gains also occurred on a standardized behavioral in-basket measure of administrative task performance under time pressure following CASMT. In addition to overall positive changes in performance across phases of the switching-replications design, and in accordance with Fiedler's (1995) cognitive resource theory, performance increments following stress management training were greater for candidates who reported high boss stress than for low-stress candidates. Whereas high-stress candidates in the delayed Oregon treatment condition performed at a significantly inferior level compared with their trained counterparts during the first (nontraining) interval, high-stress candidates in both groups improved significantly and performed as well as low-stress candi-dates following training.

Finally, the intervention was related to changes in correlations between fluid intelligence and scores on time-pressure in-basket performance tasks.

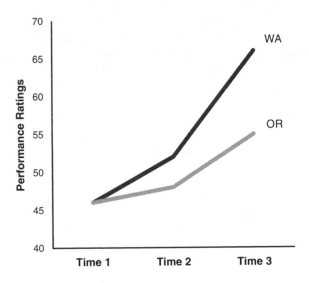

FIGURE 2.4. Changes in experts' performance ratings of prospective military officers at two Officer Candidate Schools. The Washington (WA) school received CASMT between Time 1 and Time 2, whereas the Oregon (OR) school was administered CASMT between Time 2 and Time 3. Data from Jacobs, Smith, Fiedler, and Link (2013).

In high-stress candidates, negative correlations between fluid intelligence and performance were eliminated in the Washington OCS group (going from $r = -.65$ preintervention to $r = .06$ after CASMT) and became more positive in the Oregon group (going from a nonsignificant $r = .11$ before the intervention to $r = .59$ following CASMT).

We conclude that although high situational stress is endemic to many leadership settings and cannot be easily reduced, interventions can be applied that help individuals in those settings respond with greater resilience to the stressors. The results of this study suggest that structured coping skills training that enhances emotional self-regulation skills can be an efficacious means of maximizing the ability of leaders to utilize their intellectual abilities and thereby perform at a higher level in stressful conditions.

Heavy Drinkers

Rohsenow et al. (1985) applied CASMT with at-risk heavy college-age drinkers. Such college-age individuals frequently develop severe alcohol dependency problems over time. Moreover, drinking in this population often occurs in response to stress and is negatively reinforced by a reduction in NA, which then increases the likelihood of repeated episodes of alcohol abuse (Johnstone, Garrity, & Straus, 1997; Marlatt & Gordon, 1985). The acquisition of effective stress management skills might reduce dependency on alcohol use in the face of stress, at least in individuals who drink to reduce subjective stress. It should be noted that the participants in this study were not requesting assistance in reducing their alcohol consumption and did not necessarily view their drinking as problematic. Instead, the researchers focused on the possibility that CASMT could serve as a potential prevention program for the general population of at-risk drinkers by enabling students to acquire alternative coping skills.

Male college students who reported excessive drinking were recruited and randomly assigned to either a CASMT treatment or a no-treatment control group. So as to reduce potential demand characteristics, the treatment group was not told that the focus of the program was on reduced drinking but rather was a "study of college life and the issues that students face." They were told that they would learn methods to deal with the "stresses of college life." Daily mood ratings of anxiety, anger, and depression were collected for 6 months, as were records of "daily activities," including amount of alcohol consumed. To assess the effects of the cognitive restructuring component on maladaptive cognitions, clients also completed the Irrational Beliefs Test (Jones, 1968) before and after the study and at follow-up. Investigators assessed other individual difference variables by administering Rotter's (1966) Internal–External Scale (locus of control), the State–Trait Anxiety Inventory, a social support questionnaire, and the Alcohol Use Inventory.

Stress management treatment was associated with a significant posttreatment reduction in daily anxiety ratings, but the changes were no longer significant at the 2.5- and 5.5-month follow-ups. No significant differences were found at any period for angry or depressed moods. However, positive changes in irrational beliefs targeted by the cognitive restructuring component of CASMT were strongly correlated with reduction of NA. In participants who reported at baseline that they often drank while angry, reduced alcohol consumption was associated with a reduced belief on the Irrational Beliefs Test that people should be blamed and punished for their wrongdoing.

Although drinking was not identified as a target during the treatment, the men in the CASMT treatment group showed a significant decrease in daily drinking rates at posttreatment and at the 2.5-month follow-up, but drinking rates returned to near baseline by 5.5 months posttreatment, suggesting the need for posttreatment booster sessions to maintain treatment gains.

On the Irrational Beliefs Test, treated clients showed significant improvement on four of the 10 beliefs. Specifically, trained clients reported increased frustration tolerance, were less inclined to avoid dealing with problems, reported less need to seek perfect solutions to problems, and became less likely to believe that unhappiness is caused by external forces. In line with the latter change, treated clients shifted significantly to a more internal locus of control on the Internal–External Scale following treatment.

Finally, certain individual difference variables were strongly correlated with posttreatment changes in moods and drinking, and with maintenance of change at follow-ups. A recent data reanalysis revealed that participants who reported on the Alcohol Use Inventory that they drank to control negative emotional states exhibited the largest and most lasting reductions in daily anxiety and anger ratings. Those who drank to experience the positive aspects of intoxication or for social reasons showed no change in consumption. The extent to which participants reported preoccupation with thoughts about alcohol was also negatively related to drinking outcome at posttreatment and follow-up.

These latter findings are noteworthy, since they indicate that individual difference factors may serve as important moderator variables that influence the outcome of stress management training. There has been increasing awareness of the role that personality and other individual difference variables may play in treatment outcome (e.g., Westen, Novotny, & Thompson-Brenner, 2004). The results of this study suggest that more attention should be directed to client characteristics, including reasons for drinking, as possible predictors of outcome. In particular, CASMT treatment would best focus on those whose drinking is used to reduce NA (and who want to find other ways to reduce it), rather on those who drink to achieve positive outcomes, such as the positive "buzz" portion of the biphasic alcohol ingestion curve or for social involvement. As in this study, we would expect minimal treatment responsiveness in people who do not drink to reduce stress. Given that the intervention exhibited some degree of efficacy in a population that was not seeking treatment, it may be a promising intervention for at-risk individuals who drink to reduce NA and who are motivated to reduce their problematic drinking.

Performance Anxiety and Athletic Performance

Athletes are an excellent population for applying and testing stress management interventions, for they continuously encounter endemic stressors, their performance is known to be negatively affected by stress responses, and there are available performance outcome measures of unquestioned ecological validity. The early development and testing of the CASMT program was prompted in part by requests to a sport psychologist from several collegiate and professional coaches in elite programs for interventions with athletes whose performance was being adversely affected by performance anxiety. Early descriptions of the intervention with athletes (e.g., Smith, 1980, 1984) stimulated research by other sport psychologists, and the results suggest that athletes are a suitable target population. Meta-analytic results indicate that multimodal stress management programs, including stress inoculation training and CASMT, yield positive effects on both affect and performance (Rumbold, Fletcher, & Daniels, 2012).

Crocker et al. (1988) and Crocker (1989) investigated the effects of CASMT on cognitive, affective, and performance outcome measures in elite youth volleyball athletes. Athletes in the treatment condition received eight weekly sessions of CASMT. At posttreatment, the trained athletes reported fewer negative thoughts as they imagined themselves performing in videotaped stressful volleyball situations. They also exhibited superior volleyball performance, according to experts who rated their videotaped performance during an intense practice session just prior to an important competition. Surprisingly, no significant decreases were found on a measure of cognitive and somatic performance anxiety at the end of treatment.

Posttreatment performance gains in the CASMT condition were found at a 6-month follow-up, where state anxiety and performance measures were collected during a tournament preceding the Canada Games. Moderate to large effect sizes occurred for reductions in worry and concentration disruption aspects of anxiety (Cohen's $d = 0.85$) and in somatic anxiety ($d = 0.60$), and improved performance from baseline to follow-up ($d = 0.57$). Athletes trained with CASMT also showed significant improvement on a measure of competitive self-confidence, reflecting their perceived ability to cope with competitive pressures (Crocker, 1989). These positive changes were attributed to additional practice and refinement of coping skills learned in the intervention during the 6-month follow-up interval, although no formal booster sessions occurred. Athletes also reported using their self-regulation skills in other contexts, such as in stressful interactions with coaches and referees.

Physical Distress Tolerance

Ziegler et al. (1982) suggested that because of its focus on the control of aversive internal stimuli, CASMT could also prove useful in helping people cope with the physical stress and discomfort produced by intense physical activity. Accordingly, they compared the CASMT program with Meichenbaum's (1977) stress inoculation training and a no-treatment control condition in a study with cross-country runners, who must tolerate the physiological discomfort associated with long-distance running. The hypothesis was that increased ability to manage stress would decrease the toll of stress on cardiovascular efficiency during running. Participants in the experimental conditions met with an experimenter for stress management training twice a week for 5.5 weeks. They received either CASMT (with IA as the skill rehearsal technique) or stress inoculation training, in which no attempt was made to induce a high level of emotional arousal and covert rehearsal was used as participants imagined successfully applying their relaxation and cognitive coping skills to manage the stress of physical exertion.

Participants in the two treatment conditions and in a no-treatment control condition underwent 20-minute submaximal treadmill runs before and following the interventions. Cardiovascular efficiency was assessed by means of heart rate and oxygen consumption measures. The three groups did not differ significantly on either cardiovascular measure at pretreatment. During the posttreatment treadmill session, participants in the two treatment conditions were instructed after the first half of the treadmill run to use their "mental training techniques" to try to minimize their exertion-produced physiological stress.

The results indicated that after treatment, both stress management groups were significantly superior to the control group in cardiovascular efficiency as measured by heart rate, differing by more than 16 beats per minute from the control group during the second half of the run, but the two training conditions did not differ from one another. On the oxygen consumption measure, however, the participants who received stress inoculation training did not differ from the control group when told to use their coping skills during the last half of the run, whereas the CASMT group exhibited significantly lower oxygen consumption. On this measure, the difference between the two interventions strongly favored the CASMT condition ($d = 1.67$). The investigators attributed this result to the practice the CASMT group had received in reducing higher levels of physiological arousal produced by IA, speculating that this training gave the runners greater ability to dampen the aversive internal stimuli created by their physical exertion.

Test Anxiety Coping Skills Rehearsal:
Comparing Coping Skills Rehearsal Techniques

As noted in Chapter 2, the theoretical basis for the use of IA as a rehearsal technique departs from that underlying Meichenbaum's (1985) stress inoculation training approach. As its name implies, Meichenbaum's procedure, like medical immunization procedures, is geared toward immunizing the individual to large stresses by "learning to cope with small, manageable units of stress" (1977, p. 149). In CASMT, the emphasis is quite the opposite in that the client practices the use of coping skills to reduce levels of affective arousal that are as high as or higher than those elicited by *in vivo* stressors. The ability of participants to control this high level of arousal by applying their coping skills may result in more durable coping skills and higher levels of self-efficacy. It is assumed that the ability to control high levels of arousal will readily generalize to lower levels of affect, thus facilitating generalization of coping skills across situations, emotions, and levels of arousal.

In stress inoculation training, the primary coping skills rehearsal technique is covert or imaginal rehearsal of coping responses, in which participants who have been trained in relaxation and cognitive coping skills imagine themselves applying the responses to cope with stressful situations. No explicit attempt is made to generate high levels of affect, since the assumption underlying the inoculation model is that exposure to low levels of stress helps prepare people to deal with higher levels in the future.

Although the theoretical underpinnings of the cognitive–affective approach differ from those underlying stress inoculation training, there is no reason why the techniques of covert rehearsal and IA could not both be applied within a stress management program. There is considerable evidence that covert rehearsal is efficacious (Bandura, 1997; Meichenbaum, 1985). Moreover, the efficacy of stress inoculation training is far better established than that of CASMT in terms of the number of controlled studies. The empirical and practical questions involve the relative effectiveness of the two rehearsal techniques and the outcome variables affected by them.

Smith and Nye (1989) compared the effects of IA and covert rehearsal in reducing test anxiety and enhancing academic performance in students enrolled in a large introductory psychology course. Also of interest was the extent to which the rehearsal techniques result in generalization of treatment gains. Highly test-anxious college students within the course were randomly assigned to two treatment conditions or to a wait-list control condition. The treatment conditions were based on the six-session group format described in the CASMT manual (minus the current mindfulness–defusion component). The only difference was that in one condition, covert rehearsal rather than IA was used to practice coping responses. In this condition, participants imagined using their coping skills successfully during tests as described by Meichenbaum (1985). In the IA condition, higher levels of affective arousal were evoked using encouragement and positive reinforcement as participants imagined the test situation and then used their coping skills to "turn off" their anxiety.

Among the outcome variables were test anxiety, general trait anxiety;

state anxiety measured immediately prior to actual classroom tests in the course; academic performance on course examinations; generalized coping self-efficacy; and locus of control. With the exception of state anxiety, significant group differences were found for each of the outcome variables. On the Test Anxiety Scale (Sarason, 1975), both the covert rehearsal and IA conditions exhibited greater decreases in test anxiety than did the control condition, but the IA group showed a significantly larger reduction than did the covert rehearsal condition. On the academic performance measure (test grades on weekly tests in the same course), a significant main effect was shown in test performance in which the control group's academic performance declined over the course of the academic term, the covert rehearsal group showed no change in performance and did not differ significantly from the control group, but the students in the IA condition exhibited grade improvement over the last half of the academic term and differed significantly from the control group, but not from the covert rehearsal group.

Generalization of training effects beyond test anxiety and test performance was also assessed. In terms of general trait anxiety, the only significant group difference favored the covert rehearsal condition over the wait-list control group. Although it also exhibited reduced trait anxiety, the IA condition did not differ from either the control or the covert rehearsal condition in improvement on the generalized trait anxiety measure. Significant group differences were found on both of the expectancy generalization measures. On the Internal–External Scale, both the covert rehearsal and IA conditions exhibited significantly larger shifts toward a more internal locus of control than did the control group, but the two rehearsal conditions did not differ significantly from one another.

Bandura (1997) has cited behavioral attainments and self-perceived control of emotional arousal as potent factors in increased self-efficacy. This finding prompted a prediction that the IA condition would result in larger changes in coping self-efficacy than the covert rehearsal condition because it involved self-perceptions of control in reducing strong affect, whereas covert rehearsal did not. Results showed statistically significant differences among conditions in self-efficacy change, with both covert rehearsal ($d = 0.87$) and IA ($d = 1.79$) treatments exhibiting large effect sizes when compared with the control group (Figure 2.5). In accord with the prediction derived from Bandura's theory, however, a larger self-efficacy increase occurred in the IA condition than in the covert rehearsal condition ($d = 0.67$).

In the IA condition, improved academic test performance was highly correlated with reductions in state anxiety measures, administered before classroom exams ($r = .64$). No such relation was found in the covert rehearsal condition, suggesting that the two rehearsal techniques may

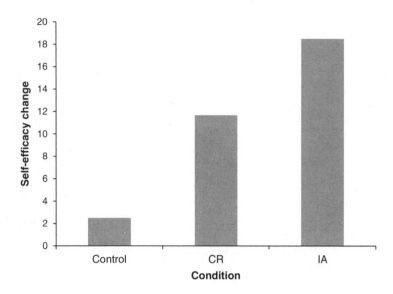

FIGURE 2.5. Changes in generalized coping efficacy, comparing the use of covert rehearsal (CR) or induced affect (IA) as the coping skills rehearsal method in the treatment of test anxiety. Data from Smith and Nye (1989).

optimally promote the acquisition and utilization of different classes of coping skills. Possibly, IA produces its salutary effects on performance by teaching people to control performance-disrupting emotional arousal and increasing their coping efficacy because of their perceived ability to reduce strong arousal in the training sessions. Some other mechanism of improved functioning may underlie the effects of covert rehearsal. For example, covert rehearsal may foster acquisition of the cognitive coping skills that are the focus of cognitive restructuring and self-instructional training, because there is little affect to which relaxation can be applied. Likewise, the covert rehearsal treatment, like the IA condition, produced positive changes in personal control expectancies, including self-efficacy and locus of control. Clearly, additional research is needed to address this treatment mechanism question.

Single-Client Experimental Studies Using Time Series Analysis

A National Institute of Mental Health (2008) research priority mandates the supplementation of group-based randomized clinical trials (RCTs) with idiographic analysis of clients: "Going forward, [National Institute of Mental Health] clinical research will not only assess overall group differences, but also individualized patterns of intervention response. The goal is a personalized approach to treatment" (p. 23). Prominent psychotherapy researchers (e.g., Kazdin, 2008) have echoed this call for more intensive single-client experimental research as a supplement to group data, which often mask important individual differences in response to treatment. Moreover, intensive analyses of repeated measures in treatments allow a unique opportunity to identify potential causal mechanisms through lagged analyses of therapeutic components and subsequent changes after they are introduced during treatment (see Boswell, Anderson, & Barlow, 2014, for an excellent example).

In recent years, we have been conducting such analyses of individual clients' responses to the CASMT intervention, utilizing the Stress and Coping Diary described above in an Internet-based assessment system to enhance an understanding of relations among stressors, cognitions, coping, and outcomes. Such data allow us to conduct collaborative therapeutic assessment with clients who referred themselves for CASMT at the University of Washington's Psychological Services and Training Center in response to advertisements offering stress management training.

To utilize the online system, clients log in to a website using a therapist-generated ID number and a client-generated password. To analyze the results of these single-client experimental studies, we use Simulation Modeling Analysis (Borckardt et al., 2008). This time series analysis program corrects for autocorrelation among repeated measures and provides significance tests of changes across phases of treatment. The diary data can be used to assess treatment changes on any of the quantitative measures in the diary.

We have now accumulated daily data on more than a dozen CASMT cases seen individually and more than 25 seen in groups. In five recent individual-client studies, we have collected 2 weeks of pretreatment diary data and 2 weeks of postintervention diary reports. A primary outcome variable has been a diary item that assesses postcoping stress level. We compared the first two sessions (coping skill acquisition) with the last four sessions in which IA is used to rehearse the skills. A within-group analysis involving all of the clients showed a significant decrease in postcoping stress level (Cohen's $d = 1.57$). Figure 2.6 shows one client's record. Time series analysis revealed a highly significant change in her perceived ability to control negative affective responses when coping skills rehearsal under IA was instituted at Session 3.

Clients varied in their reports of their extent of use and their perceived effectiveness of the various coping skills. Some clients reported relaxation as most effective, whereas others found the cognitive skills most helpful. Some clients, like the one shown in Figure 2.6, showed the strongest positive training outcome on our diary measure of perceived

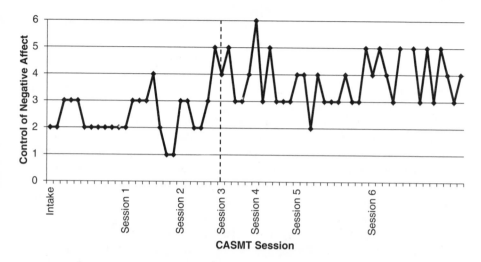

FIGURE 2.6. A client's daily ratings of her ability to control her negative emotional responses to stressors, comparing the prerehearsal and IA-rehearsal phases of CASMT. Time series analysis revealed a significant increase in self-reported negative affect regulation from the skills acquisition phase of CASMT (Sessions 1 and 2) to the IA skills rehearsal phase ($r = .59, p = .0001$). From Chen et al. (in press). Copyright by Elsevier. Reprinted by permission of the authors.

effectiveness in controlling the negative emotional responses evoked by stressors, whereas others, while reporting improved self-regulation, exhibited their largest change in general life satisfaction as training progressed. In general, we have been impressed with the notable degree of idiographic variation in response to a highly manualized treatment.

Coping skills interventions tacitly assume that the delivery of coping skills training translates into effective utilization of these skills by clients. Addressing empirical support for augmenting exposure treatment with coping skills training in the treatment of panic disorder and agoraphobia, Meuret, Wolitzky-Taylor, Twohig, and Craske (2012) have challenged this assumption and called for the independent measurement of both frequency of utilization and effectiveness of the coping skills. (We might add that situational appropriateness should also be assessed.) Where CASMT is concerned, behavioral observations of clients in their ability to reduce arousal during the IA procedure provides useful information about the level of skill acquisition the client has achieved, and such observations during IA are sometimes supplemented by physiological measures (e.g., Holmes, 1981). The trainer is also able to evaluate the quality of the client's reappraisals and self-instructional self-statements by examining the structure of the integrated coping response the client reports applying during IA. In some respects, this part of the process approaches (though not as comprehensively) the think-aloud paradigm recommended by Meuret et al. (2012) that provides a sample of the client's thinking during exposure to feared situations (e.g., Williams, Kinney, Harap, & Leibmann, 1997). Moreover, the Stress and Coping Diary provides client reports of potential reappraisals and the extent to which each coping skill is applied in real-life settings as well as its perceived effectiveness. Direct assessment of the skills taught in coping skills programs is a methodological step beyond the standard practice of assuming that training automatically translates into skills acquisition and utilization. Moreover, the data allow for mediational analyses to assess the role of specific skills in contributing to changes in distal outcome measures in both individual cases and with aggregated data from group designs.

Because nomothetic outcome research remains the gold standard for establishing treatment efficacy, therapeutic principles and procedures generally proceed in a deductive fashion, applied from RCTs to the individual client. However, the power of the individual case to illuminate therapeutic processes allows us to promote a complementary inductive process. This is described in a recent article on translational research involving the areas of personality and clinical psychology:

> We suggest that the objective and quantitative analyses of each intra-individual dynamic we described above, which might be referred to as quantitative idiography, could be a key for allowing such analyses to contribute not only to the clinician, but also to science in general. It is idiographic in that it focuses on understanding the functioning of one individual at a time. And it is quantitative in that it analyzes the pattern of intra-individual dynamics quantitatively. By creating an electronic repository of anonymized findings about each client's intra-individual dynamics captured in the way illustrated in this article and as called for by Kazdin and Blase (2011), in time, common and unique ways in which different people approach life challenges will be accumulated. The accumulated knowledge can then be culled and organized through integrative and discovery-oriented, theory-building literature reviews with a specific focus on discovering meaningful individual-to-individual variations, as well as a more qualitative "cataloguing" of the variety of processes with which different individuals address the challenge of being human, an approach some researchers already practice (e.g., Bonanno & Mancini, 2012). The result will be a cumulative science constructed with building blocks of "local knowledge" of the different ways in which individuals address life challenges. (Shoda et al., 2013, p. 565)

There is much need for additional research on CASMT's efficacy, effectiveness, applicability to various populations, and on the mechanisms that underlie positive effects when they occur. Likewise, the welcome emphasis on translational research is likely to stimulate new rapprochements between clinical science and other areas of psychology, such as personality science (Shoda et al., 2013). We believe that the importation of conceptual models such as the CAPS and research based on these models will help inform research on relevant individual differences and mechanisms of change.

CONCLUSIONS AND FUTURE DIRECTIONS

Our goal in writing this book is to acquaint clinicians and researchers with the IA procedure and to provide explicit clinical and research guidelines for conducting both IA therapy and CASMT. We hope that the reader will agree that the research evidence described in this chapter qualifies both IA and CASMT as empirically supported interventions and as foundations for evidence-based practice.

Where CASMT is concerned, we hope that the training package will help address the need for effective, time-limited interventions. It is necessary to expand the scope of both preventive and ameliorative mental health care, a theme addressed well by both National Institute of Mental Health (2008) and by leading clinical scientists (e.g., Kazdin, 2008; Kazdin & Blase, 2011). In particular, CASMT may be an efficient vehicle for prevention efforts directed at the many people who suffer from high levels of life stress (American Psychological Association, 2013). Elements of CASMT (including IA) can also be incorporated into other treatment packages to, hopefully, increase their efficacy and effectiveness. To the extent to which these objectives occur, this book will have made its intended contribution to evidence-based practice and clinical science.

WHAT'S AHEAD

In Chapter 3, we describe the technique of IA in detail and provide explicit guidelines for its use in both psychotherapy and in emotion self-regulation interventions. Our goal is to add to the ability of clinicians to elicit affective responses, teach clients how to control rather than avoid them, and to thereby increase the learned resourcefulness of clients.

CHAPTER 3

Affect Elicitation in Psychotherapy
The Induced Affect Technique

The enterprise of psychotherapy is based in part on the assumption that when people are in distress, it is good to talk with someone about their feelings. James Pennebaker (1995, 1997) conducted a series of disclosure studies in which college students talked about past traumas to an experimenter in an adjoining room, or they tape-recorded or wrote about the experiences. Participants in a control group were asked to talk or write about trivial everyday matters. A comparison of blood samples taken from the students before and after the session showed enhanced immune system functioning in those who had vented their negative emotions but not in those who had not. Moreover, the students who had disclosed the traumatic incidents had 50% fewer visits to the campus health center over the next 6 months compared with the control group.

Many subsequent studies have shown that disclosing stressful or traumatic events in these ways promotes physical health, higher levels of psychological functioning, and subjective well-being (Smyth, Pennebaker, & Arigo, 2012). In one study, Sloan and Marx (2004) used the written disclosure procedure with college students who had reported experiencing a traumatic event in their lives. The students completed measures of stress symptoms, depression, and number of days they had been sick since the beginning of the school term. In an experimental condition, participants were then asked to write about the traumatic event, whereas the control condition did an unrelated task. Physiological arousal was recorded as the participants performed the tasks. One month later, the students again completed the measures of psychological symptoms and sick days. The students had not differed on any of these measures at baseline, but they differed strongly afterward. Those who had written about their traumas showed lowered stress and depression scores, and they also reported fewer sick days at follow-up. The more physiologically aroused the participants in the written disclosure group became while they wrote about their traumatic events, the more physically and psychologically healthy they appeared a month later.

As noted in Chapter 1, emotional suppression and avoidance are among the less effective emotion regulation strategies, and they can have negative physical, psychological, and social consequences (English et al., 2013; Hoffman et al., 2009; John & Eng, 2014). In one long-term European study, people who were experiencing high stress levels but were too emotionally restrained to express negative feelings, even when appropriate, had a significantly higher likelihood of developing cancer than did highly stressed people who were not so emotionally restrained. Seeking to reduce this potential vulnerability factor, Eysenck and Grossarth-Marticek (1991) designed a treatment program to help stress-ridden and emotionally constrained people who had not yet developed cancer. The cognitive-behavioral intervention focused on teaching participants how to express their emotions in an adaptive fashion and on building stress coping skills to manage their feelings without bottling them up. A control group of similar people did not receive the training. Thirteen years later, a follow-up study revealed that 90% of the trained participants were still alive, whereas 62% of the control group participants had died from cancer and other ailments.

Given the central role that emotion plays in many behavioral disorders, as well as its relations with other psychological processes, it is not surprising that therapists of all theoretical persuasions have emphasized, and continue to emphasize, emotion elicitation as a central mechanism of therapeutic change. In-session experiencing of affect has been seen as instrumental in achieving therapeutic objectives ranging from the unearthing of unconscious psychodynamic conflicts to the extinction of maladaptive emotional responses. Conversely, both process and treatment outcome research suggests that emotional avoidance is an impediment to therapeutic process (Boswell, 2013; Cromer, 2013; Renninger, 2013).

In the next section, we briefly discuss affect elicitation in CBT before introducing the IA procedure and the ways in which it differs from other CBT techniques, such as systematic desensitization and exposure.

AFFECT ELICITATION IN CBT

Affect elicitation is an essential component of several behavioral and cognitive-behavioral approaches. In his cognitive–affective–relational behavior therapy, Goldfried (2013) uses the two-chair technique (also called the "empty-chair technique," popularized in Gestalt therapy) to elicit emotional arousal so as to reveal and change clients' personal meaning structures through cognitive restructuring. While seated in one chair, the client expresses and tries to defend the irrational and dysfunctional belief or schema, then does the same for its more rational alternative while marshalling evidence against the dysfunctional belief from his or her own life experiences. This exercise typically elicits the associated emotions and helps the client experience the consequences of the maladaptive cognitions firsthand. Research indicates that the emotional arousal elicited during this exercise is a crucial element in its success (Elliot, Watson, Goldman, & Greenberg, 2004). The two-chair technique is used in a similar fashion to analyze and change dysfunctional cognitions in schema therapy (Young, Klosko, and Weishaar, 2003).

Treatments Based on Learning Theory

Theoretical models derived from the psychology of learning view anxiety as a conditioned emotional response. By virtue of being paired with aversive or painful stimuli (unconditioned stimuli [UCS]), certain stimuli become conditioned stimuli (CS) capable of eliciting a conditioned anxiety response. Once established through direct or vicarious classical conditioning, a conditioned anxiety response becomes capable of motivating and reinforcing avoidance responses, and the resulting reduction in anxiety constitutes negative reinforcement that serves to strengthen the avoidance responses and prevents extinction from occurring (Rescorla & Solomon, 1967). Current network conceptions of the conditioning process (e.g., Foa & Jaycox, 1999; Shoda & Smith, 2004) emphasize underlying cognitive representations of the process.

The treatment technique of *exposure* refers to the general technique of exposing the individual to anxiety-provoking stimuli while preventing the occurrence of the client's customary cognitive and behavioral avoidance responses. Clinically, exposure usually involves the use of imagined scenes, although *in vivo* (real-life) exposure to the actual feared stimuli or situations could also be used, either alone or as an adjunct to the imaginal exposure. It is assumed that prolonged exposure to intense forms of the anxiety-arousing stimuli in the absence of an aversive UCS will extinguish the anxiety. A large number of clinical and experimental studies provide evidence that this does indeed occur, whereas brief exposures do not produce extinction (Antony & Roemer, 2014; Levis, 2009). Prolonged exposure is a key component of an empirically supported treatment for posttraumatic stress disorder (PTSD) in which the conditioned anxiety associated with the traumatic event(s) is viewed as part of a cognitive–affective–behavioral network that has dysfunctional consequences (Foa &

Jaycox, 1999). The goal in this treatment is (1) to extinguish the negative affect associated with the traumatic event; (2) to help the client change pathogenic elements of the memory for the event, which can involve construals of the world as a dangerous place and of him- or herself as incompetent or blameworthy; and (3) to help the client come to terms with other consequences of the traumatic conditioning, such as anger and guilt, avoidance of intimacy, lowered self-esteem, and possible suicidal tendencies.

Procedurally, the goal is to activate trauma-related fear and then modify the pathological elements that are thought to maintain PTSD. Exposure is carried out in two ways: imaginal and *in vivo*. In-session imaginal exposure is designed to elicit maximum anxiety. The client is asked to recall the traumatic event as vividly as possible, imagining that the event is happening right at the moment and allowing the feelings to be fully experienced. Outside of therapy, graded exposure is employed. The therapist and client develop a hierarchy of life situations that are avoided because of excessive anxiety. Choosing situations with a moderate level of discomfort, the client is instructed to go into those situations and remain in them for 30–45 minutes, or until the anxiety is at least 50% reduced. Care is taken to ensure that the client can succeed, and doing so not only helps extinguish the anxiety, but also increases self-efficacy and challenges construals of the situations as dangerous and of oneself as a prisoner of fear.

Much experimental evidence with clinical populations suffering from severe anxiety indicates the efficacy of exposure techniques in reducing anxiety responses (Antony & Roemer, 2014; Powers, Halpern, Ferenschak, Gillihan, & Foa, 2010). One example is the demonstrated efficacy of a massed-exposure one-session treatment for specific phobias (Öst, 1989). In the one-session treatment, a hierarchy of stimuli associated with the feared object is constructed, and the client is taken through the entire hierarchy in a session that may last as long as 3 hours and that is designed to extinguish high levels of anxiety. The one-session treatment appears to be a highly efficacious treatment in both adults and children (Ollendick & Davis, 2013).

Despite the effectiveness of exposure treatments, the mechanisms involved in fear reduction point increasingly to the importance of cognitive mediators. Recent findings of panic disorder treatment indicate that the amount of physiological activation and reduction of fear measured during exposure sessions are not related to outcome. These results are at odds with the classical noncognitive extinction model and, in conjunction with other findings, point to the role of an altered CS–UCS expectancy as a likely mechanism of change (Craske, Kircanski, Mystkowski, Chowdhury, & Baker, 2008; Meuret, Seidel, Rosenfield, Hofmann, & Rosenfield,

2012). Nonetheless, the willingness to tolerate high and sustained levels of fear during exposure is related to greater fear reduction and may therefore facilitate corrective learning mediated by expectancy violation and benign expectancy reconstruction (Culver, Stoyanova, & Craske, 2012).

Another learning-based approach is the counterconditioning model. An alternative to extinguishing a conditioned emotional response is to condition a state that is incompatible with physiological arousal responses to the anxiety-arousing cues. The general principle, according to Joseph Wolpe, the chief proponent of the counterconditioning approach, is as follows:

> If a response antagonistic to anxiety can be made to occur in the presence of anxiety-evoking stimuli so that it is accompanied by a complete or partial suppression of the anxiety responses, the bond between these stimuli and the anxiety responses will be lessened. (1958, p. 21)

According to Wolpe, through a process of classical conditioning anxious people have learned to experience excessively high levels of sympathetic nervous system arousal in the presence of certain stimuli. The goal of treatment is to replace sympathetic activity with competing behaviors that have a predominance of parasympathetic innervation, a process that Wolpe, following Sherrington's (1906) physiological model, termed "reciprocal inhibition." Wolpe's systematic desensitization treatment is designed to permit the gradual counterconditioning of anxiety, typically using somatic relaxation as the incompatible response (although other inhibitors, including carbon dioxide inhalation and vigorous motor responses, have also been employed). It is important to note that the process of systematic desensitization is carried out using a graded stimulus hierarchy designed to ensure that the client will experience little if any anxiety, a feature that differentiates this approach from exposure techniques.

More than 100 controlled studies have found desensitization to be superior to placebo or untreated controls with a wide range of anxiety-based disorders (O'Donohue & Fisher, 2009; Spiegler & Guevremont, 2003). The technique has also proven effective in the treatment of anger, which, like anxiety, has an arousal component (Deffenbacher, 2013; Rimm, DeGroot, Boord, Heiman, & Dillow, 1971).

The Coping Skills Approach

The coping skills approach is another behavioral model that utilizes affect arousal techniques and is based on the principles of emotional self-regulation. As mentioned in Chapter 1, the CASMT program detailed in

Chapters 4 through 9 is based on this model. In contrast to the extinction model underlying prolonged exposure and the counterconditioning model that informs Wolpe's systematic desensitization intervention, the coping skills model views the goal of treatment not as deconditioning maladaptive emotional responses, but rather as developing stress-reducing coping skills and replacing dysfunctional ways of coping or coping deficits with adaptive self-regulation skills and strategies. This approach encompasses a variety of techniques, including social skills training, problem-solving training, and adaptive emotion-focused strategies, such as identifying and changing irrational negative thinking, thinking in a task-relevant fashion, and learning relaxation skills to control arousal (D'Zurilla & Nezu, 2007; Meichenbaum, 1985; Mueser, Gottlieb, & Gingerich, 2014; Smith, 1980).

The coping skills approach was stimulated in part by several influential reconceptualizations of the conditioning-based technique of systematic desensitization. For example, Goldfried (1971) suggested that systematic desensitization could be reconstrued as a procedure for learning and practicing relaxation as an active coping skill for the self-control of anxiety, rather than as a counterconditioning procedure to reciprocally inhibit emotional arousal, as presented by Wolpe (1958). At about the same time, Suinn and Richardson (1971) introduced anxiety management training, based on a similar conception of relaxation as an active coping skill. In anxiety management training, clients practice using relaxation to reduce anxiety elicited by imagining stressful situations. Music designed to enhance the level of affect elicited by the imagined scenes is sometimes employed as well. Later, cognitive components such as positive self-talk and thought-stopping were added (Suinn, 1990).

In Meichenbaum's (1985) stress inoculation training, both behavioral and cognitive coping skills are taught and then rehearsed in guided imagery (covert rehearsal) and *in vivo* within relevant life situations. Clients are exposed to cues that elicit low levels of emotional arousal, on the assumption that learning to control these responses will "inoculate" them against more highly stressful situations in much the same way that a less powerful vaccine inoculates a medical patient against a more potent pathogen. Clients learn both relaxation skills to control physiological arousal and cognitive restructuring to challenge dysfunctional appraisals. Through self-instructional training, clients also develop self-directing self-statements to facilitate their coping efforts and their ability to focus on the task-relevant cues that may guide adaptive behavior.

In contrast to Meichenbaum's (1985) stress inoculation model, the IA procedure is designed to elicit high, rather than low, levels of arousal. The client's ability to control high arousal not only ensures his or her ability to control lower-level arousal responses, but also increases the client's level of coping self-efficacy—a factor that has been shown to strongly influence treatment outcome across many emotion regulation therapies (Bandura, 1997).

We now describe IA technique in some detail because this empirically supported technique is not well known among clinicians, and it is an integral part of CASMT. Moreover, IA can be used as a stand-alone treatment and can readily be incorporated into other emotion regulation therapies as well.

INDUCED AFFECT

Origin and Development

Carl Sipprelle (1967) developed the IA technique in which affect is elicited by the therapist's use of an interoceptive focus and the suggestion, encouragement, and verbal reinforcement of behavioral indicants of emotional arousal. Relaxation is used as an active coping skill to help clients gain self-control over strong emotional responses. In accord with network personality models, such as the CAPS, affect is viewed as an *entrée* into the network of associated cognitions, memories, and motives that could themselves become targets for change. Like Goldfried (1971), Sipprelle and his coworkers regarded the relaxation used to reduce the affective response as a generalized coping skill that could be applied across aversive emotional states involving arousal and that would be highly generalizable across situations

Sipprelle (1967) was strongly influenced by learning-based psychotherapies, beginning with the seminal work of Dollard and Miller (1950). As an academic, Sipprelle often treated university faculty as well as scientists from a nearby atomic energy research station. He had observed that many clients with obsessive–compulsive behaviors "don't live below the neck" and that "people who have undergone trauma often overcontrol and defend against feelings" (personal communication). Like therapists of many other orientations, Sipprelle observed that a flood of affect during psychotherapy is often accompanied by memories and thoughts that are functionally related not only to the presenting problem, but also to the amount of arousal that occurs. He became convinced that in order to change, most clients must experience arousal. He began to experiment with techniques that would allow a therapist to bypass defenses that typically controlled arousal. Earlier techniques, including hypnosis, were abandoned when studies in the 1960s showed that increases and decreases in muscle tension, cognition, and autonomic nervous system activity such as cardiac rate could be modified by operant reinforcement (e.g., Ascough & Sipprelle, 1968; Jordan & Sipprelle, 1972).

Based in part on Pascal's (1959) report that relaxation reduced the strength of defenses in his study of military veterans with battlefield trauma, and on Wolpe's (1958) demonstration that muscle relaxation could counteract affective arousal, Sipprelle's early therapeutic technique involved first training clients in muscle relaxation as in systematic desensitization. After relaxation was mastered, the next phase involved elicitation of emotional arousal through suggestion and operant reinforcement of affective increases by the therapist. The client was asked to verbalize images, memories, and thoughts that might arise during arousal while, at the same time, the therapist began instruction for another relaxation phase. After subsequent arousal and relaxation phases the client learned to "relax away" elevated affect and associated experiences. In early work the process was regarded as an abreactive uncovering technique, then as a counterconditioning technique. Later, he reconceptualized IA as a therapy to elicit feelings in a controlled manner and to teach coping responses (Sipprelle, 1967, 1981). He noted that we cannot replace a client's memories of an abusive father with memories of one who is warm, nurturing, and caring, nor can we negate a traumatic combat memory—but we *can* use the NA generated from such experiences to teach responses to deal with immediate affect and with affect in future stressful situations. The goal was for clients to leave therapy with coping skills that would allow for continued improvement in stress-resilience.

To summarize, Sipprelle's (1967) development of IA was based on three emergent assumptions:

1. It is highly useful to elicit the affective responses/behaviors that are the focus of treatment within the therapy room; *behavior* implies a response complex that includes physiological, cognitive, and musculoskeletal components.
2. Clients must face typically-avoided cues, and the use of nonspecific suggestions and instructions allows for emotional arousal that is more isomorphic with the problem than are therapist-generated hierarchies or cues.
3. Adequate behavior change must be based on more than just habituation or extinction of emotional responses in therapy. The greatest improvement will occur and the generalization of treatment effects will continue if the person learns cognitive, physiological, and behavioral coping skills that can be used in a range of stressful situations. A central goal of IA training is, therefore, the development of a "future-oriented coping response."

IA has been utilized with a variety of clinical and nonclinical populations as a stand-alone treatment. As a treatment modality, IA is in many ways a well-kept secret. In our experience, many contemporary cognitive-behavioral therapists have never heard of the technique. This is understandable for a number of reasons. First, most of the developmental and empirical activity around IA occurred from the mid-1960s to around 1980 at the University of Georgia, where Sipprelle served as Director of Clinical Training until 1967; at Purdue University, where his student Ascough established a research program; at East Carolina University, where Charles Moore, another Sipprelle student, established a research program; and at the University of South Dakota, where Sipprelle served as Director of Clinical Training and ended his career in 1980. That same year, Ascough left Purdue to assume a clinical and administrative position at a regional mental health center. The Center for Induced Affect, established at Purdue by Ascough in the 1970s, served as a repository of IA research and clinical reports. In 1981, the center published a two-volume compendium (Ascough, 1981; Ascough, Moore, & Sipprelle, 1981). The bibliographies contained a total of 113 references to published articles and chapters, papers based on convention presentations, and summaries of unpublished master's and doctoral theses. Many reports were published *in toto*.

There is no dearth of research on IA. In addition to published articles, many well-designed dissertation studies were carried out, but upon finishing their degrees, many of these students moved into clinical practice positions where there were few incentives to publish their research. Consequently, and unfortunately, many well-designed studies of meaningful scientific and practical significance never found their way into journals. We describe some of those studies later in this chapter.

IA Procedures

Specific procedures may vary among therapists who use IA, but they generally include the following sequence. The first two sessions are used for assessment, case conceptualization, and relaxation training.

Medical conditions should be assessed, as in any affect elicitation treatment, but this is seldom a concern. Where functional integrity is concerned, "adequate stability" is a criterion. Occasionally IA therapists have cautioned against employing the technique with individuals with psychoses and those with organic damage. Others have worked with such clients without adverse events occurring, and there is empirical evidence of positive therapeutic effects with patients diagnosed with schizophrenia (see the section on p. 105). One criterion, as old as European psychoanalysis, is the following question (Wolberg, 1967): Can the client step beyond his or her defenses in a session, then reestablish controls and live adequately until the next session? Most therapists have potential clients complete an extensive life history questionnaire and an objective measure, such as the

Minnesota Multiphasic Personality Inventory–2 (MMPI-2), before accepting them for therapy, and such information should provide a reasonable basis for therapeutic decisions. Moreover, an initial thorough case conceptualization helps therapists prepare rationales that are unique to individual clients, improves clients' introduction to the therapy, and connects information from the arousal phase back to the case conceptualization in the discussion phase.

The case conceptualization is typically based on a cognitive-behavioral orientation and includes relations between the presenting problem and identified stressors, supports, strengths, deficits, adaptive coping strategies, and maladaptive coping strategies (Pascal, 1959). In this model, expressed in the form of an equation, stressors, deficits, and maladaptive coping strategies (placed in the numerator) serve to exacerbate psychological problems, whereas supports, strengths, and adaptive coping strategies (found in the denominator) reduce psychological problems. The model is useful for case conceptualization and treatment planning, as evidence-based treatment strategies can be directed at any of the elements in the model. For example, the procedures described in this book are designed to reduce stress by enhancing adaptive coping strategies (and by replacing maladaptive ones, such as suppression and avoidance).

In some cases, daily measures (e.g., the Stress and Coping Diary discussed in Chapter 2) are used to track situational, cognitive, emotional, and behavioral variables and their interrelations. Additionally, personality measures may be administered; the MMPI-2 has been used most frequently as a screening measure. In addition, trait anxiety measures allow prediction of responsiveness to IA (Korn, Ascough & Kleemeier, 1972).

Relaxation training is often introduced in the first session; some therapists loan audio recordings to clients so that they can practice daily at home. Depending on each client's needs and preferences, these at-home exercises may include a general relaxation practice, a short (15-minute) body scan, a typical tension–release (progressive relaxation) guide, an active tension–release guide specifically for persons with insistent thoughts, or imagery recordings designed for either cognitive or physiological de-arousal. (A downloadable audio recording of the relaxation exercise in Appendix A, Handout A-2, is available to purchasers of this book for distribution to their clients; see the box at the end of the table of contents.) Relaxation training is continued and any needed objective measures (such as an anxiety measure or a measure of negative life events) are taken.

In the second or third session a treatment rationale is presented that involves a general explanation of purpose, assumptions, procedures, processes, and goals. This information about IA is helpful in that actual change in therapy is often stressful no matter which therapy is introduced.

Further, clients have expectancies about what may occur in therapy, and IA may differ considerably from their conceptions. The rationale and any needed objective measures suggest that the client may experience tension reduction from the release that occurs with arousal and will also benefit from learning about thoughts and other stimuli that accompany distress. However, the most important aspect of IA is the learning of coping skills. Clients are told that they will go through a series of trials in which emotional arousal is induced and they will be trained to "turn off" the arousal. Relaxation training is conceptualized as the initial step in learning a complex coping response that integrates behavior, physiology, and mental processes into measures that clients can use whenever they encounter stressful cues in future nontherapy settings.

Therapists who use IA frequently collect data throughout the sessions. Baseline data may include measures administered in the first two sessions. In treatment the session data might be state measures of emotions collected during initial relaxation, arousal, and final relaxation phases; as well as physiological data recorded on measuring devices worn by clients that provide an ongoing record of autonomic activity.

IA consists of four main phases: an initial relaxation phase lasting 6–10 minutes, an arousal phase during which affect is induced, a relaxation phase to terminate arousal, and a discussion phase. This sequence can be repeated several times within a session.

Initial Relaxation Phase

The initial relaxation phase provides contingent reinforcement upon responsiveness to the relaxation instructions. It also provides information on client compliance or resistance. It supports the therapist's suggestion that, with practice, relaxation can be achieved even when the client is emotionally aroused, and that it can be used to counteract arousal. Finally, the initial relaxation phase creates a baseline level from which the therapist will reinforce observed changes toward arousal. As mentioned above, this phase often lasts from 6 to 10 minutes; on occasion, however, this phase is skipped if, for example, a client arrives in an already aroused state that the therapist can build upon in the induction phase before relaxation is applied to dampen arousal. In such instances, the therapist works with the currently activated emotional state, whatever its nature.

Arousal Phase

In the arousal phase, the client is told to focus inwardly to experience feelings that will begin to grow stronger. In its most traditional form, IA differs from other affect elicitation techniques in that no specific cues are presented beyond the suggestion to feel feelings. Feelings are specified only after the client labels them. Several approaches are used to encourage and reinforce arousal. The therapist can continue instructions to "feel the feelings"; the therapist can make suggestions that feelings are getting "stronger and stronger"; the therapist can give specific reinforcements, such as saying "Good" as signs of arousal occur; or the therapist may note behaviors, such as "Your hands are trembling and the feelings are becoming stronger . . . that's great, just let them grow." In general, the therapist will reinforce any overt signs of arousal, whether directly observed or, in a research setting, based on shifts shown in psychophysiological data. As arousal begins to wane, or if the therapist judges that the arousal is becoming too strong, the therapist asks the client to verbalize feelings, thoughts, and images being experienced (if she or he has not done so spontaneously). The therapist can use that material to further arouse the client, elaborate the material, or terminate the arousal phase. In early sessions the therapist may administer relaxation instructions to "bring the client down." In later sessions, the arousal phase is terminated with instructions to "turn it off" with self-applied relaxation.

Relaxation with Arousal Phase

With termination of the arousal phase, relaxation is reinitiated as the therapist reiterates the material noted during the arousal phase while simultaneously applying relaxation instructions. The relaxation initiates the process of learning to cope. Statements might include "You can recall all the things you said, but you can continue relaxing"; "Agitation and anxiety are reversible, and you can become more comfortable still"; and "You can cope with this emotion." It is not unusual for the therapist to reiterate relationships between cognitive statements, autonomic nervous system activity, and current muscle tension or recalled behaviors. Increasingly-rhythmic abdominal breathing, reduced muscle tension, and calm affect signal arousal reduction. The therapist may ask for occasional self-reports from the client using SUDS ratings such as the scale shown in Appendix B (Figure B-4).

As noted above, over the sessions the therapist fades out and simply asks the client to apply his or her relaxation skills to reduce arousal, as will be required outside of the therapy context. The simultaneous presentation of instructions to relaxation with suggestions to focus on affect and content, continued over sessions, allows the client to learn to dampen the level of emotionality in the presence of internal cognitive and physiological cues. The fact that internal affective cues are common across a variety of emotions and stressful situations helps create generalizable coping skills.

The coping skills model conceptualizes the role of relaxation as a future-oriented emotion regulation skill. The goal is for clients to control affect and enhance self-efficacy. In the first few inductions, therefore, arousal is kept at a moderate level so that the therapist can be confident that relaxation skills will successfully counter the arousal. In later inductions, given confidence that the client has adequate coping skills, no limit is set on how high the arousal can become, as the focus here is on showing the client that levels of arousal even higher than what he or she is likely to encounter outside of therapy can be controlled. Such demonstrations help establish high levels of coping self-efficacy (Smith & Nye, 1989). In most sessions, the therapist will present several arousal–relaxation sequences, the objective being to provide multiple coping skill trials.

Discussion Phase

The discussion phase is a highly significant part of IA therapy. After arousal has been reduced and the client is relaxed, the therapist asks the client to describe feelings, thoughts, memories, and other content experienced during the arousal phase. The therapist can offer reassurance, clarification, reflection, support, and interpretation. The intent is to facilitate the integration of the experience, to explore with the client its significance and meaning, and to engage in cognitive restructuring that will allow the client to perceive future situations with similar cues in a more adaptive manner.

This phase may begin with the therapist saying, "You said/felt/recalled _____. What does that mean to you?" At times a therapist may suggest several hypothetical directions and allow the client to further explore his or her own perceptions. Later, the therapist might ask the client how the material fits into the current and evolving case conceptualization. Discussion not only allows review but may also elicit additional memories, which in turn provides an opportunity to enhance (1) the client's recognition of his or her emotions, leading the client (2) to further integrate and understand the relations between cognitions, autonomic nervous system activity, and behavior. IA may thus facilitate treatment within other therapies (including psychodynamic and humanistic approaches) when the client would profit from access to emotional material. Again, we emphasize that IA is a therapeutic tool as well as an approach to treatment in its own right.

When is the decision made to end an IA phase of therapy? Therapy may be terminated when arousal phases begin to level out, there is no significant physiological or somatic arousal in response to previously emotional situations, and there is a decrease in negative thoughts. Other indicators may include low arousal during the arousal phase, cognitions that are not related to any significant difficulties, and the appearance of positive affect during the arousal phase. The therapist and client may decide to use positive arousal in several sessions to teach and elaborate positive feelings. In treating clients with depression (or other conditions), it can be very helpful to use IA as a vehicle for eliciting positive affect. This can be accomplished by (1) asking clients to imagine happy events from the past, (2) inducing affect by suggesting a rising intensity of the feelings, and (3) reinforcing physical or verbal indications of increasing positive emotion. In clients with depression, this approach can serve as a personally experienced demonstration of their continued capacity to feel positive emotions and help counter the anhedonia and hopelessness concerning future happiness that is so often part of the disorder. Of course, the most important outcome criterion is evidence of improved coping outside of the therapy room.

To illustrate the phases of IA, we present excerpts from a transcript (adapted to ensure anonymity) of a tape used by Sipprelle to train therapists in IA (Ascough, 1975). It is based on a training case demonstration done by Sipprelle at a psychiatric hospital. The client was an unmarried rural Protestant minister who had been hospitalized with what was termed "a total emotional collapse" featuring comorbid anxiety, depression, and vegetative symptoms such as gastrointestinal distress, loss of appetite, and insomnia. He exhibited classical stress-induced burnout symptoms in response to unremitting demands on his time and personal resources. In Pascal's (1959) case conceptualization model, used by Sipprelle, the most pronounced elements were a high level of life stress and NA (anxiety and depression) created by the many emotional and time demands to which he was subjected. He also exhibited a deficit in emotion regulation skills and maladaptive coping responses involving emotional constraint that contributed to a low level of emotional support from others who were unaware of his torment. The initial treatment goal was the development of coping skills to reduce NA.

Notice how Sipprelle uses the client's self-reported reactions to intensify the IA and elicit associated thoughts and situational factors through restatement, encouragement, and reinforcement, and how he later uses this material during the discussion phase to help reassure the client and set the stage for additional therapy.

The client was seated in a comfortable recliner chair. Sipprelle first did progressive relaxation to create a low baseline level of arousal, then began IA.

DR. S: Mr. A, I want you to lie there very quietly and I want you to feel how relaxed you are. It's a good, peaceful, comfortable feeling. That's good. Now I want you to turn your attention deep down inside. Just keep your eyes closed and lie there quietly, and I want you to turn your attention deep down inside. A feeling down inside of you is going to start to grow . . . and that feeling is going to get stronger and stronger. The feeling is getting bigger now; bigger, bigger, bigger. That's fine. Let it grow. Just let the feeling get as big as it wants to. I want you to just let it happen. No matter what the feeling is, you're just going to let it come. (*Mr. A begins to exhibit muscular tension, increased respiration, and facial frowning.*) That's good. That's fine. Just let it grow stronger now. Bigger and bigger . . . stronger and stronger . . . that's good. You're doing fine. That's good . . . let it grow bigger and bigger. You can feel it more and more. Good, let it get bigger and bigger. It's getting very big now. Good. Okay, I'd like you to keep your eyes closed, but I'd like you to tell me what your thoughts are. What are you feeling, Mr. A?

MR. A: I'm getting all tense again . . . and I think I could cry!

DR. S: You're getting all tense and feel like crying. That's good, just feel the feeling. You feel tense and feel like crying. Just let that feeling get stronger. That's fine. You're doing good. Just let that feeling come out now. That's fine . . . just let the feeling come out now. It's okay. Just let the feeling come out now. Just let the feeling get stronger. That's good. All right now. Just let the feeling get stronger. (*Mr. A begins to sob and exhibits tension with clenched fists and stiffened legs.*) The feeling is getting stronger and stronger. Just let it get stronger and stronger. It's okay. You're doing fine. Let the feeling grow. Just forget everything outside you and let the feeling get stronger. Stronger and stronger, and you feel it more and more now. Your whole body has that feeling. How do you feel now?

MR. A: Why do I have to go through this?

DR. S: Why do you have to go through . . . you feel that you have to go through a lot, don't you? Does it seem you have to go through a lot? Just think now in your mind of all the things you have to go through. Think of them now and get that feeling. It's a terrible feeling when you think of all the things you have to go through. The feeling is getting stronger and stronger now. Tell me what you're thinking now, Mr. A. What thoughts do you have?

MR. A: (*crying*) I put in so many hours of work. . . .

DR. S: You feel you have to work awfully hard? All right, just think of all the hours of work you've had to do. How hard you've had to work. Has your work worried you?

MR. A: Oh. There's so much of it . . . really . . . so much work itself. It's grinding me down.

DR. S: You feel it's more than you can handle? That's good. Just picture all the work you've had to do. And the feeling that it's more than you can handle, that it's grinding you down. Just let the feeling get stronger and stronger. That's good. Just let it come out. You're doing fine, Just think of all the work you've had to do . . . it's more than you can handle . . . let the feeling grow. Just let the feeling grow. Just picture all that you have to do. What are your thoughts now, Mr. A, what are you thinking?

MR. A: Ah, ah . . . just . . . uh. So many depend on me and nobody will help me.

DR. S: You don't feel anybody helps you. Are you saying that you have helped everybody else, but nobody helps you?

MR. A: Uh . . . huh . . . uh-huh . . . that's it exactly.

DR. S: It's kind of a lonesome feeling, isn't it? You're all alone and you have to help others, but nobody takes care of you. That's good. Just let the feeling grow now. Let it get stronger. That's good, let it get bigger. You have to take care of everybody, but nobody takes care of you. Let the feeling get stronger now. . . . Okay, now, Mr. A, I want you to lie there and I want you to think about the things you've told me today. About the feeling that you wanted to cry, you get depressed, you're all bottled up and tense and anxious, you feel that you have to work awfully hard, everybody's depending on you, and nobody's taking care of you. It's a hard life and a lot is required of you. Think about that. I want you to hold all that in your mind and I want you to start to relax. I want you to take a deep breath, a great big one. Fill your lungs up . . . and let it out. That's good. . . . Fill your lungs up . . . and let it out. That's good. Now take another great big, deep breath. Let it out. There, that's good. And every time you let a breath out, you're getting more and more relaxed. That's fine. More and more relaxed every time. It's fine to feel nice and relaxed and comfortable now. That's good . . . that's good, you're doing fine. I want you to think of all the things you've told me today. I want you to relax. I want you to think of how you feel like crying, I want you to think of how it feels that you've been all bottled up, how hard you have to work, how people depend on you but nobody takes care of you. This is a terrible feeling that you get but I want you to think about it and relax. That's good. Just think about it and relax.

All the tension goes out of your body, that's good. I want you to think of your toes and let them relax. A wave of relaxation is going from your toes—that's good, up through your feet . . . you're doing fine . . . to your ankles . . . your calves . . . good . . . your knees . . . thighs. That's good . . . your stomach . . . your fingers are starting to relax. You feel real good and peaceful. Your fingers and arms and chest are relaxed . . . your shoulders are relaxing. Your neck is relaxed. That's good. I want you to lie there very relaxed. . . . Keep your eyes closed. I want you to think about what you've told me today. I want you to think about all the tension you walk around with and this need to cry. . . . I want you to think about how good it is to let it out, but you don't have any place to let it out. Just think about that and relax. I want you to think about how hard you have to work and all the demands that are made on you. You have to take care of people . . . but no one takes care of you . . . you don't feel they do . . . and relax. Just think of this and let all the tension go out of your body. Let yourself be nice and relaxed and comfortable. That's good . . . just take nice, deep, even breaths now and let them out . . . and every time you let that breath out, you get more comfortable.

The client reports feeling better and less burdened after the relaxation. During the subsequent discussion phase, Sipprelle summarizes the themes that emerged during the IA process:

Dr. S: What happened today when we relaxed you and had you tune in to your feelings? What sort of feelings did you get? . . . What happened to you? Can you tell me about it?

Mr. A: Well, this tension and desire to cry came back rather strongly . . . and uh . . . I told you about the overwork and uh . . . uh . . . uh. . . .

Dr. S: You're a minister and you've got the whole community riding on your back, and nobody is doing anything for you, are they? Is that the way it feels?

Mr. A: That's it.

Dr. S: That's what it's like to be a minister. You have everybody riding on your coat tails and no one is looking out for you. That's a kind of occupational hazard, isn't it?

Mr. A: Yeah . . . it is.

Dr. S: You've been around the ministry long enough to know you get pretty drained. You're like a cow that gets milked too often and doesn't get fed enough. That's what your problem is.

Mr. A: Yeah.

Dr. S: So that's an occupational hazard of our business, and we all feel that way if we try to work too much. We think we have to take care of everybody and nobody gives a damn for me . . . and we have to go around with a stiff upper lip and everybody else is crying and carrying on and we have to be old toughies. You and I aren't any different from anyone else. . . . We have to take care of people, but somebody has to take care of *us*. Who takes care of you? Huh? Who looks after you? Who hears your troubles? Who? (*long silence*) No wonder you get all tense and depressed inside. This is a natural feeling under the circumstances, isn't it? Well, today we relaxed to show you that when you relax, you feel good . . . and when you think about your troubles, you feel terrible. You get tense. You can do this . . . it would be nice if you had someone to tell your troubles to, but you can do this alone. You can learn to relax. If I could work with you, I'd help you learn to relax completely, and then we'd practice using it to control that tension. Unfortunately, I live in another state. However, if you think that what we did today would be helpful to you, we can get you a therapist here in the area who is trained to do this kind of stress management work, and you can continue working on developing some good coping skills, plus have someone to talk with about the challenges you face in your work and life. Whether or not you decide to go in that direction, however, we can send you home with some relaxation training tapes so you can teach yourself to relax very quickly and get as deeply relaxed within a few breaths as I got you to feel. And then when things are getting stressful and the tension starts developing and you get to feeling overwhelmed, you can use your relaxation to tone things down a bit so that you don't get overwhelmed by all the demands on you. It's sure better to handle stress at the time and tone it down than to bottle it up until you crack under all the stored-up pressure. [adapted from Ascough, 1975, pp. 132–145]

IA as an Uncovering Technique

Particularly with emotionally constrained clients, the use of IA can elicit emotional responses that clients have avoided or suppressed. In the three sections that follow, the first two clients represent coping styles involving repression and denial, whereas the third client exhibits a pattern sometimes seen in obsessive–compulsive clients whose compulsions successfully shield them from negative emotions. These cases illustrate the diagnostic potential of IA in helping emotionally avoidant clients access feelings and their associated psychological issues. For purposes of brevity, the session excerpts are condensed to present their relevant features.

The Mentally Tough Marine

Mr. B was trained as a medical corpsman and served successfully for months on a Navy ship in the South Pacific. Then he was suddenly deployed to serve a Marine unit in Afghanistan. He spent the tour under fire caring for severely injured Marines. The client received commendations for his performance under fire and was described as unusually "mentally tough." Part of this label came from his ability to function despite bouts of severe back pain.

Mr. B completed his 4-year commitment and was discharged, after which he became a fireman, again performing admirably in stressful situations. Following a harrowing escape from a burning house in which he found the burned remains of a mother and two children, he experienced debilitating back pain. A series of medical examinations, including scans, failed to find a physical basis for his pain. Faced with the negative medical results, the client steadfastly resisted any implication that psychological factors were involved. A psychiatric evaluation, including a MMPI–2 profile that contained a marked peak on the Hysteria scale, resulted in a DSM-IV diagnosis of conversion disorder and a psychotherapy referral. After an initial interview and case conceptualization, Mr. B was trained in relaxation. As often occurs, the material elicited in arousal surrounded traumatic events, but in this case, they had occurred a decade earlier. The therapist introduced a deep state of relaxation and then began arousal.

THERAPIST: Now turn your attention inward and feel the feelings that begin to grow. The feelings become stronger and stronger. That's good. [Therapist reinforces behaviors above a baseline of relaxation: a small hand movement, a grimace, a change in breathing.] Feel the feelings. They're growing. Feel what's happening inside. It's coming out now . . . stronger and stronger. That's good.

MR. B: (*Makes a gurgling sound.*)

THERAPIST: Let it come . . . let it grow.

MR. B: Oh, God!! The blood and guts! So much . . . so much. So many guys.

THERAPIST: Focus on those feelings. Study them. What happens in your muscles? Your insides? Your head? Feel all of that.

(The induction continues and Mr. B writhes and begins to weep. At one point, he sobs, "I thought I was past this 10 years ago—it's like it happened today!")

THERAPIST: You've been carrying this around for a long time, but it's okay to let it out so we can work on helping you handle these feelings. To show you how, I want you to begin to relax. And now again begin to relax. Turn off the feelings and thoughts. Notice how they decrease. Notice how you can control the feelings. That's good. Continue relaxing. Just letting go and allowing that wave of relaxation to flow through your body. . . .

(The therapist presents relaxation instructions, with nearly 10 minutes being required for Mr. B to return his emotional arousal to a baseline level.)

MR. B: Wow! This is the most relaxed I've been in months.

THERAPIST: You got into some pretty loaded stuff, it seems. Can you tell me about it? What came to you?

MR. B: A vivid memory came to me, something I hadn't thought about for years. On my first day we were moving down a street and bullets started hitting walls. I ducked into an alley to my right. Two Marines were waving to me from the alley across the street, so I ran hard and got into the alley as bullets hit the building beside me. A lower leg was lying in the alley. Not far away they were propping up the guy who lost his leg. He was hit in the shoulder too. I bandaged him and gave him morphine and we made him ready to transport. I felt someone put his leg in my pack—we don't leave parts. Then someone was yelling for us to move forward. Down the street there was a guy shot badly in the gut and he was bleeding out. All I could do to help was give him enough morphine to stop the pain. For a second I thought, "Will this much kill him?" but my mind said he's about dead now. I don't want to go on with this. Several hours later I thought, "What a first day indoctrination. Will more days be like this? No, for the most part they were worse."

THERAPIST: How did you handle the feelings that these experiences caused?

MR. B: I guess I just blocked them. I've always prided myself on being a tough guy. In my family, we learned early on that feelings are weakness. My dad didn't even cry when my mother died, and I didn't either. In Afghanistan, I just kept a stiff upper lip and pushed them out of my mind, both during the action and afterward. I had to be strong and tough to do my job. That was no place for an emotional weakling. After I was discharged from the service, I honestly thought Afghanistan was no longer bothering me. The doctor who treated my back pain asked me about that, but I honestly believed that those experiences were past history and not bothering me. I'm sure he didn't buy that, or he wouldn't have sent me to you. But today, they all flooded back.

THERAPIST: I think that perhaps they've been buried in your gut for years, eating it away. Some folks have an uncommon ability to block out and suppress bad feelings, but that doesn't mean those feelings aren't still alive inside, doing unseen damage. I wonder if the awful scenes you saw in the burning house, which was an awful source of stress, finally broke the dam that's held back the feelings and helped you survive.

With many individuals who have repressed and avoidant defensive styles, shifting the focus to "handling" external stressors that the client is facing makes the possibility of psychological factors more palatable and can serve as an *entree* to a coping orientation that the client can tolerate. Note that at this point, the therapist did not attribute the back pain to suppressed feelings, but therapy eventually moved in that direction.

Displacement of Sacrilegious Anger

Mrs. W was a young mother who consulted with her minister because she inexplicably felt compelled to hit her 6-month-old daughter. The client had not actually struck her child, but the impulse had stunned and alarmed her because she considered it sinful and was concerned that she might be demon-possessed. She belonged to a fundamentalist sect that eschewed the expression of anger and hostility. The sect was also uncomfortable with mental health services but appeared to regard the mother's impulse and her agitated state as an emergency. Her minister therefore brought her to a community mental health center in the hope that she might obtain medication. The therapist witnessed an agitated state that made it difficult for the client to converse and decided that relaxation might reduce her distress, but to no avail. Without the usual relaxation training, he then implemented IA.

THERAPIST: I'd like for you to lie back in the recliner and get comfortable. That's good. You seem to be having so many feelings, so just focus on them. Let them grow . . . let them become stronger. They begin to affect your breathing, the tension in your shoulders and chest . . . let them come out. Stronger and stronger. (*Mrs. W's body begins to shake.*) Feel that . . . stronger still.

MRS. W: (*Abruptly screams.*) You son of a bitch!! You son of a bitch!!

THERAPIST: (*Thinks, "Not church-like . . . she can't mean me—she doesn't know me well enough."*) Good! Feel the feelings . . . let them go . . . let them come out.

MRS. W: (*Yelling*) You didn't need her, God! I needed her! I got a baby. I don't know what to do . . . how to take care of her! What to teach her. I need my mom! Who will teach me? You took her away, damn You!

THERAPIST: Let it out . . . feel it . . . let it out.

MRS. W: I'm so angry! Why did You take her . . . what will I do?! Who will help? Oh, God, I'm angry! Have mercy on me!

The therapist continued to reinforce Mrs. W as she expressed her anger until the affect began to decrease in intensity, then introduced relaxation, which she was able to achieve. Discussion revealed that Mrs. W. was also furious with two physicians who had hospitalized her mother but then sent her home with what Mrs. W regarded as a wrong diagnosis, only to have her die precipitously within 24 hours. The therapist induced arousal again and finished with a longer relaxation phase.

Mrs. W was seen once more the following week. She reported no further urges to hit her daughter. Her minister strongly supported her apparently displaced anger toward the doctors and told her that he could understand her distress over being abandoned by God. He assured her that God would forgive her. In addition, several church members had been kind and supportive, and far less NA occurred during the next arousal phase. The client continued in therapy to resolve her feelings of anger. A combination of relaxation and cognitive therapy, focused on the acceptability of experiencing even negative feelings, proved effective in this case.

Affective Antecedents in a Compulsive Client

Mr. H was a graduate student who worked compulsively at many tasks and developed an extensive set of "checks." Before he left for class each morning, *all* electrical plugs had to be pulled from their outlets: clocks, computer and printer, toaster, coffee pot, toothbrush, radio, TV, etc. If he did not switch off the breaker for the electric stove, he checked the burners repeatedly. It was not unusual for him to head to the university, only to return home to recheck some appliance, compelled by the obsessive question "Did I pull the plug?" Often he was late for class or meetings. He was unusual in that in the first session, he did not describe any recent emotional experiences, but under IA recalled anxiety-provoking events from about 5 years of age.

Mr. H had two sessions of relaxation training and practiced six separate relaxation audio recordings for 3 weeks.

THERAPIST: As we begin today, I'd like you to relax quietly for several minutes. Just do the things you've been practicing at home. That's good. As you become more comfortable, your muscles loosen and your breathing becomes more even. You scan your body and feel calm. . . . Now, from this level of relaxation, as you turn your attention inward, you will notice that feelings from deep inside and feelings are stirring. Slowly, these feelings begin to bubble up and grow. As they grow, your breathing changes a little . . . your fingers tightening [observations]. That's good . . . stronger and stronger. Your chest becomes full. Muscles shift in your face. Let the feelings grow . . . stronger and stronger. Study the feelings . . . let them out. What is happening for you?

MR. H: I'm getting angry . . . pissed . . . but . . . I'm anxious . . . or scared . . . yet I keep getting angrier. I want to fight . . . but that makes me scared and I want to run. Oh, God! I don't know what . . . now I'm getting more scared!

THERAPIST: Stay with the feelings. How do they affect your body?

MR. H: The fear gets in my guts and my head reads it. When I'm angry I feel . . . tight . . . tense . . . in my shoulders, arms and thighs.

THERAPIST: Study those feelings and let them grow. . . . That's good.

MR. H: Wait! I see my dad. He's like the big sergeant that came back from Viet Nam. He's got a machete and all around him what look like saplings are cut down. He looks young again and strong. He's standing there looking at me. He's got an evil grin, and the sharp edge of the machete shines in the sunlight. He terrifies me. He'll use it or beat the shit out of me if I don't do things right.

THERAPIST: Feel how the fear goes through you . . . what muscles tense. . . . Remember any words or thoughts that come to you so we can talk about them. What labels or words come to you? (*Pause*) Now, take a deep breath. As you let it out, think *calm* and begin to relax. Letting go in your muscles . . . breathing more regularly. Notice how the arousal begins to decrease. (*Continues relaxation until Mr. H is deeply relaxed, then introduces the content for discussion.*) When the feelings bubbled up, with all of the arousal, your father came to mind. What do you make of that?

MR. H: It's like I'm still scared of him even though now he's a funny-looking, little old guy now. I'm still scared of doing anything wrong.

In subsequent treatment sessions, Mr. H worked through his fear-based internalization of perfectionistic standards. IA inductions in which he imagined situations in which he violated these standards, together with *in vivo* prevention of the compulsive acts, reduced his anxiety. Combined with cognitive therapy, in which he challenged these unrealistic "oughts," the multifaceted treatment resulted in a marked reduction in his compulsive behavior.

It is not unusual for clients to show fight–flight responses in initial IA sessions. Having used various strategies to avoid experiencing their underlying feelings, clients are often surprised by the affect that occurs and the content of their underlying cognitions.

IA was developed as a stand-alone behavioral therapy, but it can be employed as a component of other interventions as well. As shown in the preceding cases, it could be applied when indicated within insight-oriented and experiential treatments to elicit affect and associated cognitions and motivational states in clients who are out of touch with their feelings. IA's demonstrated ability to elicit affective arousal also makes it an ideal method for rehearsing coping skills developed through cognitive restructuring and self-instructional training in cognitive therapies. As we have seen, IA is used as the primary coping skills rehearsal method in the CASMT intervention described in subsequent chapters of this book. In CASMT, it is now being used to practice mindfulness and acceptance skills as well.

Therapeutic Issues

The preceding descriptions of how IA is conducted with clients are a beginning, and other IA transcripts are presented in the chapters to follow. This section addresses some therapeutic issues, frequently asked questions, and procedural aspects of IA administration.

Clinicians are drawn to therapeutic endeavors because they want to be helpful. Sipprelle (1981, p. 2) observed that it "goes against the grain to make a patient deliberately anxious." There may be concerns that the therapy could overwhelm a client or weaken defenses that mask psychotic processes, or even that excessively high levels of arousal may have adverse medical consequences. These concerns require typical caution and assessment, as mentioned earlier.

One of the most frequent questions is the following: Can arousal ever get out of hand? Clinicians new to this process are often concerned that the client might achieve an especially high level of arousal that cannot be easily terminated. Sipprelle (personal communication) contended that clients have a "built-in safety valve" and will plateau before the arousal becomes too great. Nonetheless, it is perhaps best to refrain from reinforcing a very high level of arousal in the first few sessions so the client can learn and become somewhat comfortable with the process of feeling, then relaxing. Further into the therapy some individuals will reach very high levels of arousal. They may not verbalize clearly and may strike out. One client ruined a file cabinet by slamming it with his forearm, and another tore an arm off the recliner chair during a rage response. Nevertheless, deep relaxation was easily reestablished in these cases.

On very rare occasions, a client may continue with a high state of arousal and even bodily shaking, with relaxation having little dampening effect. This persisting arousal may reflect the effects of long-term chronic tension—although for some personality-disordered clients, the gyrations appear much like sexual activity. Less experienced therapists may become alarmed if events like this occur, but it is easy to simply go with the behavior: "You are very tense and your body is shaking all over . . . just continue with that . . . feel that." The client cannot keep it up for very long, and as the behavior begins to subside, the therapist can institute relaxation instructions. The calmness of the therapist and the outcome of the event can communicate to the client that even the strongest feelings are transitory and can be controlled. Such a message can serve a valuable purpose for affect-avoidant clients, who often fear that if powerful feelings are released, they may never regain control of them.

It is best to be prepared for unexpected content to emerge. The client who tore the arm off the recliner chair was a meek business student being treated for test anxiety. While imagining taking an important professional certification exam under IA, he suddenly shouted "You son of a bitch!," ripped off the arm rest, threw it across the room, then sobbed, "You won't love me unless I'm just like you. But I don't want to be like you, you bastard!" The therapist instructed the client to stay with that feeling, and the client expressed rage toward his father for forcing him into a business career when he wanted to be a teacher. Needless to say, this event opened up a new issue to be worked through in treatment.

Once affective arousal occurs, the client might introduce material from recent events, from school days, or even from preschool days. Material surrounding anxiety is typical, and depression and anger are also common. Depression often has a strong unexpressed anger component, so a person who presents with a depressive affect may shortly thereafter express anger concerning a loss as well, as in the case of Mrs. W. described above. Physical (medical) complaints may also mask anger. Some clients with obsessive–compulsive components may have feelings for which they have no cognitions or cognitions that suggest emotions for which they have no arousal. A professor may show little muscle tension but show "nonstop" thoughts. One professor, told that there are people with muscle tension from working a metal lathe but with little going through their minds, countered, "You can't be serious." He could not imagine a quiet mind. Further, a client may show a generalized anger that becomes discriminated in levels, from miffed irritation to rage, and in variations, such as anger–bitterness or anger–loneliness. Under conditions of arousal, the emotionality and thoughts that involve autonomic nervous system activity become better integrated, and the total underlying pattern may appear for the first time. As the CAPS personality network (Mischel & Shoda, 1995) stresses, individual identity is represented in excitatory and inhibitory links between cognitive–affective units within the network system. Affective arousal can initiate a spread of activation throughout the system, eliciting memories, appraisals of situations, self- and other-representations, situational schemas and scripts, and behavior tendencies. Individual differences in affective dispositions are thus important aspects of personality and are therefore highly relevant to therapy.

Arousal induction in IA can be nonspecific or focused in nature. To initiate the arousal phase, most IA therapists begin in much the same way, with statements such as, "Turn your attention inward and focus on feelings that will begin to grow." In the transcript provided earlier, Sipprelle did not initially suggest any particular feeling or situation. Unlike therapies such as systematic desensitization or imaginal exposure, where cues or images are prepared for sessions, IA generates its cues with non-specific instructions. However, specific cues can also be used when a particular situation is the focus, but this specificity often emerges further into therapy, based on information from earlier arousal phases, from recent experiences, or from the case conceptualization. This specificity allows for the practice of coping responses to deal with highly relevant emotionally provoking situations. The transcripts presented in later chapters illustrate this focused variant of IA.

One concept elaborated through the years is that coping should be future oriented. A person with posttraumatic stress disorder (PTSD) may report a difficult father and a demanding drill sergeant. After service and therapy, he may encounter a stern boss or a critical professor. Can he cope by modifying cognition, behavior, and autonomic nervous system activity to be at an optimal level for necessary tasks? Statements that would begin to initiate future-oriented coping may be included in the relaxation phase: "Just as you're now controlling the strong feelings associated with that memory from your childhood, you will be able to do so when you encounter distressing events in the future."

Research and Applications

IA therapy has been applied to a wide variety of nonclinical and clinical populations. Below, we summarize research trials in which IA was the primary therapeutic modality. Though many of the studies are unpublished for reasons described above, we believe that they meet current methodological standards and establish IA as an empirically supported treatment.

Does IA Treatment Result in a Generalizable Coping Capability?

A central assumption is that IA provides an opportunity to learn a relaxation coping response that can be used to control physiological responses that are part of aversive emotional states. This capability, which also yields salutary cognitive effects such as enhanced self-efficacy and changes in self-construal, is assumed to be generalizable across situations and across emotions that involve arousal because the rehearsal focuses on the control of internal arousal responses that are common to a variety of emotional states (Sipprelle, 1967). A study by Boer (1970) tested this central assumption. Boer hypothesized that greater generalization would occur with IA than with systematic desensitization, which focuses on deconditioning anxiety responses to specific stimuli and minimizes in-session anxiety arousal.

Eighty undergraduate college students were randomly assigned to one of four experimental conditions: an IA condition, a systematic desensitization condition, a verbal discussion condition, or a no-treatment condition. Participants in the three treatment conditions were seen individually on a weekly basis for a total of three training sessions. The verbal group discussed the challenges and stresses experienced as a college student with a supportive interviewer. Systematic desensitization using progressive relaxation training was administered to participants based on hierarchies derived from one of three items from a 62-item fear survey that they rated as most anxiety arousing for them. Care was taken to minimize affective arousal, as in traditional desensitization (Wolpe, 1958). The IA condition was administered with a baseline relaxation phase (identical with that used in the desensitization condition), an IA phase with no specification of the affective state that the participant might experience, and a second relaxation phase in which the participant was told to use the relaxation to "make the feeling go away." Affect was induced once during the first session and twice during the second and third sessions for a total of five inductions.

A week after treatment ended, participants in the four conditions returned for an experimental session designed to test their responses to a laboratory stressor. While their physiological responses (heart rate, galvanic skin response, and respiration) were measured, they were exposed to a 16-minute motion picture that showed in vivid detail an aboriginal puberty rite involving a crude surgical subincision in the adolescent male's penis. This film's ability to elicit subjective distress and strong physiological responses has been well established (e.g., Speisman, Lazarus, Mordoff, & Davison, 1964). Participants were told that they would see a "somewhat stressful" film and were asked to "try to be as relaxed as possible" while watching it.

The conditions did not differ in mean ratings of the film, with participants in all conditions rating the film as highly unpleasant, but they differed in their physiological responses to it. Participants in the IA condition exhibited significantly lower heart rate and galvanic skin responses sampled at 60-second intervals during the film. The largest difference occurred for heart rate. As shown in Figure 3.1, the mean of the IA condition was 24–30 beats lower than the means of the other three conditions, which did not differ from one another.

Boer's results supported the potential value of IA for developing a generalizable coping response that enhances emotion regulation in response to novel stressors. Boer concluded that IA is a potentially useful preventive technique that could enhance people's ability to cope with future aversive events.

In another study that assessed generalization effects, Ingram (1981) found that students treated for speech anxiety with IA showed significant reductions not only on a self-report measure of speech anxiety, but also on Cattell's (1965) IPAT Anxiety Scale, a measure of general trait anxiety. No significant decreases on this measure were found for conditions that received relaxation training alone or no treatment. Results suggested that IA treatment had anxiety-reducing generalization effects beyond that obtained for relaxation training alone.

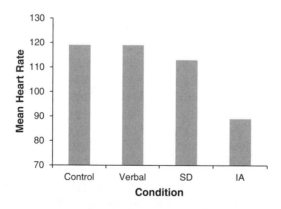

FIGURE 3.1. Mean peak heart rate during the viewing of a stressful subincision film as a function of previous verbal treatment, systematic desensitization, or IA treatment. Data from Boer (1970).

Clients with Fears and Phobias

In its original formulation (Sipprelle, 1967), IA was called "induced anxiety." Not surprisingly, therefore, much early research was done with individuals who had anxiety-based problems. Several studies testing different variations of IA treatment focused on test anxiety, a widespread problem among college students. Holmes (1981) assessed the effectiveness of IA by direct versus vicarious experience with test-anxious female college students who scored above the 75th normative percentile on the Test Anxiety Scale (Sarason, 1958). After the initial assessment, subjects were assigned to one of five conditions. The first condition experienced *in vivo* IA treatment with general arousal instructions and no reference made to test-taking anxiety unless verbalized by the participant. In a second condition, participants watched an IA videotape of the treatment of a female test-anxious student; and in a third condition they listened to the same IA treatment via audiotape. The fourth condition received relaxation training, and the fifth served as a no-treatment control condition. Participants in the treatment conditions were seen individually for 10 weekly sessions, and physiological measures were obtained for cardiac rate, blood volume fluctuation, and respiration rate in the IA conditions to study changes in physiological arousal over time as a process variable.

Results revealed significant decreases in Test Anxiety Scale scores ($p < .01$) for both the *in vivo* and the two vicarious IA groups, but not for the relaxation and control groups. There were no differences between the three IA groups in improvement, suggesting that vicarious exposure to IA may also be an efficient method for reducing test anxiety. Although the participants in the IA conditions reported decreased test anxiety, physiological data did not show an expected decrease in heart rate arousal over sessions in any of the IA groups, even though the participants became increasingly able to reduce it in the second relaxation phase. Holmes suggested that "time on task," experiencing emotional stimuli and reducing arousal, is more important than changes in physiological arousal itself across treatment sessions, and that cognitive changes in coping efficacy may be a key mechanism of improvement.

Childers (1981) assessed another IA variation: the role of massed versus spaced IA sessions in the treatment of test-anxious students. The dependent measures included scores on the Test Anxiety Scale as well as measures of heart and respiration rate. One condition received an individual session each week for 8 consecutive weeks, with IA elicited as participants imagined concerns about taking a test. A second condition received two identical IA treatment sessions per week for 4 consecutive weeks, and a third condition was treated over 8 consecutive days. A fourth group served as the control and was administered the pretreatment and posttreatment measures, as well as the clinical interview and explanations given to the other groups. The spaced IA condition exhibited a significant decrease in test anxiety scores and differed significantly from each of the other treatment groups, supporting the greater efficacy of weekly over massed treatment. Childers suggested that perhaps the extended time period allows for greater consolidation and opportunities for application of coping skills in actual test situations.

Ingram (1981) investigated the effectiveness of IA in reducing performance anxiety associated with public speaking. The subjects were matched on speech anxiety scores and randomly assigned to one of four groups. An IA group received one treatment session per week for 8 weeks, and a progressive muscular relaxation training group received training for an equal amount of time. They were compared with two no-treatment control groups. Both the IA and relaxation groups decreased significantly in self-reported speech anxiety in comparison with the two control groups, but the two treatment conditions did not differ significantly. The control groups showed no decrease in anxiety.

A study by Maxwell (1981) involved snake-phobic participants. One aim of the study was to assess whether a generic IA treatment without reference to snakes would generalize to phobic fear reduction. Thirty-six students who scored highly on a snake anxiety questionnaire used by Lang and Lazovik (1963) to identify snake-phobic individuals were randomly assigned to receive a nonspecific IA treatment; a systematic desensitization treatment involving a snake hierarchy used by Bandura, Blanchard, and Ritter (1969); or to a no-treatment control group. Results showed that both IA and systematic desensitization conditions exhibited significantly greater reduction in snake anxiety scores than did the control group, indicating targeted symptom efficacy for systematic desensitization and generalization effects for the IA condition. The two treatment conditions, though superior to the control condition, did not differ significantly from one another on posttreatment snake anxiety scores, and the IA and systematic desensitization conditions did not differ from the controls on posttreatment physiological arousal measures collected while the participants watched an innocuous informational film about snakes. This film elicited much lower levels of arousal in all conditions than did the subincision film used by Boer (1970), which may have masked potential differences among conditions. Unfortunately, the design did not include a behavioral approach test to a snake, which would have provided more convincing evidence for phobic improvement, or an IA condition that was explicitly focused on snake stimuli.

We should note one other anxiety-based application of IA therapy. As the treatment was being developed in the late 1960s and applied in the early 1970s, IA was used to treat World War II, Korean War, and Vietnam veterans with PTSD. Clinicians trained by Sipprelle and Ascough have continued to use it in the intervening years because it appears clinically efficacious. Unfortunately, no formal outcome studies were conducted, so that the stand-alone efficacy of IA and its comparative efficacy in relation to other PTSD treatments remains an empirical question. From a theoretical and mechanism perspective, however, a comparative study would permit a test of the coping skills model underlying IA in relation to the extinction model represented in the current front-line prolonged-exposure CBT treatment (Foa & Jaycox, 1999).

Mixed-Diagnosis Outpatient Clients

Most of the studies described above involved clients with specific fears or phobias and were conducted in experimental settings. In a study done in a large university outpatient clinic with a general clinical population, Moore (1981) assessed anxiety reduction in 26 self-referred college students. Sixteen exhibited a fairly even distribution of anxiety disorders and depression and 10 were diagnosed with DSM-II personality disorders with mild to moderate deficits.

Female–male ratio and diagnostic category were equated across groups, and clients were randomly assigned to three conditions: IA treatment, relaxation therapy, or a wait-list control group. In an introductory session all participants were administered the IPAT Anxiety Scale (Cattell, 1965) and were given a treatment rationale concerning the role of anxiety in many life problems. Beginning the second week, clients in the IA condition were individually administered a nine-session treatment consisting of baseline relaxation, IA, and a second relaxation phase on a weekly basis. There was no discussion phase surrounding behavior or affect to avoid adding an element not present in the progressive muscle relaxation condition. The latter was individually administered to the students for the same amount of time and in the same room as the IA sessions. Session-by-session physiological measures were obtained during the IA and relaxation sessions. Clients assigned to the wait-list control group were told after this session that service demands prevented them from being seen immediately and they would be called for further testing. At 10 weeks they entered therapy at the clinic.

After the 10-week treatment all clients completed the IPAT Anxiety Scale a second time. The IA group showed significantly greater reduction in trait anxiety scores compared to the other two groups. The in-session physiological recordings did not show arousal differences between the IA condition during its relaxation phase and that exhibited in the relaxation-alone condition. Moore observed that the students diagnosed with personality disorders did not show as strong cardiac changes in arousal phases as those with "neurotic" diagnoses but that some did exhibit notable changes in anxiety scores. Commenting on the latter observation, Sipprelle (1981) suggested that IA can be applied appropriately to any disorder that generates internal and autonomic cues of psychological distress, including personality disorders, in order to treat the arousal aspect of the disorder.

Clients with Obesity

Obesity is a complex phenomenon that is influenced by a host of biological, psychological, environmental, and behavioral factors. Among the psychological factors is a large body of evidence that compulsive overeating is related to NA, as well as deficits in emotion regulation capabilities (Berg et al., 2014; Gianini, White, & Masheb, 2013).

Bornstein and Sipprelle (1973a) published a preliminary case report on the treatment of obesity. Two instrumental conditioning procedures were used to help a female graduate student achieve weight loss: (1) IA was used to elicit and control affective arousal, and (2) verbal shaping and reinforcement of reduced food intake were administered over a 15-week treatment period. The client lost a total of 41.5 pounds over the period and maintained the loss over a 60-week no-contact follow-up period. There were also indications of improved adjustment in coping with daily stresses, heightened feelings of self-worth, and no evidence of "symptom substitution."

Building on this promising outcome, Bornstein and Sipprelle (1973b, 1981) conducted a clinical trial on the use of IA in a group-administered intervention for obesity. Forty participants were randomly assigned to four stratified blocks based on percentage overweight, and to one of four experimental conditions: IA administered on a group basis, a relaxation training group, a nonspecific therapy group that discussed psychological reasons for their overeating, and a wait-list control group. Treatments occurred over eight weekly sessions.

Weekly sessions occurred in two phases: weigh-in, followed by a discussion of causal factors in loss or gain. The experimenter recorded the weight of each subject, which was visually displayed, and provided positive reinforcement for accumulated weight loss. The relaxation group was told that they would be taught a response antagonistic to anxiety, since people often overeat in response to anxiety, and that they could apply their relaxation skills to situations in which they felt tense or anxious. The IA group was provided with a similar rationale. In the IA group, participants were given a sequence of relaxation, arousal, relaxation, arousal, and relaxation, with each phase lasting 4 minutes.

Results of the trial are shown in Figure 3.2. The four conditions had virtually identical mean weights at baseline. At posttreatment the IA group's weight loss was significantly greater than the control group's, but the other treatment conditions, although exhibiting some weight loss, did not differ from the control condition. At 3- and 6-month follow-up weight measurements, the IA group differed significantly from all of the other groups in amount of weight loss, and posttreatment IA treatment gains were being well maintained, whereas all other groups immediately regained weight and returned to their baseline weights following the experimental period.

Results were interpreted as supporting a mechanism of learned emotion regulation of internal NA cues as an adaptive substitute for overeating as a coping response. Another possibility is that increased general sensitivity to internal cues as a result of treatment made the IA-treated patients with obesity more sensitive to cues accompanying satiety, which resulted in greater regulatory control over eating cessation.

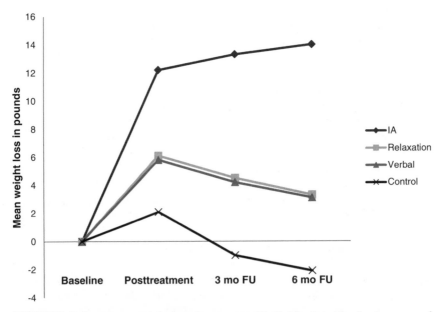

FIGURE 3.2. Mean weight loss in groups of individuals with obesity equated for body weight at baseline and then assigned to a nonspecific verbal intervention, relaxation training, IA therapy, or no treatment. Adapted from Bornstein and Sipprelle (1981) by permission of the Center for Induced Affect.

Clients with Schizophrenia

Many therapists would hesitate to use a procedure such as IA with patients with schizophrenia for fear that high levels of affect elicitation would overwhelm their poorly established emotion regulation skills. Sipprelle (1981) maintained that if such patients were well trained in relaxation techniques, their self-perceived ability to control affective arousal might yield salutary results, including badly needed confidence in their coping efficacy. Additionally, the presence of a therapist to "turn off" arousal that might overwhelm the patient using relaxation instructions would be a protective therapeutic factor.

To assess the suitability of IA with such patients, Friedberg (1969) applied IA to a sample of chronic, hospitalized patients diagnosed with schizophrenia at a Veterans Administration (VA) hospital. The research was designed to assess a process variable, a verbal versus nonverbal condition in the arousal and discussion phases, as well as to provide outcome data. Twenty-one chronic patients were randomly assigned to three conditions in which each patient was seen individually for 6 weeks. One condition received standard IA treatment with patient verbalization of experiences and discussion, whereas the other IA condition occurred without client verbalization or discussion. A third attention-placebo control group received discussion without IA. Dependent measures included the Psychotic Inpatient Profile (PIP; Lorr & Vestre, 1968) to evaluate decreases in withdrawal as rated by psychiatric nurses and ward attendants, and a sentence completion test to assess changes in affective verbal response. Results indicated that the IA group that verbalized showed significant decreases in staff-rated withdrawal on the PIP, whereas the nonverbal IA and control groups showed no change. A 60-day follow-up revealed that 14 of the 21 patients had been released from the hospital. Only two of the released patients were control-group patients, whereas 12 of the 14 patients in the two IA conditions had been released. This difference was statistically significant ($p < .01$).

In a follow-up study, Cockshott and Ascough (1981) assessed IA efficacy with a sample of female patients with chronic schizophrenia who had been hospitalized an average of 13.7 years. Thirty-six patients were randomly assigned to an experimental group that received individual IA treatment for eight weekly sessions, a contact-control group that received eight sessions with the same phases as the IA group except that a rest period was substituted for the arousal phase, and a no-contact control group. The three groups were equated for age, IQ and, where practical, length of hospitalization, previous therapy, recreation, and other concurrent activities. Medication levels were held constant throughout treatment. Anxiety, ward behavior, and physiological responses were focal outcome variables.

The IA condition exhibited significant reductions scores on the Manifest Anxiety Scale (Taylor, 1953) compared to the other conditions. In contrast to Friedberg's (1969) results with a less chronic population, however, no differential behavioral improvement was shown on the PIP in this more chronic cohort. Physiological measures obtained during IA treatment sessions showed that the IA group exhibited little arousal initially, but this pattern was changing when the predetermined eight sessions ended, suggesting that the arousal phase must be long enough to achieve actual arousal and the number of sessions needed for therapeutic gains must be determined for a chronic population. Significantly from a clinical perspective, the 26 patients in these two studies tolerated IA treatment without loss-of-control incidents. Again, however, we should note that they were well trained in relaxation coping skills before IA was applied.

Clients with Substance Abuse

Although substance abuse involves numerous causal factors, many theorists and researchers have emphasized the use of alcohol and other substances for emotion regulation purposes. There is a wealth of evidence to support the principle that substances can create positive affective states and reduce negative ones (Kober, 2014). A number of efficacious CBTs (e.g., Carroll, 1998) have been developed that involve identification of high-risk situations and development of coping skills for dealing with cravings and high-risk interpersonal situations. Although little research on the use of IA with substance abuse problems exists, we suggest that its success in promoting the development of affective coping skills in other populations indicates its applicability to substance abuse populations as well, particularly to the subset of abusers who use substances to reduce NA. IA could also be used as an ancillary procedure in other efficacious treatments.

Bereika (1976) conceptualized substance dependency as a learned tension reduction coping response for some abusers and evaluated the incremental efficacy of IA to ongoing group treatment at a VA hospital. Forty-five patients with drug dependency issues were assigned to three groups: an IA condition, a relaxation training condition, and a contact-control group. The subjects were also engaged in group treatment as part of the center's treatment regimen. Pre- and posttreatment self-ratings as well as objective ratings of ward behavior and behavior during the therapy groups were obtained. Anxiety measures were administered weekly and IA group members also responded to a within-session subjective arousal measure for phases of the IA procedure.

Clients in the IA condition exhibited the largest reduction in weekly anxiety scores. The self-report measures clearly indicated greater effectiveness for the IA condition in lowering trait anxiety and in improving quality of interpersonal relationships. Objective behavioral ratings made during the encounter groups offered substantial support for the effectiveness of IA in decreasing staff-rated anxiety level, improving interpersonal relationships, increasing emotional awareness, and increasing ability to cope with stress and conflict. Although IA treatment was confounded with the ongoing group therapy and is best regarded as an incremental ancillary treatment, Bereika concluded that IA can be useful in the treatment of substance abuse either as a stand-alone treatment or as an ancillary intervention that can enhance emotion regulation skills.

Boer and Sipprelle (1969) described a unique application of IA in a case study in which they used IA to obtain operant control over LSD flashbacks in a college student who was referred from the university hospital. He had used LSD on 11 occasions and marijuana on a longer basis. The last LSD episode resulted in a "bad trip," and the client was having flashbacks with anxiety, panic, and fears of loss of control and becoming insane. He reported intermittent muscular rigidity, tension, frightening somatic and visual sensations, unusual afterimages, general restlessness, an oppressive feeling induced by bright colors, and an almost constant obsession that he had damaged his chromosomes or brain. The client was scheduled for a psychological evaluation and treatment at the campus psychological clinic but disappeared for 5 months. During that time he married and his wife became pregnant, but thoughts surrounding chromosomal and brain damage intensified so he reentered therapy and was treated with IA.

Treatment included 16 sessions. The first four were used to build rapport and teach relaxation, the next eight involved IA treatment, and the final four were used to consolidate gains and monitor the client to ensure a positive outcome. Under IA, he exhibited intense anxiety and verbalized bizarre feelings of pressure and splitting in his brain, panic, fears of loss of control or nothingness, and other strange feelings that were characteristic of his "bad trip" on LSD. However, he was able to achieve control of these symptoms by applying his relaxation coping skills, and they quickly began to subside. By the end of treatment, he had been free of all symptoms and bizarre experiences outside of therapy for several months.

Although IA is far less researched than many other cognitive-behavioral treatments, the level of efficacy it has demonstrated in studies involving varied nonclinical and clinical populations in multiple independent laboratories and clinical settings meets established criteria for an empirically supported treatment. It is unfortunate that much of this work has not been published, for many of the studies reflect the level of methodological rigor that is required for a doctoral thesis at major universities having a clinical scientist emphasis, and most of them met prevailing publication standards of their era.

In this chapter, we have considered applications and research on IA as a stand-alone intervention. As noted earlier, however, the technique is readily applicable to other treatment modalities as well. For example, it can be utilized in dialectical behavior therapy (Linehan, 2015) to help clients rehearse emotional dysregulation coping skills. Likewise, it could be applied within Barlow's unified protocol, which contains an emotion elicitation module that is used to enhance emotional awareness and control of coping skills (Barlow et al., 2011). Given the high degree of current interest in emotion regulation and the transtheoretical focus on countering emotional avoidance and eliciting emotional arousal, we believe that IA has the potential to advance current therapeutic practice. IA's demonstrated ability to elicit affect can facilitate emotional processing, help produce insight, and permit the application of coping skills ranging from relaxation to acceptance and defusion within the therapy room. IA is an essential component of CASMT, the emotion regulation intervention that is described in the remainder of the book.

The next six chapters (Chapters 4 through 9) provide guidelines in how to conduct the CASMT intervention and how to use the IA procedure to help clients practice cognitive–affective coping skills in the presence of emotional arousal. We describe the six-session group format that has been used in most of the outcome studies discussed in Chapter 2. We believe that group administration is not only efficacious, but that it also helps address the significant, largely unmet needs of the large population reporting a desire to manage stress more effectively. However, we also recognize that the intervention may be even more effective when used in individually administered treatment, where it can be personalized and monitored closely by a therapist. Therefore, we also provide guidance for administering CASMT on an individual basis. Likewise, we emphasize that there is nothing sacred about the six-session format aside from its efficiency, and that therapists could easily expand the treatment by extending the number of sessions and injecting new elements into it.

CHAPTER 4

Preparation, Assessment, and Session 1

PREPARING TO CONDUCT CASMT

As noted in Chapter 2, CASMT can be presented in either an individual or a group format. Most of the CASMT experimental outcome studies described in Chapter 2 have followed the manualized six-session format (minus the more recently added mindfulness and ACT components) presented in this and the next five chapters. Sessions are typically held once a week for 6 weeks, with each session lasting an hour, but successful outcomes have been reported in some of the studies cited in Chapter 2 using two sessions per week. The weekly format obviously provides more out-of-session opportunities for skill building.

CASMT has been administered to groups ranging from fewer than 10 participants to over 50. We find the optimal group size to be 8–12 because it allows for give-and-take between the group leader and participants, as well as some level of attention to individual needs, questions, and concerns. Participants are asked to respect the privacy of group members who disclose information about themselves.

Who Is Qualified to Conduct CASMT?

Both the individual and group formats require previous graduate-level practicum training in clinical methods. Clinical and counseling psychology graduate students have administered the program in their second year of graduate training under supervision, often as part of their normal clinical caseload. The same criteria apply to other health or mental health professions that provide the requisite background training, such as social work or psychosocial nursing.

Who Is an Appropriate Client for CASMT?

As noted in Chapter 1, there has been an increased emphasis on the construct of neuroticism in relation to problems involving negative emotionality in both clinical and nonclinical populations (Barlow et al., 2014; Lahey, 2009). The CASMT program is appropriate for both clinical and nonclinical clients who are reacting to high levels of life stress with distress, anxiety, and anger responses. The cognition–arousal relations in these emotions are well suited to the emotion regulation skills in CASMT. Though not the treatment of choice for depression on either conceptual or empirical grounds, the intervention may be applied to clients with comorbid depression and anxiety as an anxiety reduction adjunct to other depression treatments. The demonstrated efficacy of CASMT with a variety of nonclinical populations (e.g., athletes, medical students, military officer candidates, test-anxious students) suggests its applicability within a prevention orientation.

Options for Tailoring CASMT for Particular Clients

When administering the program in a traditional therapist–client mode, a therapist can tailor it to that person's particular circumstances, coping strengths, and weaknesses, and can expand the scope of the program or the number of sessions to be sure that every element is mastered by the client. For example, a therapist may choose to devote additional sessions to cognitive restructuring or to the mindfulness skills taught in the later sessions. However, we recommend that clinicians follow the general guidelines and sequencing of training experiences we spell out here, for they build upon one another. Some therapists use CASMT to build foundational emotion regulation skills, then switch to other modes of treatment to address issues in other life domains. For example, whether in an expanded group format or in the treatment of individuals, CASMT can also include acquisition of problem-focused coping skills that can be applied to dealing directly with problematic situations. Examples of such skills are cognitive problem-solving strategies in which people learn how to systematically analyze problems, set specific goals, consider alternative approaches to attaining the goal, evaluate their potential value and applicability, choose the most promising strategy or response, implement it, and evaluate the outcome (e.g., D'Zurilla & Nezu, 2007). Indeed, to the extent that the individual views his or her stress responses as a problem to be solved, much of what is done in CASMT can be viewed as problem-focused as well as emotion-focused. Other problem-focused elements could include training in social skills, communication and conflict resolution, assertiveness, time management, parenting practices, behavioral marital skills, team building, and systematic time management.

INITIAL ASSESSMENT

In many clinical settings, an initial telephone or screening interview is conducted. A decision to consider CASMT as the treatment modality in our setting is typically based on a presenting problem of difficulties in dealing with stressful situations, anxiety, or anger-related problems. In our settings, panic disorders, PTSD, or depression are treated with other evidence-based interventions, sometimes augmented with IA.

If the client is deemed suitable for CASMT, it is useful to get relevant information before the first interview. A useful screening (and outcome) measure is the Perceived Stress Scale (PSS; Cohen et al., 1983), which assesses the degree to which situations in one's life are appraised as stressful. The PSS has both college student and community norms, which can be useful in identifying clients who could profit from stress management. We also use an online version of the Stress and Coping Diary measure to collect at least 1 week of data before the first session, using HIPAA-compliant collection procedures to maintain confidentiality, including password-protected access to the diary. Alternatively, we recommend mailing clients copies of the diary form to be completed and brought to the first session. Clients can also be asked to keep a daily log, in which they simply describe stressful experiences.

SESSION 1: CLIENT ORIENTATION, COLLABORATIVE ASSESSMENT, AND RELAXATION TRAINING

About Session 1

Therapists of all persuasions have emphasized the importance of orienting the client to the therapeutic assumptions and methods that underlie an intervention (Addis & Jacobson, 2000; Mumma, 2011). When clinician and client have a common frame of reference concerning the nature of the problem, the factors that contribute to it, and the means that will be taken to remediate it, treatment goals are easier to establish and compliance with therapeutic procedures is more likely to occur. Accordingly, CASMT begins with an introduction to the conceptual model of stress and coping and the presentation of a rationale for the skills training that will be the focus of the intervention. The objectives of this first session are to engage clients in analyzing and understanding their stress processes and to reframe clients' stress-related complaints from being overwhelming, hopeless, and uncontrollable into problems amenable to solutions within the clients' spheres of personal control. The trainer should create a positive expectancy about the program—that it is appropriate to the clients' problems and that it will increase their stress resilience *if* they commit themselves to acquiring the skills.

A demonstration of relaxation training sets the stage for out-of-session assignments designed to develop competency in this coping skill. We begin with this skill because it is more quickly and easily mastered than are the cognitive skills, and so it provides clients with some quick accomplishments and stress-reducing tools. In this and subsequent chapters, we focus first on the group format and then on the individual format. Again, we note that the session-by-session format could also be seen as a *phase-by-phase* protocol involving additional sessions if the client's needs and rate of progress require a more extended intervention.

Overview

TRAINING OBJECTIVES

1. Use a stressful incident to help the client "discover" the underlying model of stress.
2. Explain the rationale for the training program.
3. Seek client buy-in and commitment.
4. Present the "personal scientist" concept.
5. Introduce the client to relaxation training.
6. Explain and obtain commitment to out-of-session exercises.

SESSION OUTLINE

- Welcome and orientation to CASMT
- Definition of stress: Situation, response, and transaction
  - Examining a stressful incident
- Presentation of the stress model
- Ways to reduce stress
- Description and rationale for the program
- Breath and somatic relaxation training
  - Abdominal breathing
  - Muscle relaxation
  - Yoga breathing exercise
- Ending Session 1: Homework assignments and handouts

MATERIALS NEEDED

- For groups: Whiteboard or poster board (or computer, if using Power-Point slides)
- Graphics of stress and CASMT models—either hard copies, overheads, or PowerPoint slides (Appendix B, Figures B-1 and B-2)
- Copies of orientation and program overview (Appendix A, Handout A-1)
- Breath and relaxation training instructions (Handout A-2) and instructions on how to download an audio recording of this training aid
- Stress and Coping Diary (Form A-1)

HOMEWORK ASSIGNMENTS

- Read orientation materials in Handouts A-1 and A-2.
- Practice breathing and progressive muscle relaxation training on a daily basis (Handout A-2).
- Complete Stress and Coping Diary entries on a daily basis (Form A-1).

Group Administration

WELCOME AND ORIENTATION TO CASMT

Leader introduces him- or herself, as does each member of the group. Any other business is covered at this time (e.g., fees, deposits). Confidentiality is emphasized and clients are reassured that the trainer will keep any information expressed in the group strictly confidential. It is important that group members do likewise so that members can feel free to disclose their experiences.

In the following material in this chapter, we provide suggested scripts to guide trainers and therapists in presenting the material. In practice, however, trainers should present the material in their own words and not read the scripts.

"I want to welcome you to the stress management workshop. I'm looking forward to working with you over the next 6 weeks. I'm guessing you're here for a common reason. We live in a very stressful time, and we know that stress takes a tremendous toll on people's physical and psychological well-being. Fortunately, all of us can learn skills that make us more stress-resistant, and that is the goal of this stress management program. It has been used successfully for over 30 years with many different kinds of people in all walks of life who are experiencing excessive stress. It is an educational program designed to help you master coping skills that have been shown to be effective in managing stress. The goal is to help you gain greater personal control over your body, mind, and behavior in the face of life stress. Some have described it as a 'mental toughness' program. The skills you'll learn in this program are important life skills that you will use for the rest of your life. They can increase your resilience in the face of stressful life events.

"Each of you is a unique individual with your own specific background, life experiences, and current situation, including your own personal sources of stress. But whatever the sources of stress involved, we'll see that they have some things in common. Our goal is to teach you how to analyze the stressful situations in your life and to use body–mind skills that will give you greater control over your emotional responses to them. We will provide you with a buffet of proven coping strategies that you can fit to your own personal needs so as to become more resistant to the challenges we all face in life. By the time you complete the program, you'll have selected for yourself a personalized set of skills for coping more effectively with stressful life events. The goal is not to eliminate stress from your life. That's not possible. Instead, the goal is to help you become more resilient in the face of stress.

"Before we go on, however, let's talk about stress. It's a term that is used all the time. But it can have different meanings to different people. Can someone tell me what you think of when you hear the word *stress*?"

Define Stress: Situation, Response, and Transaction

On a whiteboard or poster board, list the definitions clients volunteer (or enter them on a new PowerPoint slide if you're using a computer). Try to elicit both situational (stressor) and personal (stress reaction) definitions. Verbally reinforce participants' contribution. For example:

CLIENT 1: I think of stress as situations that are upsetting, like having your flight cancelled so you're stuck in another city overnight.

THERAPIST: Great example. Anyone have another slant on what stress means?

CLIENT 2: I think of stress as feeling all tense and anxious, or irritated.

THERAPIST: Ah, another way of looking at stress. Let's analyze those two definitions. We have a nice range of meanings for the term *stress*. Do these meanings seem to fall into different classes?

Hopefully, the participants will detect the categories of *stressor* and *personal reactions*. Either way, proceed:

"As your answers illustrate, we typically use the term *stress* in two different ways:

"First, we use it to refer to certain *situations* (or, to use the technical term, *stressors*). Your example of missing a flight and being stuck away from home overnight fits that one very well. Or, 'There's a lot of stress at work—too much work, too little time, and people at each other's throats.' In this case, the term is being used to refer to time pressure, certain tasks, interpersonal problems. Physical stressors, such as suffering a painful injury or medical procedure, fit here as well, as do dangerous situations like being physically assaulted and robbed. In fact, a good summary definition of a *stressor* is anything that places excessive demands on us and threatens our well-being in some way.

"Second, we use the term *stress* to refer to your *personal reactions* to such situations—for example, 'I'm feeling a lot of stress.' Your example of feeling tense and irritated fits this way of defining stress. Here, we're talking about stressful thoughts and feelings, such as anger, frustration, anxiety and sadness.

"There is not always a perfect relationship between the two ways the term is used—between a situation and a reaction. We tend to say 'That makes me angry,' but it's not really true. Different people can react to the same situation in different ways, which would not be possible if a situation could really cause us to be angry. Examples: A driver cuts in front of you: Some people get furious, whereas others shrug it off. When asking someone for a date, some of us are tongue-tied and anxious, others are suave and confident. A skydiver easily steps out of a plane at 10,000 feet, whereas I (and probably most of you) would be terrified.

"What is the reason for the differences among people in their reactions? [Elicit the beliefs or attitudes or previous life situations that cause the reactions.]

"Actually, there's also a third way of thinking about stress, which combines the first two meanings, to refer to an ongoing back-and-forth transaction between the person and the stressor. The features of the stressor may cause us to react in various ways, both emotionally and in terms of our behavior. These ways of responding may feed back into the situation and change it in certain ways that elicit a new response, and so on."

EXAMINING A STRESSFUL INCIDENT

THERAPIST: Now, let's go a little deeper into the nature of stress. Can someone please share with us a stressful situation you've experienced recently? Please describe what happened and how it affected you.

CLIENT: [female group member] I had one just the other night that I can talk about. I was driving on the interstate in that rainstorm we had when my engine started to sputter and then died. Fortunately I was able to coast over to the shoulder, but there I was in the dark with cars whizzing by. I got out my cell phone and saw that the battery was just about dead. I had just finished a 9-1-1 call when it went out. Then a car stopped and this really seedy-looking guy came over, leered at me when he saw I was a woman, and offered me a ride to the next gas station, which I declined. Fortunately, he left when I told him that I had made a 9-1-1 call and they were sending someone. A police car arrived in a few minutes. My car had to be towed and repaired. That was one of the worst experiences I've ever had.

Ask questions to evoke the following elements:

- In addition to the description of what occurred (the situational stressor), what was it about the situation that made it demanding? (Note that names used in case examples are pseudonyms.)

  THERAPIST: Thank you, Lisa. I think all of us can feel for you going through that. What was the worst thing about that situation?

  CLIENT: Just feeling so helpless and at the mercy of whatever happened. I was really scared.

- How did the person react emotionally? What was the emotion? What was the physical reaction?

  THERAPIST: You say you were scared, and understandably so. Do you recall how your body felt?

  CLIENT: I was all tense, my heart was pounding, my stomach felt queasy. My hands were trembling. I started to sweat under my arms. I was afraid I'd hyperventilate.

- What were the person's thoughts when the event occurred?

  THERAPIST: What did you think when that happened. Can you recall any thoughts you had?

  CLIENT: I thought that it was horrible. I also thought I could be hit by another car, that I could be there for a long time with no help, and I did not like the looks of the guy who stopped; he looked creepy.

- How did the person cope with the situation (e.g., "What did you do to deal with that situation?"; "How did you deal with your feelings?")?

THERAPIST: What did you do to try to cope with that situation?

CLIENT: I locked myself in the car. I called 9-1-1. Also, I turned down the ride from that guy.

THERAPIST: And how did you cope with the feelings you had of being scared?

CLIENT: I told myself to stay calm, but that didn't work too well. I was still scared to death.

THERAPIST: Thank you for sharing that experience, Lisa. It's one that would probably challenge any of us. Now that we've talked about a specific instance of stress, I want to share with you a model that has been developed by scientists who study stress and that captures much of what we've talked about so far.

Present the Stress Model

Present the graphic of the stress model without interventions, as shown in Appendix B, Figure B-1.

"This model contains four elements that Lisa just described in her stressful experience:

1. "The *situation* or *stressor* was being marooned in her car on a dark interstate on a rainy night. Also, encountering a rather ominous character.
2. "The way the situation was perceived and interpreted, which we call the *cognitive* (or mental) *appraisal*; Lisa said that she thought it was a horrible situation, that she could be hit by another car, could be there for a long time with no help, and she appraised the man who offered help as kind of creepy.
3. "The 'feelings' portion of the stress response, the so-called *fight-or-flight response* that arouses and mobilizes our bodies to respond to emergencies; in Lisa's case this included increased heart rate, breathing, sweating, queasy stomach, and muscle tension.
4. "What Lisa did to try to *cope* with the stressor: a combination of trying to get the help she needed and to control her feelings and stay calm.

"Our schematic also shows some of the negative consequences of the stress reaction that are linked to our thoughts, emotional reactions, and behaviors. Although we know that stress can sometimes have positive effects by motivating us to respond to a situation in ways that can have positive outcomes, such as escaping physical danger, we also know that excessive and unnecessary stress over the long haul can have negative effects on our physical health and on our psychological well-being. So, what we want to be able to do is to control stress responses in ways that enhance our physical and emotional health. We can't always avoid stressors, but we can gain greater control over how we respond to them.

"Let's summarize what we've discovered so far in our discussion. According to this model, stress involves an imbalance between the demands forced on us by the situation and the resources we have to deal with them. Resources can include everything from knowledge, money, social support, technical or communication skills to coping skills. The stress response is especially likely to occur when we appraise our resources as insufficient to deal with the demands, when the perceived consequences are negative and seem likely to occur, and when these consequences have important meaning to us, such as threatening our physical well-being, important goals that we have, personal relationships, or our feelings about ourselves. Then our bodies react with an emotional response and we usually try to do something to cope with the demands of the situation and with our feelings.

"Does this analysis make sense to you? Do you have any questions or comments so far?"

Address any questions or comments.

Ways to Reduce Stress

"Let's say that we want to think of ways to reduce stress. It follows from this model that there are a number of different ways we could do it. Can you think of places in the model where changes could be made that would affect the stress process?"

In groups, wait until you get suggestions for all four elements (situation, appraisal, emotional response, behavior). Then elaborate on client responses in the order they are given with examples like the following:

"First, you can change the situation: An overloaded student could decide to take a lighter course load in school. A worker could learn some additional skills that would increase her efficiency or help her get a job she'd like better. One could do something to resolve a conflict, defuse a confrontation, or break off a stressful relationship. Lisa called 9-1-1 to get help.

"Second, even if you can't change the stressful situation, you can control the way you react to it. You could do something to reduce or control the emotional *arousal* portion of the stress response: People can engage in responses that are incompatible with the stirred-up fight-or-flight response. Here are some things that are incompatible:

1. "Muscle relaxation: You can't be uptight or enraged while deeply relaxed.
2. "Vigorous exercise, such as jogging: Helps drain off tension and afterward, you become more deeply relaxed.
3. "Sexual behavior: We're not going to teach that coping skill here, but the incompatibility of anxiety and sexual performance is one reason why sexual dysfunctions are often related to anxiety about sex.
4. "Eating: Some people overeat when they are under stress, because eating makes them feel more relaxed. This response can lead people to gain weight when under stress.
5. "Substance use: Some people control their stress responses by turning to alcohol or drugs that reduce their arousal. Obviously, we don't recommend overeating or substance abuse.

"Third, you could change the cognitive appraisal of the situation, that is, you could rethink it. The brain is continuously having a conversation with itself, often below the level of awareness—a kind of internal monologue. We like to call these self-statements, things you're saying to yourself. These self-statements create our appraisals. Our thoughts and perceptions are a key place to influence stress. In a very real sense, we react to the situation *as we perceive it* rather than the actual situation. Some psychologists refer to this as the 'psychological situation,' or the situation as interpreted in our minds. Fortunately, you can do things at the appraisal level. You can learn to identify your automatic thoughts or beliefs about a situation, and counteract these beliefs with more productive appraisals and self-statements. A different interpretation of the situation by rethinking or reappraising it can change your emotional response and how you respond behaviorally. You can also 'talk yourself through' a stressful situation, giving yourself prompts or instructions on how to handle it.

"It's important to understand that our thoughts and perceptions often operate as well-learned habits. They are as automatic as driving a car or riding a bicycle is. For example:

"A car runs a stop sign in front of you. You slam on the brakes, swerve, and your heart's up in your throat, all before you have time to think. You must have believed that the situation was dangerous for you to react as you did, even though you may not have been aware of thinking 'This is dangerous' at the time.

"You greet an acquaintance who seems to look right through you as he or she walks by. You react by feeling hurt instantly. But what must you have believed about your friend's reaction in order to react by feeling hurt? If you thought your friend was so preoccupied that she didn't even see you, you'd react differently than if you thought she was rejecting you.

"Fourth, you can change your behavioral response: That is, you can change the situation through more effective problem-solving behaviors or you can leave or avoid the situation. It also follows that you can make the situation worse by responding in a way that makes the situation even more demanding, as when a student decides to avoid the anxiety connected with a test by going to a party instead of studying, or when someone drinks too much to blunt his or her emotions."

Description and Rationale for the Program

"Now I want to return to our stress model and to look at it in light of the stress solutions just described. In this program we concentrate on what goes on inside the brackets of the model, that is, in your thoughts and feelings. Here's an expanded model that shows what we're going to be doing."

Present the stress model with the interventions as shown in Appendix B, Figure B-2.

"Part of the stress response involves physiological arousal that is part of the so-called fight-or-flight response, which nature has built into all animals to deal with emergencies. In actual emergencies, that arousal can increase the chances of survival. But most of the stressors we encounter on a day-to-day basis do not involve running away from or fighting tigers, and prolonged arousal from psychological stressors can take a toll on both our bodies and our minds. At the level of physiological responses, you are going to learn to increase your sensitivity to your body's signals so you'll more quickly recognize tension and use it as a cue for coping. You're also going to learn breathing and muscle relaxation skills that you can apply to prevent or reduce the physical arousal aspect of the stress reaction. You'll also learn some meditation and mindfulness techniques that have stress-reducing effects.

"At the level of cognitive appraisal, you will develop a set of mental coping responses tailored specifically for you. You will learn to recognize your stress-producing beliefs or self-statements and replace them with stress-reducing self-statements. You will also learn how to talk yourself through stressful situations in ways that keep you focused and able to manage your feelings and the situation more successfully. In later sessions, I'll teach you some ways to separate yourself psychologically from stress-producing thoughts so that they're not taken literally.

"Stress management skills are no different than physical skills like playing a sport or a musical instrument. They have to be practiced so that you can master them. So, once you learn these skills, we'll help you to practice them while imagining yourself in stressful situations.

"You will be given out-of-session training materials and assignments to help you acquire these skills. These exercises are very important to do, because we don't have the time during our sessions for you to achieve mastery of the coping skills. I'm like a coach who shows you how to do the skills, but you have to master the skills by working on and practicing them, like athletes do. That means that you have to decide whether this is important enough to you to do what it takes to profit from it. It may mean having to plan your time so that you set aside a specific time to do your out-of-session work. Like other things in life, you will only get out of this program as much as you put into it. I want all of you to be successful, and I'll do all I can to help that happen."

Breath and Somatic Relaxation Training

"So, let's get started. We'll begin with some breath and relaxation training today. Relaxation is a stress management skill that you can quickly apply in stressful situations to prevent and control excessive arousal. Additionally, it will increase your body sensitivity, making you more aware of low levels of arousal, when it is easier to control. I might add that as people practice relaxation training, they often tell us how they were never really aware before of how much tension they carried around with them even when they thought they weren't stressed.

"In the relaxation training we use, you will tense your muscles, slowly relax them to the halfway point, and then completely relax them while paying close attention to your levels of tension. This focus of your attention helps increase your tension sensitivity and in the end allows you to create a state of muscle relaxation. The key principle here is that you can't be tense and relaxed at the same time, and so relaxation can be a powerful weapon to control and prevent tension. We are also going to add a word, such as *relax* or *calm*, as you relax. After repeated pairings, just thinking or saying the word will help trigger relaxation. To start, I want to show you how the way you breathe can influence your state of tension or relaxation."

ABDOMINAL BREATHING

"Breathing comes naturally, so it may surprise you that it plays an important role in stress control. There are two breathing patterns that have very different effects. One involves breathing into the chest, and it is often shallow and rapid. This is technically called *thoracic breathing* and it is part of the stress response. Hyperventilation involves rapid thoracic breathing that decreases levels of body-calming carbon dioxide and increases muscle tension in the chest, shoulders, and neck.

"The other form of breathing is called *abdominal breathing*. The breath is taken into the stomach instead of the chest. This type of breathing is seen in sleep or relaxation. It has a calming influence on the body. It is easy to learn. Next, we are going to practice each kind of breathing so you can experience the difference."

You might dim the lights and suggest that clients close their eyes during the breathing and muscle relaxation portion of the session so they can concentrate closely on internal sensations. If anyone is uncomfortable with eyes closed, they can simply look downward with their eyes open and concentrate on their muscles. Ask the clients to put one hand over their chest and the other over their abdomen.

"Now, inhale so that the hand on your chest moves while the hand on your abdomen does not. Do this five times. [Allow time for five breaths.] Next, inhale so that the hand on your chest does not move, and only the hand on your abdomen moves. Imagine there's a bright red balloon in your stomach. Breathe in slowly and feel the balloon fill. Then slowly let the air out as you exhale. Feel the balloon slowly, slowly deflate. . . . And when the air is gone, take another slow, natural breath into your stomach, filling your stomach, and then as you slowly exhale, think the word *relax* to yourself as the balloon slowly deflates."

Ask clients about their experience with the two types of breathing. Where they able to do both? What was their experience?

Explain that the word *relax* is typically suggested to pair with the exhalation, but clients can choose any word that connotes a calm, relaxed, or desired state to them. One professional baseball pitcher used *oily* to help himself relax while performing because it denoted for him the fluid, lubricated feeling of a smooth, tension-free throwing motion. Another person used *calm* and another *melt* to reference the longer version of the "tension melting away." The chosen word is paired with relaxation as part of the cue-produced relaxation training that occurs during somatic relaxation training. This breathing exercise, which can be relatively brief (about 3 minutes), will become an important component of the integrated coping response.

MUSCLE RELAXATION

Next, go through the somatic relaxation training procedure.

"Next, I'm going to teach you a form of progressive muscle relaxation. We're going to pair the word *relax*—or whichever word you choose— with your voluntary relaxation of muscles. We are going to divide the body's muscles into three groups: (1) feet, legs, and buttocks; (2) hands, arms, shoulders, chest, and abs; and (3) back, neck, jaw, and face. For each group, we're going to first tense the muscles. When you tense, do not make it so extreme that you risk pulling a muscle; a healthy tension is sufficient. Then slowly let the tension out halfway and think the word *relax* as you exhale and completely relax the muscles.

"Generally it's best to do the relaxation exercises with your eyes closed so that you can focus your attention totally on your internal sensations of tension and relaxation, but it's your choice. Before we begin, I'm going to demonstrate the specific muscle tension movements we're going to go through so you can see how they're done. [Sit in a chair as you demonstrate.]

"First, we're going to tense feet, legs, and buttocks. We do this by curling our toes and bending our feet downward. Tense the calves, straighten the thighs to tense the leg muscles, and tense the buttocks. Like this. [Demonstrate while sitting.]

"Next, we'll move to the upper body: arms, shoulders, chest, and abs. Make a fist with both hands; bend your hands down while tensing your upper arms, your biceps and triceps muscles. Press your arms against your body to tense your shoulders and chest while at the same time tensing your stomach muscles. Sounds like a lot to do, but it's easy to remember once you've done it a few times, and it gets the major muscles in your torso and arms. Here, let me show you the whole combination. [Demonstrate while sitting.]

"Finally, I'll have you tense your back, neck, and head. Thrust your jaw out, scrunch your eyes, and wrinkle your forehead. [Demonstrate.] By the way, it's best to do these movements in private, not in public places, unless you're starved for attention.

"Okay, let me quickly demonstrate the tension movements again."

Repeat the sequence. This exercise demonstration will take less than 10 seconds.

Over the years, we have reduced the specificity of the muscle groups

tensed and relaxed. At first, we used a 16-step progressive relaxation protocol used with traditional 1970s systematic desensitization. Clients find
the current three-muscle-group procedure nondemanding, and we have
observed much better compliance with the training. The process takes
only a few minutes, so clients can also practice several times a day if they
wish. However, we continue to emphasize the sequence of tensing fully,
slowly releasing halfway, and then slowing releasing completely as a way
of increasing sensitivity to arousal level and localizing tension. With a
week of practice, most clients are able to utilize the breathing-relaxation
response successfully. They can then practice by tensing the entire body
and releasing if they wish.

"Now, I'm going to take you through the exercise you'll be practicing
at home. Again, we're going to tense the muscles, slowly let the tension out halfway, then let it out all the way and completely relax the
muscles."

As we take clients through the process, we have found the images
in the suggested script useful in enhancing the experience. A soft, relaxing voice (as in hypnosis) is also helpful, especially during the relaxation
phase.

Full Tension

"As you tense the muscles of your buttocks, legs, and feet, pay special
attention to the feelings of tension, the way the muscles contract and
bunch like rubber bands; making those muscles become tense and taut
. . . the tension making the muscles feel a bit shaky . . . the muscles
tightening like ropes, with tension flowing into the muscles."

Halfway Tension Release

"Now, slowly let that tension out halfway. Notice the difference as the
tension slowly decreases. You may be surprised with how many stages
it goes through even to get to the halfway point. Notice the difference
between full and half tension, but be aware that there's still tension
there in your buttocks, legs, and feet."

Complete Tension Release

"Now slowly let the tension out all the way, and notice the sensations at
the different levels of tension you go through. . . . And now you can let
the muscles relax completely. Just letting go . . . letting the tension flow
away . . . the tension draining away as the muscles become limp and

loose and relaxed. You might picture an actual wave of relaxation that slowly flows downward from your waist through your hips, into your thighs, down through your calves and into your feet. As it moves, the wave slowly flows into the muscles and flushes out the tension. [Don't describe the wave as *warm, cool,* or having a color unless you have first asked clients and make sure that any description matches their sense of tension and relaxation.] The muscles become limp and loose and relaxed; your body is supported totally by the chair. And each time you exhale, say the word *relax* to yourself and feel your body obey. When you inhale, you draw the tension out of the muscles, and when you exhale, you breathe the tension away. Notice the difference between the relaxation you now feel and the tension that was there at the full and halfway points. Notice also how saying the word *relax* to yourself while exhaling helps deepen the relaxation."

YOGA BREATHING EXERCISE

When muscle relaxation is complete, teach the yoga breathing exercise. This exercise (Step 4 of the relaxation instructions) is well received by clients, who report that it deepens relaxation. It is an excellent way to end the session and demonstrate how relaxed a person can become.

"Now we're going to top off your practice with a simple breathing exercise that will deepen your relaxed state even more. Many people really like this one, and you can use it anywhere to quickly relax. Here's how it works:

"Take a series of short inhalations into your chest, one per second. When you've filled your lungs, hold that for a bit and then very slowly release the air as you exhale and say a long, slow "relaxxxx" to yourself, and let your body completely relax, as if you're sliding slowly down a hill. Then, breathe softly down into your stomach."

Purchasers of this book can download this recording for use with their clients (see the box at the end of the table of contents).

The following script (or one in your own words) can enhance clients' commitment to doing the relaxation homework assignment:

"Did you feel relaxed after going through the exercises? If so, you experienced how different it is than tension. How would you like to be able to produce that kind of relaxation at will within a few breaths? That's our goal. This skill will give you a powerful weapon against stress when you can produce the deep relaxation with one or two breaths and your cued-relaxation word. Most people can master this skill with about a week of committed practice. I often tell people that if you'll give yourself a week's investment in this training, you'll have a skill that will serve you for a lifetime.

"Let me tell you why we practice purposely creating the various levels of tension and ask you to pay attention to them. It's to help you become more sensitive to your own unique state of tension, especially to low-intensity levels. Many people walk around with a high tension level and don't become aware of it until it is too high to control effectively. If you can detect low levels of developing tension, it will be much easier to apply your relaxation skill and keep tension under control. So throughout your practice, I'd like you to be attentive to low levels of tension. As people learn to relax, they often report that they never realized how much tension they have been carrying around with them in their neck, shoulders, or other areas. As you develop awareness of your personal tension points, you can focus special attention on learning to relax those areas using these procedures."

Ending Session 1: Homework Assignments

Instruct clients to practice abdominal breathing paired with their cue word as often as possible during the day and the muscle relaxation exercise twice a day during the next week. Make sure they pair the cue word with each exhalation. Emphasize the fact that what they ultimately get out of the program depends on the extent to which they practice the skills. By the end of the program, they should have much greater control over their stress if they do the necessary work outside of sessions, for that is where the real skill acquisition occurs.

HANDOUTS

Give clients the handouts describing the program, the schedule of sessions, and the stress models (Handout A-1) and the breathing and muscle relaxation handout (Handout A-2). Encourage clients to keep the handouts and forms they receive in a dedicated folder or loose leaf binder. We provide a three-hole binder and punched materials. At the end of training, we provide a fresh set of resource materials for the clients' future reference, as they are likely to have underlined, highlighted, and written on the handouts and forms provided during training.

STRESS AND COPING DIARY

Distribute copies of the Stress and Coping Diary (Form A-1) with an orientation like the following:

"Part of mastering stress is understanding how you personally react to certain situations, how you think and feel when exposed to them, and what you do to cope with them. We've developed a Stress and Coping Diary to help you become your own Sherlock Holmes in learning about your process. The diary, which is based on the stress model we've talked about today, will help you gain greater awareness of your own stress process and help you identify the places where you could make changes. Over a period of time, the completed forms will help you understand the active ingredients of the situations that you find stressful, provide you with greater awareness of your internal appraisals, and help you figure out how you could change problematic ones. The diary can also give you greater insight on your possible use of 12 different coping strategies—some of which you use often, some of which you rarely or ever use, some of which might be stress reducers, and some of which are not.

"I'd like you to take a packet of forms home and complete one of them each day. It's especially important to fill out a form on days when you have a stressful experience. You will not be asked to hand them in; they are for your use. However, you should retain the forms you complete. I'm happy to discuss them with you if you wish. Please take one of the forms out so we can go over it. [Review the diary with clients and answer any questions.]

"You can use a collection of completed forms to see if any patterns emerge. Your responses on the forms may provide valuable information on your typical positive and negative emotional states, the themes in stressful situations that bother you—for example, feeling incompetent or let down by others. Pay special attention to the coping strategies you favor and how effective they are for you. See if you increase the use of the coping skills you learn here, and how well they work. The diary form will give you insights into how you function. We will be discussing all of the elements of the diary in the sessions to follow."

Individual Administration

When administering CASMT to an individual client, the first session is conducted in basically the same sequence as in the group format. The difference is that it is possible to personalize the intervention in terms of the client's personal stressors, stress responses, and coping behaviors and to establish a personal collaborative relationship, as illustrated in the case example described on page 128. As in any intervention, relationship factors are of paramount importance to the success of the program, for it is within the context of the therapist–client relationship that coping skills are developed and nurtured.

Initial Assessment

When working with an individual client, a personalized assessment is carried out, as would be the case in any other treatment. One goal in the initial sessions is to initiate an empathic, supportive, collaborative relationship with the client and to discuss the client's stress-related problems and symptoms. The therapist wishes to identify the external and internal events that trigger stress reactions with an eye to selecting intervention targets and procedures and providing an overview and rationale for the intervention. Session 1 begins with a standard interview in which the client is asked to describe the nature of the problem, its duration, how and how severely it impacts the client's life, the situations under which it occurs, and conditions that either intensify or alleviate the problem behaviors. How has the client dealt with the problem in the past, and how effective were these attempts? If the client has completed pretreatment Stress and Coping Diary forms, the therapist will have a sample of stressful encounters. The PSS (Cohen et al., 1983) can provide normative information on the client's level of life stress.

Therapist style plays an important role in establishing a therapeutic relationship in which the client feels free to explore and disclose thoughts and feelings. Warmth, acceptance, and compassion facilitate such a relationship. Statements such as "I can understand how that situation could be upsetting to you" can convey understanding, and statements like "It sounds like you handled that quite well; clearly you already have some skills we can build on" help increase a sense of self-efficacy and capacity for change. Likewise, to convey an atmosphere in which the client exercises personal control that is part of the collaborative relationship in the intervention, it should be communicated that whereas self-disclosure of sensitive material can facilitate treatment, the client can do so at his or her own pace.

The following clinical case example illustrates a typical first session of an individual administration of CASMT.

Harlan, an unmarried 35-year-old office worker, referred himself for treatment because of strong social-evaluative and performance anxiety. His anxiety manifested itself in several domains, including dating relationships and nearly any kind of public performance, particularly speaking before groups. The precipitating event that led to his self-referral was a recent job interview in which he reported failing to get the job, "probably because I came across as terrified and incompetent." On the basis of a clinical intake interview in which he reported long-standing problems of this kind, he received a diagnosis of social anxiety disorder. He was judged to be an appropriate candidate for CASMT, to be directed at his social anxiety, the major source of stress in his life.

Harlan completed a Stress and Coping Diary (Form A-1) on three occasions in the week preceding his first session of CASMT. His responses on portions of one report are shown in Figure 4.1.

Harlan's diary responses indicate that he is experiencing a good deal of negative affect (Items 1 and 2). The situation he describes involves an unexpected opportunity for a blind date with an attractive woman. This proposal creates intense anxiety and triggers an impulsive avoidance response of lying to his coworker and saying he will be out of town. Item 4 shows that the elements of the situation that were especially prominent were his feeling incompetent, helpless, confused, and rushed. The situation also felt as if expectations were not met and his goal (presumably, meeting an attractive woman) was blocked by his avoidance. He feels little control over either the situation or his emotional response to it (Item 6).

The thoughts that seem associated with his intense anxiety (Item 7) involve concerns about not being good enough for the woman, making a fool out of himself, and causing the woman to be bored and unwilling to date him again, thus reinforcing a sense of inadequacy. He has difficulty thinking of an appraisal that would have prevented or reduced his anxiety. In terms of coping strategies (Item 8), the most prominent pattern is problem solving—in this case, through avoidance. He does not endorse using the coping skills that will be the focus of training, namely, relaxation and rethinking the situation. Finally, he reports a relatively low level of current life satisfaction on Item 10.

The collection of pretreatment data sometimes reveals a particular recurring stressor that can be the subject of the orientation to the stress model. In Harlan's case, two of the three stressors he reported involved some aspect of his social anxiety. In the absence of such data, the therapist can ask the client to select the most meaningful recent stressor for analysis: (1) "What happened?"; (2) "How did you respond emotionally?"; (3) "What thoughts did you have about the situation?"; and (4) "What did you do to try to cope with it?" You can also ask the client how characteristic this instance is of his or her stress experiences, hopefully to detect a recurrent pattern that may represent a chronic problem.

Orientation to CASMT

The therapist can then begin to orient the client to the CASMT intervention:

"It sounds like you have some significant stress in your life that's been with you for quite some time. Much of what you describe fits a problem category called *social anxiety*. We think you are a good candidate for a relatively brief stress management program that we offer in which you

Stress and Coping Diary

1. **Please respond to the following question based on how you have been feeling since your last diary entry.**

	Not at all stressful		Somewhat stressful		Extremely stressful	
In general, how stressful have your life circumstances been since your last diary entry?	○	○	○	○	○	●	○

2. **To what extent do these terms describe how you have been feeling since your last diary entry?**

	Not at all	A little	Some- what	Moder- ately	A fair amount	Quite a bit	Extremely
Optimistic	○	○	○	●	○	○	○
Irritable	○	●	○	○	○	○	○
Tense	○	○	○	○	○	●	○
Unhappy	○	○	○	○	●	○	○
Relaxed	○	●	○	○	○	○	○
Angry	●	○	○	○	○	○	○
Anxious	○	○	○	○	○	●	○
Enthusiastic	○	○	●	○	○	○	○
Discouraged	○	○	○	○	●	○	○
Resentful	○	●	○	○	○	○	○
Contented	○	○	●	○	○	○	○
Afraid	○	○	○	○	●	○	○
Depressed	○	●	○	○	○	○	○
Energetic	○	○	○	○	○	●	○

3. **Please describe a stressful event you experienced since your last diary entry.**
In the box below, please indicate what happened. Please describe the event in enough detail so that when you read it later, you'll be able to reexperience the event. Please do the best you can to describe what made this event stressful to you.

> One of my coworkers approached me to arrange a blind date with her cousin over the weekend. She showed me a picture, and the woman is very attractive. I got really nervous and said that I'd like to do it in the future, but will be out of town this weekend (which is not true). I'm not sure she believed me or that I'll have another chance unless I arrange it later. I'd love to date this woman, but feel afraid to take a chance, so I feel stuck.

FIGURE 4.1. A Stress and Coping Diary report submitted by Harlan.

4. Please respond to the following questions based on the situation you just described.

	Not at all		Somewhat				Extremely
To what extent did you **feel incompetent** in this situation?	○	○	○	○	○	●	○
To what extent did you **feel exhausted** in this situation?	○	●	○	○	○	○	○
To what extent did you **feel excluded** in this situation?	●	○	○	○	○	○	○
To what extent did you **feel helpless** in this situation?	○	○	○	○	○	●	○
To what extent did you **feel irritated** in this situation?	●	○	○	○	○	○	○
To what extent did you **feel confused** in this situation?	○	○	○	○	○	●	○
To what extent did you **feel rushed** in this situation?	○	○	○	○	○	●	○
To what extent did you **feel as though your time was wasted** in this situation?	●	○	○	○	○	○	○
To what extent did you **feel betrayed** in this situation?	●	○	○	○	○	○	○
To what extent did you **feel bored** in this situation?	●	○	○	○	○	○	○
To what extent did you **feel as though your expectations** were not met in this situation?	○	○	○	○	○	○	●
To what extent did you **feel as though your goals were blocked** in this situation?	○	○	○	○	○	○	●
To what extent were you **afraid of letting others down** in this situation?	○	○	○	○	○	●	○

5. How stressed did you feel?

	Not at all intense		Somewhat intense			Extremely intense	
How intense was your emotional reaction to this stressful event?	○	○	○	○	○	●	○

(continued)

6. Please respond to the following questions based on the stressful event you described at the beginning of this diary entry.

	I felt I had little or no personal control		I felt I had some personal control		I felt I had a great deal of personal control
To what extent did you feel you had **personal control** over this situation?	○ ● ○	○	○	○	○
To what extent did you feel you were able to **control your emotional reaction** to this event?	○ ● ○	○	○	○	○

7. We tend to have thoughts or perceptions that occur more or less automatically when we encounter certain situations. The following two questions ask you to describe what you may have mentally "said to yourself" about the stressful event.

A. In the box below, please indicate what you may have automatically "told yourself" about the event that could have contributed to your emotional reaction.

> *She's out of my league. I'll be so nervous that I'll make a fool out of myself. I won't know what to say and she'll be bored stiff. She'll reject me and I'll feel like a schmuck.*

B. Instead of what you told yourself about the **event**, what could you have told yourself in order to prevent or reduce your emotional reaction?

> *Can't think of anything except maybe, what do I have to lose, and maybe it will go okay.*

8. The following questions ask you to indicate what you did in response to the event you described at the beginning of this diary entry.

	Not at all		Somewhat		A great deal
Rethinking the situation involves reevaluating the situation and its meaning in ways that counteract stress-producing thoughts and thereby reduce the stress response. To what extent did you engage in rethinking the situation?	○ ● ○	○	○	○	○
If you engaged in **rethinking the situation,** to what extent did it help you reduce your stress response?	○ ● ○	○	○	○	○

FIGURE 4.1 (*continued*)

	Not at all		Somewhat			A great deal	
Relaxation techniques involve attempts to reduce emotional arousal using muscle relaxation, meditation, or breathing techniques. To what extent did you engage in relaxation techniques in this situation?	●	O	O	O	O	O	O
If you engaged in **relaxation techniques**, to what extent did they help you reduce your stress response?	O	O	O	O	O	O	O
Seeking social support involves seeking or finding emotional support or advice from loved ones, friends, or professionals. To what extent did you seek social support in this situation?	●	O	O	O	O	O	O
If you engaged in **seeking social support**, to what extent did it help you reduce your stress response?	O	O	O	O	O	O	O
Direct problem solving involves thinking about solutions to the problem, gathering information about the problem, or actually doing something about the problem. To what extent did you engage in direct problem solving in this situation?	O	O	O	O	●	O	O
If you engaged in **direct problem solving**, to what extent did it help you reduce your stress response?	O	O	O	O	●	O	O
Blaming yourself involves being critical of yourself for the problem. To what extent did you blame yourself in this situation?	O	O	O	O	●	O	O
If you engaged in **blaming yourself**, to what extent did it help you reduce your stress response?	O	●	O	O	O	O	O
Blaming others involves criticizing and/or getting angry with the people you view as most responsible for the situation. To what extent did you blame others in this situation?	O	O	O	O	●	O	O
If you engaged in **blaming others**, to what extent did it help you reduce your stress response?	O	O	●	O	O	O	O
Wishful thinking involves daydreaming, fantasizing, or just **hoping** that things would be better or that the event will turn out differently. To what extent did you engage in wishful thinking in this situation?	O	O	O	O	O	●	O

(continued)

	Not at all		Somewhat			A great deal
If you engaged in **wishful thinking**, to what extent did it help you reduce your stress response?	○	●	○	○	○	○	○
Distraction involves diverting your attention from stressful thoughts and feelings by thinking about or imagining more pleasant things. To what extent did you engage in distraction in this situation?	●	○	○	○	○	○	○
If you engaged in **distraction**, to what extent did it help you reduce your stress response?	○	○	○	○	○	○	○
Avoidance involves doing things to sidestep confronting the problem or thinking about it, doing things to evade experiencing negative emotions, or not letting others know what is happening or how you are feeling. To what extent did you engage in avoidance in this situation?	○	○	○	○	○	○	●
If you engaged in **avoidance**, to what extent did it help you reduce your stress response?	○	○	○	○	○	●	○
Counting your blessings involves focusing on the good things in your life or reminding yourself that, no matter how difficult things might be, you are still better off than many people. To what extent did you count your blessings in this situation?	●	○	○	○	○	○	○
If you engaged in **counting your blessings**, to what extent did it help you reduce your stress response?	○	○	○	○	○	○	○
Physical activity includes any form of exercise (e.g., jogging, swimming). To what extent did you engage in physical activity in this situation?	●	○	○	○	○	○	○
If you engaged in **physical activity**, to what extent did it help you reduce your stress response?	○	○	○	○	○	○	○
Acceptance involves simply allowing the presence of stressful thoughts and feelings and waiting for them to pass away rather than trying to control them. To what extent did you engage in acceptance in this situation?	●	○	○	○	○	○	○
If you engaged in **acceptance**, to what extent did it help you reduce your stress response?	○	○	○	○	○	○	○

FIGURE 4.1 (*continued*)

9. Please respond to the following questions based on the stressful event you described at the beginning of this diary entry.

	Not at all stressful			Somewhat stressful			Extremely stressful
How stressful was the event **at the time you experienced it?**	O	O	O	O	O	O	●
How stressful was the event **after engaging in coping behaviors?**	O	O	O	O	●	O	O

10. Current life satisfaction

	Most unhappy									Most happy
Overall, how would you rate your general life satisfaction at this time?	O	O	●	O	O	O	O	O	O	O

Thank you for completing today's entry.

can learn some emotion control coping skills that have helped many people with issues like yours. We'll be especially targeting your social anxiety, but the skills you'll learn are really life skills, applicable to lots of different kinds of stressful situations.

"One way to explain how the program works is to consider the nature of stress through a situation that you described in one of your diary entries. Do you recall the incident in which your coworker tried to arrange a blind date with her cousin? Could you describe what happened?"

EXAMINING A STRESSFUL INCIDENT

One useful procedure, if clients are comfortable doing it, is to have them sit back, close their eyes, and relive the experience while describing the situation and whatever thoughts and feelings occurred before, during, and after the event. Based on the client's description, the therapist can help the client identify the parts of the stressful experience that match the stress model.

We believe that training and compliance with the program are most successful when the therapist can lead the client to "discover" the stress and coping model and the measures that might be taken to reduce stress. Rather than a didactic presentation, we favor leading questions based on the situation described by the client, as illustrated above. Fitting the client's description into the model and then asking what might be done to modify its elements before presenting the intervention schematic help the client to view the solutions as his or her own. This approach is consistent with the "personal scientist" orientation of the program. Therapists can ask questions like the following:

THERAPIST: Did you have any sense that this was going to be an upsetting experience? If so, did you try to prepare for it? How?

CLIENT: Chelsea [Harlan's coworker] had asked me a few times if I had a steady. I told her no. But I had no idea this was coming. It caught me completely off guard, and I was unprepared for it.

THERAPIST: How did your body react? Tell me about your physical response to her asking you to date her cousin.

CLIENT: It was like a hot flash went through me, especially when she showed me a picture of this really attractive woman. I could feel myself tense up and my heart started going a lot faster. I just stood there kind of immobilized, wondering what to do. By the time it was over, my underarms were pretty wet.

THERAPIST: Did your bodily responses affect your thoughts about what was happening or how serious the situation was?

CLIENT: I guess so. I mean, the way my body reacted let me know that this was a really tough situation. I was afraid Chelsea would notice my panic and wonder what kind of screwball I am.

THERAPIST: What was it about that situation that made it so demanding for you? Can we get a handle on the "active ingredients"?

CLIENT: Like I said in that diary form, I was worried that I would make a fool out of myself on the date, that the woman wouldn't like me or would be bored with me, and that she'd probably be mad at Chelsea for fixing us up. Chelsea would also think I'm a dud if that happened.

THERAPIST: So, what did you do to deal with that situation?

CLIENT: I felt so overmatched that I told Chelsea that I was going to be out of town over the weekend. She seemed to accept that, and said, "Maybe another time."

THERAPIST: How did that affect your feelings?

CLIENT: On one level, I felt a sense of relief. I also felt guilty about lying to Chelsea. But most of all, I was really frustrated with myself because I blew a chance to get a date with a really attractive woman, which I've wanted for a long time. Now I don't know if I'll get another chance. And if I have to ask this woman out, it'll be a lot harder than it would have been if Chelsea had set it up.

THERAPIST: So, by avoiding the dating situation, you got some immediate relief from your anxiety, but at the cost of endangering an important longer-term goal of meeting a nice woman. That's how avoidance often works—a short-term gain in relief, but longer-term negatives. Is this avoidance pattern characteristic of how you cope with your anxiety?

CLIENT: Yeah, I think pretty much so. That's why I haven't asked anyone out for over a year. I can't stand the possibility that I'll get rejected.

THERAPIST: Are there any other situations that you avoid?

CLIENT: I really get nervous when I have to speak to a group, especially one that will be evaluating what I'm saying. I worry that I'll freeze up, stammer, and look stupid or incompetent. About a month ago, I declined my pastor's invitation to speak to the entire congregation about a funding drive in which I'm involved.

THERAPIST: Social anxiety can affect lots of things people do, or don't do. But let's back up a bit. As you think about the blind date situation now, is it still as upsetting as it was when it occurred?

CLIENT: Well, if I could do it over, I'd be more likely to go on the date, especially feeling now that I blew a good opportunity.

THERAPIST: What's changed? Are you looking at the situation any differently now that you've had some time to reflect on it?

CLIENT: One thing is that she might have been easy to talk to and that we might have had some common interests. Also, as I thought about the question on the questionnaire [diary] about what I could have told myself instead. I probably was overly critical of how I'd come across. I'm really not without some social skills. Finally, if you think in the long term, I had little to lose even if she didn't like me. I wouldn't see her again, and as it stands now, I might not anyway unless I can get another chance to meet her.

THERAPIST: Would your current mind-set have been helpful if you had applied it when that situation occurred?

CLIENT: Yeah. It would have gotten me a date with a woman I might have liked a lot.

THERAPIST: Well, I think it's been helpful to go over what you reported in your diary. We'll be doing this a lot when we meet for several reasons. First, we want to see what patterns we detect in your stress and coping, and to also see what kinds of changes occur over time. Second, lots of clients tell us that as they become more aware of the thoughts and feelings and answer the question about what they could have told themselves instead, they begin to think differently and in ways that short-circuit the stress response. In this program, you're going to learn ways of talking to yourself in stressful situations that are more like how you're thinking about the dating situation now. For now, however, let's talk about what stress is and how we can handle it more effectively.

Define Stress and Present the Stress Model

At this point, using the client's description, discuss the nature of stress. Start by asking the client what he or she means by stress. Use leading questions (e.g., "Yes, frightening or irritating situations qualify as stress. Is there any other way we use the term?") In the end, present the three uses of the term as (1) high-demand situations (stressors), (2) responses to those situations, and (3) an ongoing transaction between the person and the situation, with each influencing the other. Then, using the situation described by the client in the diary entry, show how the description is captured in the portions of the model that address situational factors, appraisal, physiological arousal, and coping efforts. Present the model of stress (Appendix B, Figure B-1). Reinforce the client for "discovering" the scientific model of stress in his or own experience.

Follow this discussion with a presentation of the CASMT intervention model (Figure B-2), fitting the client's descriptions into the elements of the model and discussing the relations among them that your leading questions elicited from the client. Show the client how the treatment addresses the cognitive and physiological elements of the stress model.

"There are many instances in which we can't directly change the situation, but we do have control over how we respond to it. We're going to concentrate on your gaining greater control over the thoughts and feelings that contribute to your stress. In this program we concentrate on what goes on inside the brackets of the model—that is, on your thoughts and feelings. Here's an expanded model that shows what we're going to be doing."

Present the stress model with the interventions as shown in Figure B-2.

"Part of the stress response involves physiological arousal that is part of the fight-or-flight response that nature has built into all animals to deal with emergencies. In actual emergencies, that arousal can increase the chances of survival. But most of the stressors we encounter on a day-to-day basis do not involve running away from or fighting sabre-tooth tigers, and prolonged arousal from psychological stressors can take a toll on both our bodies and our minds. At the level of physiological responses, you are going to learn to increase your sensitivity to your body's signals so you'll more quickly recognize tension and use it as a cue for coping. You're also going to learn breathing and muscle relaxation skills that you can apply to prevent or reduce the physical arousal aspect of the stress reaction. Finally, you'll learn some meditation and mindfulness techniques that have stress-reducing effects.

"At the level of cognitive appraisal, you will learn a set of mental coping responses tailored specifically for you. You will learn to recognize your stress-producing beliefs or self-statements and replace them with stress-reducing self-statements. You will also learn how to talk yourself through stressful situations in ways that keep you focused and able to manage your feelings and the situation more successfully. In later sessions, I'll teach you some ways to separate yourself psychologically from stress-producing thoughts so that they're not taken literally.

"Stress management skills are no different than physical skills like playing a sport or a musical instrument. They have to be practiced so that you can master them. So, once you learn these skills, we'll help you to practice them while imagining yourself in stressful situations.

"I'll be giving you out-of-session training materials and assignments to help you acquire these skills. These exercises are very important to do if you want to achieve mastery of the coping skills. I'm like a coach who shows you how to do the skills, but you have to master the skills by working on and practicing them like an athlete does. That means that you have to decide at the outset whether this is important enough to you to do what it takes to profit from our work together. It may mean having to plan your schedule so that you set aside a specific time to do your out-of-session work. Like other things in life, you will only get out of this program as much as you put into it. I want you to be successful, and I'll do all I can to help that happen."

EXPLORING AND RESPONDING TO CLIENT EXPECTATIONS AND CONCERNS

With an individual client, it is advisable to assess the credibility of the CASMT rationale as presented and to address any questions and concerns he or she might have. This is important to determine because client reservations about the underlying rationale could affect compliance with the coping skills acquisition and rehearsal procedures. Here are some questions that sometimes arise:

THERAPIST: I wonder if the approach we're taking meets your expectations about the kind of treatment you'd receive when you contacted us.

CLIENT: It sounds reasonable, but I'm surprised that it only goes for six sessions. Is 6 weeks long enough?

THERAPIST: We've found that much can be accomplished in 6 weeks, though we can always be flexible if we need more time for you to acquire a skill. However, it's important to realize that the treatment does not consist of just the six sessions. It includes 36 other days when you'll be actively working on acquiring and refining the skills outside of our sessions. I'm going to give you lots of self-training materials whose value is supported by research studies. Our relationship is a bit like a coach and an athlete. As your stress management coach, I'll be guiding you through some self-awareness, learning, and skill rehearsal exercises when we meet, but as the athlete, you need to work on the skills through your hard work and practice. Even the most brilliant coach depends on the athlete's commitment to learning and practicing. Do you think you can make that commitment?

CLIENT: It says in this schedule that I'm going to be controlling emotional responses from imagining stressful situations. Am I going to be experiencing a lot of stress as I do this?

THERAPIST: An important part of the program is for you not only to learn stress reduction skills, but also to practice them to reduce emotional responses. We use a procedure called *induced affect*—*affect* is another term for *emotion*—to help you experience fairly intense emotions right in the session, but not until you have acquired the skills to turn off the emotional response. You can be confident that you will be able to turn it off. What you can do in here, you'll be able to do out in the real world. The rehearsal of your coping skills to turn off emotional arousal in this safe environment is one of the most important features of what we'll be doing. Experiencing strong negative feelings is no fun, but you might look at that experience as an investment, as a way to master some stress management skills that can serve you for the rest of your life. Think of how your life would change if you were able to reduce your social anxiety. Keep that long-term goal in mind as we proceed.

CLIENT: I've had this problem all my life. Can I hope to get rid of it at this point in my life?

THERAPIST: I hear what you're saying, and it's a legitimate question. In particular, the ways you think about situations, yourself, and your abilities—the mental appraisals that help create your stress—are well-practiced thought patterns that go back a long way. We aren't going to search for the historical factors in your thinking; our focus is going to be on changing them in the present and future. I can only tell you that people have a capacity to change at virtually any age, and the techniques we're going to teach you have a lot of scientific support. I should also tell you that you will not be a stress-free "finished product" when we're done here. First, no one is ever completely stress-free. However, if you're like most people we treat, you will be much better at managing your feelings. More importantly, you won't be a finished product in 6 weeks any more than 6 weeks of tennis lessons will make you a tennis pro. However, like the tennis player, you will have a skills foundation that works for you, and those skills will get even better as you use and refine them in the weeks, months, and years to come. Our plan is to jump-start that process and give you the coping skills you need to live a happier and less stressful life.

Clients are often self-critical because they feel that they should be able to cope more effectively. It is helpful to reassure them about the universality of stress responses, and that nature has wired us to respond to stressors with fight-or-flight responses. It is true that some people are more reactive than others either because they are simply more physiologically reactive or because they've had different learning experiences. These experiences may have created attitudes that make them more or less likely to be emotionally reactive to certain kinds of situations. This does not mean, however, that they cannot learn or strengthen coping skills that will increase their resilience. And that's exactly what this program is designed to help them accomplish.

Breath and Relaxation Training

Proceed to breath and relaxation training, relating it to the model. Using the format applied in the group administration, take the client through the breathing exercise to show the difference between abdominal and thoracic breathing. Ask the client to put one hand over the chest and the other over the abdomen to feel the difference in abdominal and thoracic breathing. The goal is abdominal breathing, which is more relaxing. Follow the same procedure as in the group administration and in Handout A-2. Explain that the word *relax* is typically suggested to pair with the exhalation, but that clients can choose any word that connotes a calm, relaxed, or desired state to them.

"Next, I'm going to take you through a procedure called progressive muscle relaxation. We're going to pair the word *relax*—or which other word you choose—with your voluntary relaxation of muscles. We are going to divide the body's muscles into three groups: (1) feet, legs, and buttocks; (2) hands, arms, shoulders, chest, and abs; and (3) back, neck, jaw, and face. For each group, we're going to first tense the muscles. When you tense, do not make it so extreme that you risk pulling a muscle; a healthy tension is sufficient. Next, you slowly let the tension out halfway, and then think the word *relax* as you exhale and completely relax the muscles."

Demonstrate how to tense each muscle group and then take the client through the process using a soft, relaxing voice. When the relaxation exercise is complete, finish with the yoga breathing exercise—a series of quick, short inhalations to fill the lungs, followed by a long, slow exhalation while saying the cue word. If desired, give the client instructions on how to download the audio recording of the relaxation exercise.

Follow up the relaxation training by assessing the client's experience. How relaxed, on a scale from 1 (deeply relaxed) to 100 (as tense as one could be), did the client become? Were there any difficulties in relaxing certain muscle groups? Could the client distinguish the levels of tension as it was released halfway and then all the way? How many tension levels did the client experience?

If the client experienced deep relaxation, end this discussion with a statement such as the following:

"You can see how the state of relaxation is the exact opposite of what happens when the body gets emotionally aroused. It follows that since it is impossible to be tense and relaxed at the same time, being able to voluntarily relax yourself will help reduce or prevent emotional arousal. If you had been relaxed instead of emotionally aroused with anxiety when Chelsea asked you to date her cousin, you might have handled the situation more easily.

"With about a week of practice, most people can induce relaxation even in stressful situations in the space of a few breaths. Many also tell us that until they learned to experience deep relaxation, they never realized how much tension they were carrying around in their bodies. It's really important that you do the practice every day this coming week, because it lays the foundation for what we'll be doing in future sessions."

Promoting Realistic Expectations

Two varieties of unrealistic expectation may occur in clients. The first is an overly positive one that, as a result of treatment, the client will become stress-proof. More typically, however, clients tend to selectively embrace information that supports their existing belief that they are powerless in their ability to handle stressful situations. Any setback will help confirm this aspect of their self-image. As Marlatt and Gordon (1985) demonstrated in their work on relapse prevention, it is important to counter this tendency so that lapses in coping success do not confirm perceived helplessness or cause clients to discount the value of learning the skills. For relapse prevention purposes, one should emphasize that the various coping skills are not guaranteed; clients should not expect themselves to control their stress responses in every stressful situation:

"Although you're going to learn a set of coping skills that have proven to be generally effective in dealing with stress, we can anticipate that they're not going to work for every stressful situation you encounter, even once you master them. This program will make you stress-*resistant*, not stress-proof. Sometimes we can be overwhelmed by the demands of a situation, or sometimes a different coping strategy would have worked better in a particular situation. The important point is how you respond when a setback happens. It's important not to conclude that the coping skills 'don't work' or to get down on yourself because you weren't as successful in dealing with the situation as you would have liked. The goal is to learn from the less successful experiences and make adjustments that increase the likelihood of dealing more effectively with similar situations when they recur in the future. That's also an important part of becoming a better personal scientist. Thomas Edison was once asked if he was discouraged by his more than 700 failed attempts to create the incandescent light bulb. He replied, 'Certainly not. Every wrong step discarded is another step forward. I've now learned 700 ways not to make a light bulb.' I'm not implying that you're going to have 700 unsuccessful coping attempts, but if you're like most people I work with, you can be sure you'll have a few along the way. View them as opportunities to learn how to increase your effectiveness."

Fostering Compliance with Homework Assignments

As in the group procedure, it is important to obtain commitment to doing the out-of-session training assignments, because this is where most of the skill acquisition will ultimately occur. Most clients will not be used to doing structured self-monitoring, practicing relaxation, or preparing anti-stress self-statements. Some don't read the client resource handouts. To the extent that you can enhance compliance and remove barriers to doing the outside work, the program can proceed efficiently. When a client comes back for a second session without having practiced the relaxation because "I just couldn't find the time to do it," it's frustrating to the therapist and impairs the coping skills learning sequence as the client is already a session behind.

Meichenbaum (1985) described a number of ways to forestall non-compliance. One is to communicate your understanding that a fair amount is being asked of the client and that there may well be challenges to getting the out-of-session activities done.

THERAPIST: The success of this program depends as much upon what goes on between our sessions as it does upon what goes on in them. That's because the out-of-session training activities, including the Stress and Coping Diary, are where we learn more about your stressors and your ways of coping, and where you learn and practice the coping skills. I also have skills training assignments for you to do. The things I'm asking you to read and practice don't take a lot of time, but we all have very busy lives with lots of competing commitments. I am wondering what problems, if any, that you might see in practicing your relaxation exercises?

CLIENT: One of the reasons I'm stressed is because I'm overwhelmed with demands from my work, and I'm spending a lot of time with my parents because my mother has cancer treatment. I'm a bit worried that I will forget to do some things or not get to them.

THERAPIST: That's a very common challenge. I can see how, with so much going on, one might forget. Can you think of any ways you could build in reminders in your schedule?

CLIENT: I guess I could put reminders into my smartphone. Another thing that should work is to put up some Post-it notes at home where I'd see them, such as the refrigerator door or bathroom mirror.

THERAPIST: Those are some great ideas. I can see you have some well-developed problem-solving skills. I can also relate to your busy schedule; sometimes I think there are not enough hours in the day to do everything I should do. So I understand your concern that given a schedule that is already overwhelming at times, plus unanticipated things that come up, it could be hard to find the time. Can you think of any ways to block in the needed time to make sure you can do the readings and practice?

CLIENT: I guess the best thing would be to set aside some times during the day to do the stuff. Maybe I could get up a half hour earlier or block in some time in the evening—maybe right after dinner—instead of reading or watching TV.

THERAPIST: Another good idea. Getting up a bit early guarantees the needed time. Scheduling time and committing yourself to using that time slot is a very effective way to do it. I also like your idea of doing your activities right after dinner because then you can use what you enjoy—reading or watching TV—as a reward for doing your training activities. Creating a routine also helps a lot. I should add one more point. This week you'll be doing relaxation training, which should place you in a pleasant and relaxed state that you will enjoy. So, there is another built-in reward.

End-of-Session Summary and Homework Assignments

End the session by giving the client a verbal summary of what transpired and Handouts A-1 and A-2, Handout plus a set of seven Stress and Coping Diary forms (Form A-1) for self-monitoring.

"As we end today's session, let me do a quick summary of what we talked about. First, using the example of the blind date situation you described in your Stress and Coping Diary, I shared our model of stress with you and we discussed the model's elements: situations, appraisals, emotional responses, and coping behaviors. Then, we examined the model's implications for how you might achieve greater control over your stress responses, and we discussed the stress management program. We saw that we're going to concentrate on the parts of the model inside of the brackets—that is, on the appraisals that are the true causes of the emotional response and the physiological arousal that are the problem—by developing mind–body coping skills that you can use to reduce or prevent these stress responses. That brought us to our first coping skill, designed to help you control high physiological arousal. I took you through our breathing and relaxation training procedure. Then we discussed some questions that you had about what we are doing. Have I missed anything, or are there any questions or issues that you might want to bring up?

"Then I passed out the materials for you to read and to work on at home. During the next week, we want to get a good jump on your relaxation skills, so I gave you the assignment to practice the abdominal breathing paired with your cue word as often as possible during the day and the abbreviated relaxation training twice a day during the next week. Again, make sure you pair the cue word with exhalation and muscle relaxation, as the training instructions direct you to do. If you can get this foundation skill down quickly, you can begin using it in your life situations, and we'll be able to work smoothly through the program. I look forward to working with you, and I anticipate a positive outcome."

As did this chapter, those to follow provide specific guidelines for the next five phases of the CASMT program. In each instance, group and individual formats are described. The specificity of the guidelines is designed to foster treatment fidelity for both clinical and research applications while also allowing therapists the latitude to adapt the program to their therapeutic style and the needs of their individual clients.

CHAPTER 5

Session 2: Cognitive Coping Skills

*Introduction to Cognitive Restructuring
and Self-Instructional Training*

ABOUT SESSION 2

Session 2 is one of the most critical and challenging in the program because cognitive coping skill acquisition is inherently more difficult than developing somatic relaxation skills. Here, we are dealing with cognitive processes and schemas that are deeply ingrained and operate in a more or less automatic fashion. Because clients often have minimal awareness of these cognitions, they tend to find it challenging to uncover the appraisals that trigger their stress response. It is even more challenging to replace maladaptive appraisals with adaptive reappraisals. It is not uncommon for traditional cognitive therapy (Beck) or rational–emotive therapy (Ellis) to extend well beyond 40 sessions in clinical settings, and around 15–20 sessions in clinical trials (Hollon, Thase, & Markowitz, 2002; Morrison, Bradley, & Westen, 2003).

As discussed in Chapter 2, our goal is far more modest than the widespread revision of cognitive schemas sought in traditional CBT. We cover some basics of this approach in this second session, but we supplement our in-session efforts with bibliotherapeutic materials on cognitive restructuring and self-instructional training (Handout A-3). Our experience is that CBT-based handouts that are used to guide cognitive coping skills acquisition enable clients to create sets of stress-reducing self-statements. Consistent with a recommendation by Hope, Heimberg, and Turk (2006), we find that a few global "rational responses," such as "It's not that big a thing" or "I may not like this, but I definitely can stand it," can be applied in numerous situations. Such statements can be useful to clients in countering catastrophizing or magnifying cognitions and emotional overreaction. Component analyses of CBT interventions indicate that decreases in catastrophizing cognitions is an important mediator of outcome (Meichenbaum, 1985; Turner, Holtzman, & Mancl, 2009), so we target tendencies (1) to exaggerate the demands and aversiveness of stressful situations, (2) to expect highly negative outcomes, and (3) to feel helpless in coping with them. Such reappraisals should be highly generalizable across a variety of stressors even if they do not involve the confrontation of core beliefs, as would be the therapeutic goal in rational–emotive or cognitive therapy.

Stress-reducing cognitions can also be developed using a self-instructional training approach that does not involve logical refutation of maladaptive cognitions (Meichenbaum, 1974). Even clients with educational, intellectual, or logical thinking limitations can make use of these. We therefore place major emphasis on written handouts designed to develop stress-reducing reappraisals and self-instructions. As in other brief programs such as stress inoculation training (Meichenbaum, 1985), we find that effective cognitive coping skills can be acquired, rehearsed, and applied in life settings so as to enhance emotion regulation. Cognitive coping skills training is accomplished through didactic instruction and take-home reading materials (Handout A-2). Form A-2, Analyzing Thoughts and Feelings, can be used instead of the Stress and Coping Diary (Form A-1), and vice versa. Alternatively, both forms can be used.

Training Objectives

1. Review relaxation training compliance.
2. Introduce the ABCD cognitive model.
3. Discuss automatic thoughts that produce stress.
4. Discuss guidelines for challenging and replacing stress-producing thoughts using cognitive restructuring and self-instructional training.

Session Outline

- Review relaxation training progress; confront noncompliance
  - Relaxation exercise
- Mental control of emotions
  - The ABC model of emotion
  - Characteristics of automatic thoughts
- Irrational core beliefs
  - Application to the stress model
- Identifying stress-producing automatic thoughts

- Identifying stress-reducing thoughts
  - Reappraisal: Stress-busters
  - Self-instructional training: Performance-enhancing thoughts

Materials Needed

- Stress and CASMT models (Figures B-1 and B-2; hard copies, overheads, PowerPoints)
- Mental Control of Emotions and Stress (Handout A-3)
- Stress and Coping Diary (Form A-1, multiple copies)
- Analyzing Thoughts and Feelings (Form A-2)
- Challenging and Replacing Stress-Producing Thoughts: Where's the Evidence? (Form A-3)
- Anti-Stress Log: Stress-Reducing Statements (Form A-4)

Homework Assignments

- Continue to practice relaxation, now once a day, and practice breathing, pairing cue word with exhalation and general relaxation often during the day (Handout A-2).
- Read Mental Control of Emotions and Stress (Handout A-3).
- Complete Stress and Coping Diary (Form A-1) or Analyzing Thoughts and Feelings (Form A-2) on a daily basis.
- Work on evidence-based worksheet Challenging and Replacing Stress-Producing Thoughts (Form A-3).
- Begin developing Anti-Stress Log (Form A-4) with stress-reducing self-statements derived from cognitive restructuring and self-instructional training materials and the two forms: Analyzing Thoughts and Feelings, and Challenging and Replacing Stress-Producing Thoughts.

GROUP ADMINISTRATION

Review Relaxation Training Progress

Elicit feedback on how the relaxation training is going. If the computerized daily diary has been used, comment on any notable things you've seen in reviewing the diaries. Ask clients if they've detected any patterns that seem important in completing the diary. Ask the same question if they've done a printed version of it.

Gently and supportively confront those who haven't practiced the relaxation. Communicate your understanding that you're asking them to add to an already busy schedule where things can come up unexpectedly, but emphasize how critical it is not to fall behind in skill acquisition. They must find a time and a place to practice. It soon will take much less time *if* they practice, but they won't get there if they don't do the steps. Tell them that if their goal is to manage stress, it's important not to deprive themselves of getting everything they can from the program.

Troubleshoot for problems or reservations. Ask group members if they've found any helpful strategies to deal with potential blocks to doing the out-of-session relaxation training. Frame the situation as a problem-solving exercise in getting the critical homework activities done. Suggest creative times and places. For example, many participants have reported that a good strategy is to set their alarm 15 minutes earlier than usual and practice then. Another good time is when they return home after a busy day and prior to dinner. Other participants simply block out a specified time interval during the day.

Relaxation Exercise

Take 5 minutes to go through the relaxation routine with the group.

Full Tension

"As you tense the muscles of your buttocks, legs, and feet, pay special attention to the feelings of tension, the way the muscles contract, stretch and bunch like rubber bands; letting those muscles become tense and taut; the tension making the muscles feel a bit shaky; the muscles tightening like ropes; tension flowing into the muscles."

Halfway Tension Release

"Now, slowly let that tension out halfway. Notice the difference as the tension slowly decreases. Notice the difference between full and half tension, but be aware that there's still tension there in your buttocks, legs, and feet."

Complete Tension Release

"Now slowly let the tension out all the way, and notice the sensations at the different levels of tension you go through. . . . Now you can let the muscles relax completely. Just letting go; letting the tension flow away; the tension draining away as the muscles become limp and loose and relaxed; and each time you exhale, say the word *relax* to yourself and feel your body obey. Notice the difference between the relaxation you now feel and the tension that was there at the full and halfway points. Notice also how saying the word *relax* to yourself while exhaling helps deepen the relaxation."

Proceed through the other two groups of muscles in the same fashion, with full tension, halfway tension release, and complete tension release:

Hands, Arms, Shoulders, Chest, and Abs

"Make fists with both hands, bend your hands downward to tense your forearms, and tense your upper arms (biceps and triceps). Then, press your arms in against your body, tensing your shoulders and chest and crunching up your abdominal muscles."

Back, Neck, Jaw, and Face

"Push your shoulders back to tense your back muscles while thrusting your jaw outward, tensing your neck muscles, and scrunching your forehead and facial muscles."

"Now, let's do the yoga breathing exercise. Take a series of short inhalations into your chest, one per second. When you've filled your lungs, hold that for a bit and then very slowly release the air as you exhale and say a long, slow, *relaxxxx* to yourself, and let your body completely relax, as if you're sliding slowly down a hill. Then, inhale softly down into your stomach."

End this phase with this kind of message:

"If you've been practicing your relaxation exercise regularly, you should be pretty good at it by now. Continue practicing in the coming week. If you haven't been practicing, you really need to do so in the coming week because we're going to start using it to reduce arousal that I'm going to help you experience. If you have practiced, you may be ready for a shortened version of the exercise. In the shortened version, you tense all of the muscle groups at once, then slowly release the tension while thinking your cue word, such as *relax*, as you exhale. This shortened exercise only takes 10–15 seconds, so you can get lots of practices in each day. Remember to practice the exhalation, accompanied by the word *relax* (or whatever other word you've chosen). When you get good at this, you'll be surprised how effectively you can turn off physical stress reactions."

Mental Control of Emotions

"Last time, we talked about relaxation and how it can be used to control the physical aspects of stress. If you've been practicing the breathing relaxation skill, you may already be more aware of tension as it starts to develop, and, if you've applied the skill in some stressful situations, you may already be capable of tuning down arousal. Has anyone had any experiences like that? [Ask any positive responders to describe their experiences so that they become models for compliance and success.]

"Today, we're going to talk about other active ingredients of the stress response—specifically, the mental triggers for stress. As we'll see, where emotion is concerned, thoughts and feelings are intimately related to one another.

"Over the years, we have collected lots of accounts of stressful experiences. I'm going to read one of them from several years ago, and then we'll analyze it."

Read the following:

" 'My boss's secretary called me yesterday and told me the new manager they just hired to run our division wanted to see me. When I hung up, my first reaction was to get really nervous because I had a good idea of what was going to happen. The company has been downsizing, getting rid of senior people like me who have contributed to its success over the years, and my sales figures have been down because I lost a major client. After a while though, I began to also get really angry about this situation. In a few minutes, I got totally stressed out. My guts were churning, my heart was pounding, and my underarms were wet, all of which made the situation seem even worse.' "

We recommend having Figure B-1 (the stress process and its potential consequences) displayed in the room for repeated reference. With the stress model visible to the participants, ask them to put themselves into the same situation. First ask what it was about the situation that made it stressful (i.e., the specific demands). Ask which emotions were triggered. Then ask what kinds of appraisals the man might have made that would produce those emotions. Start with anxiety, then anger. Go through the four kinds of appraisal in the model in each instance. Where anxiety is concerned, the threat is the possibility of being let go, a sense that the man doesn't have the power to prevent it, the possibility that he thinks losing his job would be catastrophic and is likely to happen, and possible implications for his future and his view of himself as a person. For anger, the key cognitions involve a sense that he is being treated unfairly and that his past and present contributions to the company are not being acknowledged or appreciated. Try to elicit stress-producing self-statements. Push members to finally arrive at the distressing beliefs by continually asking them, "Yes, but *why* is that so upsetting?"; "Yes, but *why* should/shouldn't the company do that?"; "*What* would somebody have to say to themselves to react in that fashion?"

Relate the reported experience to the model, stressing the appraisal–emotion links. Reinforce participants for their insights. Then, give them the punch line for this episode: The man went to the manager's office filled with anxiety and outrage, only to find that the manager wanted him to take charge of an important new account because "I need someone with your knowledge and experience on this. I wouldn't trust anyone else with it." The man realized that he had created needless stress based on a misappraisal of the situation. He made assumptions without checking out the evidence. You can refer back to this vignette in the later discussion of catastrophizing based on jumping to conclusions.

The rest of the hour is didactic, related to Handout A-3, Mental Control of Emotions and Stress. Tell participants they do not have to take notes, as they will get a handout related to this session.

The ABC Model of Emotion

"How often have you said things like, 'That situation really stressed me out,' or 'He really made me mad when he said that'? Or 'I felt awful when she put me down'? It's very common to hear such statements, and to think them. We have a common tendency to view situations as the causes of our feelings.

Situation → Emotion

"But, as we have seen, that's not really the case. The reality is that events trigger *thoughts*, which in turn trigger the emotion. Even the amount of physical pain that people experience when injured depends on what they think about the sensations. Thoughts that interpret physical sensations as very hurtful and having dire implications increase subjective pain. We call these interpretive thoughts *appraisals*. Many of the most effective treatments for pain and for emotions such as anxiety, depression, anger, and guilt on are based on the proposition that emotions are typically preceded by thoughts, however fleeting and out of awareness they might be. These thoughts actually cause the feeling. This is known as the ABC model of emotion:

Situation (A) → Appraisal (Thought) (B) → Emotion (C)

"Thus, two different people can react very differently to the same situation. Why? It's because each appraises or interprets it differently. People can also change their feelings over time. For example, who among us has not looked back at a situation (as the executive mentioned earlier did) and said, 'I overreacted emotionally'? Who among us has not had a change of attitude about something or someone who seriously upset us in the past? In both cases, the original situation had not changed. What did change was *your view of it*, what we refer to as a *reappraisal*.

"The good news is that we can change emotion by changing how we think—that is, by changing our appraisals. The goal is not to get rid of all unpleasant emotions; that would be impossible. The goal is to reduce the frequency and intensity of needlessly distressing emotional reactions to situations.

"Let's talk more about the relationship between thoughts and feelings. A key idea is that you simply cannot experience anything without interpreting it, without deciding what it means. Look at this. [Hold a pen up.] How long did it take you to decide what this is? Did you carefully consider its appearance, texture, and dimensions and say, 'Let's see now . . . it's oblong and has a button at one end, a point at the other, and a clip. After careful reflection, I do believe that is a black pen'? Of course, not. Your recognition was instantaneous. Electrochemical impulses were instantly flashed from your eyes to your brain, there to be matched with a circuit of neurons representing a concept ('pen'), and this object matches that concept, so you immediately recognize it. You were totally unaware of this process as it occurred, which tells us some important things about how our minds work. Now, if I had held up some object you had never seen before, you would have been more aware of the interpretive process, which might have started with a thought such as 'What in the world is that?' followed by some pretty explicit (conscious) thinking about what it could be.

"Scientists who study mental processes have established that a great deal of our thinking occurs outside of our awareness. Behind the veil of awareness, our brain is engaged in an unending monologue that tells us the way things are. This monologue creates the psychological reality that we experience. Various theorists have referred to this internal monologue as 'self-talk' or 'automatic thoughts.' We like the term 'automatic thoughts' because that's how they are experienced. We also like the term 'self-talk' because we have the power to change the monologue in ways that benefit us and reduce stress.

"Over the past 60 years, research on emotion has revealed a lot about our automatic thoughts. One thing we have learned is that thoughts or images we rarely notice can trigger powerful emotions. We have also learned that certain specific "hot thoughts" lie behind each emotion. People differ in their hot thoughts as a result of past learning and life experiences. For example, anxiety is triggered by thoughts that tell us that an actual, possible, or future situation could harm us.

Anger-inducing thoughts have to do with others deliberately hurting us or treating us or others unjustly. Chronically depressed people are tyrannized by thoughts of irreplaceable loss, their own flaws, or a hopeless future."

Characteristics of Automatic Thoughts

"Let's take a look at what these automatic hot thoughts are like.

"First, they run instantaneously in a kind of mental shorthand. They are rarely complete sentences, although when we discover what they are, we can turn them into complete sentences. The thought can be expressed in a single word—*lonely, terrible, failure*—or as a fleeting visual image, a recollected smell, or a physical sensation. It may be a momentary flashing of a traumatic memory or a past humiliation. It likely is not even expressed in words but triggers a 'gut feeling.' Whatever form hot thoughts take, they are experienced as spontaneous and believable. They are rarely questioned because they seem compellingly true.

"Because they run in a mental shorthand largely out of awareness, our automatic thoughts tend to be persistent and to form chains of similar thoughts. What starts as a relatively neutral thought such as 'What is he doing?' may trigger increasingly more intense thoughts on the same theme—for example, 'He can't do that! This is unfair.' The person cycles from mild annoyance to full-blown rage. I think all of us have experienced that kind of emotional escalation.

"Because we are generally unaware of automatic thoughts, they may be very different from our conscious view of ourselves or our public statements. This discrepancy can create major differences between how people see themselves and how other people see them. For example, some people project an air of superiority and arrogance, whereas underneath, they may be terrified of failure or rejection. Research on automatic or 'implicit' attitudes finds that most people who believe that they are not prejudiced actually harbor subconscious negative attitudes toward certain groups of people. You can go to a website called 'Project Implicit' to take the test and see for yourself.

"Automatic thoughts are often extreme and out of proportion to the actual state of affairs. They turn up the volume, 'awfulizing' events and producing inappropriately strong emotional reactions. They help us prepare for the worst-case scenario, but extreme negative appraisals trigger emotions that are also extreme in intensity. They may predict dire consequences and tell us that we are powerless to deal with the situation. We can therefore react to a minor stressor as if it were a catastrophe, concluding that 'This is awful and I can't stand it.'"

Irrational Core Beliefs

"A great many automatic thoughts are surface manifestations of underlying core beliefs that we have internalized based on what our culture, parents, teachers, peers, and other important social influences have told us to be true. Basic beliefs can be extreme. According to Albert Ellis, a pioneer in cognitive therapy for emotional disorders, basic beliefs are full of 'shoulds,' 'oughts,' and 'musts.' When we, events, or other people do not act in accordance with these standards, we can respond with a full range of negative emotions, including anxiety, anger, fear, guilt or shame, self-loathing, sadness, and depression. In his usual colorful style, Ellis labeled such thinking 'musturbation.' He believed these extreme, absolute, widely held core beliefs underlie much needless emotional distress. Here are some examples of the core beliefs identified by Ellis. [Display the following list; see Table B-1.]

1. "To be a worthwhile person, it is essential that one be loved and approved of by virtually everyone.
2. "In order to be worthwhile, one must be perfectly adequate, achieving, and competent in all possible respects.
3. "Some people are bad, wicked, and villainous and therefore should be blamed and punished for their deeds.
4. "There are right and wrong solutions to every problem, and it will be catastrophic if the right one is not found.
5. "Unhappiness is caused by external and past circumstances, and we must accept that the individual has no control over it.
6. "Dangerous or fearful things are causes for great concern, and their possibility should be dwelt upon continually.
7. "One must have someone stronger upon whom to rely for support and guidance.

"You can think of automatic thoughts as whisperings in your brain from a little gremlin. Most people don't embrace all of them, at least in their extreme form, but most of us buy into at least some of them without realizing it.

"Now, let's take a look at Ellis's list of irrational beliefs and see if we can figure out which emotions they are likely to evoke."

Go over the list one at a time, inviting group members to identify the resulting emotion. A PowerPoint slide that allows you to present them sequentially works very well.

Plausible answers: (core belief 1) fear of disapproval, self-deprecation, social anxiety, easily hurt by criticism; (2) performance anxiety, fear of failure; (3) anger, outrage, hostility, punitiveness; (4) anxiety; (5) feelings of hopelessness and resignation to unhappiness; (6) needless worry about possible misfortunes and an exaggerated sense of their likelihood of occurrence; generalized anxiety; and (7) helpless dependence and fear of taking personal control and responsibility.

" 'Should-based' thinking has another negative effect. It leads to what is called polarized thinking, which is the tendency to think in black-and-white terms about what is right and wrong, worthwhile or not worthwhile. As we see in instances of political and religious dogmatism, things can be represented as either right or wrong, good or evil. This thinking is also seen in perfectionistic people, who tyrannize themselves trying to meet unattainable standards. If there are only two categories, there can be no middle ground. It's either perfect or totally defective. A person is either for or against you. You are either worthwhile or worthless, happy or miserable, totally successful or a failure, lovable or unlovable.

"Let's take this one step farther. One can make the case that almost all of these beliefs find expression in one master stress-producing self-statement. [Display this statement, if possible.]

> It's terrible, awful, and catastrophic when things (life, other people, the past, or me) are not (or are certain not to be) the way that I demand that they be, and I can't stand it when things are this way.

"Can you find any irrational elements in this statement that could cause a person distress?"

Most groups or individuals can isolate the irrational elements. Ask the participants what is irrational about each one. They should identify these elements:

> It's terrible, awful, and catastrophic . . . (catastrophizing)

"Most things are not catastrophes; they're inconvenient, threatening, annoying, or unpleasant. When we turn up the appraisal volume by awfulizing in this fashion, we also turn up the emotional intensity, which usually means overreacting.

"It is important to emphasize that the goal of what we're doing is *not* to deny or distort reality by means of 'positive thinking.' We're not about unrealistically turning negative thoughts into positive thoughts. Rational thinking is not the same thing as rationalizing. Some events are, in fact, objectively awful, such as the death of a loved one or a destructive tornado. The goal is to recognize that negative events and consequences fall along a range that extends from a bit negative to truly catastrophic. The tendency to overreact with appraisals like 'It's awful' and 'I can't stand it' results in an escalation of negative emotions. Putting events and consequences into perspective, based on the evidence, reduces needless distress.

. . . are not . . . the way that I demand that they be. . . .

"There's no reason the world must be as you would prefer that it to be. People have their own ideas of how things should be, and they have their own needs and interests. It's perfectly rational to prefer that events or people (including ourselves) be a certain way, and to take action to change things to our liking, but none of us is the center of the universe, and there's no reason for the world to bow to our demands. God is *not* a special agent of yours or mine. By turning preferences into dire necessities, people set themselves up for all of the emotions we've just discussed.

. . . (or are certain not to be) . . .

"Do we know for certain that the awfulized outcome is going to occur in the future?

. . . and I *can't stand* it . . .

"Actually, people can and do stand all manner of things, including true catastrophes. They suffer but endure. We may not like something, but we can definitely stand it. If we think we can't, we may find that something we could easily tolerate or even shrug off triggers an extreme emotional response that would not occur with a more realistic reappraisal."

Application to the Stress Model

"Now, let's apply this idea—'It's terrible, awful, and catastrophic when things (life, other people, the past, or me) are not the way that I demand that they be, and I can't stand it when things are this way'—to our model of stress. [Show the model.] Look at the appraisal part. Recall that it lists four different levels of appraisal that we can make: of the situational demands, of the resources we have to help us cope, of the consequences that could occur, and of the meaning of those consequences for our personal identity. Catastrophizing can occur at any of those levels, and may occur in all of them.

"Let's take as an example a young man whose girlfriend just ended their relationship. First, he could catastrophize about the situation's demands: 'This is horrendous, awful, terrible, and I can't stand it.' Next, he could catastrophize about his resources: 'I'm helpless. I can't deal with this.' He could also catastrophize about the consequences, both in terms of how awful the consequence is and how likely it is to occur: 'I'll never, ever, *ever* find another woman who could love me. I'll be miserable and alone forever.' And, finally, catastrophic appraisals can occur at the level of personal meaning: 'This proves that I'm a worthless person—revolting and totally unlovable.' Any of these appraisals, alone or in combination, are capable of triggering negative emotional responses."

Identifying Stress-Producing Automatic Thoughts

"Automatic thoughts are, by definition, largely out of our awareness. That being said, we should not conclude that they are beyond our reach. The good news is that we can, with some effort and guidance, tune in to the gremlin and become aware of our automatic thoughts. That is the first step in eventually replacing them with alternative appraisals that we refer to as "stress busters." And that is exactly what you are going to be doing. When you have a better idea of the kinds of hot thoughts involved in your experience of stress, anger, and other negative emotions, you will be ready to go to work on them.

"One way to gain access to the automatic thoughts is to stop whenever you find yourself getting upset and ask yourself what you are saying to yourself that is causing the distress. Another way is to recall a past stressful event of importance, especially one to which you now think you overreacted; try to recreate the thoughts that must have occurred in order for you to experience the emotional upset. In the weeks to come, you'll be doing some journaling about the stressful events you experience and your reactions to them that will assist you in identifying your particular hot thoughts.

"When you do this, you will find that in most instances the hot thoughts take forms such as 'Isn't it *awful* that . . . ?' or 'Wouldn't it be *terrible* if . . . ?' or 'What an (awful) (lousy) (rotten) thing for (me) (him) (her) (them) to do.' In most cases you are either telling yourself that it is awful that things are not the way you are demanding they be, or you are condemning yourself or someone else because your demands are not being met.

"We use the term 'catastrophizing' to describe the kind of thinking that leads to needless stress and emotional disturbance. Relatively minor frustrations, inconveniences, and concerns are mentally blown up so that they become, for the moment, catastrophes that you emotionally react to. Much of our distress-producing thinking sounds like some or all of these protestations: 'I don't like this situation! This is terrible! I can't stand it! It's driving me crazy! It shouldn't be this way! It's simply got to change or I can't possibly be happy!' By systematically tuning in to our own internal statements about troublesome situations, we will find that we can pretty quickly pin down the thoughts that are producing our distress. We can then stop and ask ourselves, 'How is it terrible that . . . ?' or 'Why would it actually be awful if . . . ?' or 'Who am I to demand that things be exactly the way I'd like them to be?' In other words, we can dispute the catastrophic thought. We can then add a *D* (for *dispute*) to the ABC model of emotion we talked about earlier. When we dispute hot thoughts, we often find that we quickly get over being upset because we can see the irrational aspects of what we are telling ourselves. You will probably find the following links between your thoughts and your emotions:

"*Anxiety* often involves a tendency to catastrophize—a sense of some awful impending doom, like the executive who thought he was about to be fired. The dreaded result is often left vague, unspecified. 'What if *X* happened?' is left unanswered, but still considered terrible. Added to this is a sense that the awful event is bound to occur.

"*Anger. Shoulds* are usually at the root of anger; I expect that people or the world should be the way I want them to be; the world should be fair. *Demands* are made on people and life. People (including yourself) are *condemned* for not being the way they 'should' be. *Catastrophizing* is also involved in that it seems terrible or awfully important. Thoughts of injustice triggered the executive's anger.

"*Depression.* Again, *catastrophizing* is involved in that it seems awful that things aren't going the way I want them to go; events are seen as *hopeless. Shoulds* are often turned against the self: 'I should be successful all the time, and if I am not, I am worthless.' *Self-condemnation* may occur.

"Any questions or comments?

"As we have seen, catastrophizing can cause us needless stress, and it is probably the most frequent cause of emotional overreaction. However, several other illogical thinking patterns, often found in automatic hot thoughts, can cause us to make distorted appraisals of ourselves, situations, and other people. They often feed into catastrophizing as well. You'll find examples in today's handout. It's good to look out for these five tendencies in ourselves.

1. *"Polarized (black–white) thinking* is the tendency to think of people or events in terms of two extreme categories, such as good or bad, for me or against me, moral or immoral, wonderful or horrible, success or failure, worthwhile or worthless, strong or weak. It's easy to see how this kind of thinking would lead to extreme appraisals, and it is particularly problematic when applied to how you judge yourself.
2. *"Overgeneralization* is the tendency to draw sweeping conclusions based on a single experience or one piece of evidence. A single failure or rejection may lead to the conclusion that a person is incompetent or unlovable. One sign of overgeneralization occurs in the use of words such as *always, everybody, never, none, total jerk,* and *nobody.*
3. *"Mind reading* occurs when you assume you know how others are feeling, what they are thinking, or why they did something. It often is sometimes based on a mental process called 'projection,' whereby we project our own characteristics onto others and assume they think and feel as we do. Thus, a person with a negative self-image might assume, 'She thinks I'm unattractive' when that is not the case.
4. *"Selective perception* occurs when we latch onto information consistent with our beliefs and filter out or discount nonsupportive information. This can cause us to miss the big picture as we focus only on the negative while ignoring positive aspects of the situation.
5. *"Personalization* is the tendency to relate everything to oneself by comparing oneself endlessly with others or viewing their behaviors as somehow directed at oneself. Social comparison may result in unfavorable self-comparisons or 'taking things personally' that are not directed at oneself."

Identifying Stress-Reducing Thoughts

"Now we're ready to talk about two kinds of replacement self-talk that people have found helpful in dealing with stressful situations. One kind is designed to help you reappraise and reinterpret situations in more rational ways and replace the hot thoughts that create stress responses. We call these reappraisals *stress-busters.*

"The second kind of self-talk is an instruction to yourself that guides your behavior. These are performance-enhancing thoughts. Intense emotion can often have a disruptive effect on how well we function. We can become so upset or angry that it is hard to function effectively. For example, we've worked with students who become so anxious and pre-occupied with negative thoughts during tests that they can't concentrate on the questions and so cannot answer them correctly, even though they know the material. We can become so bound up in self-defeating thoughts about how terrible a situation is that we cannot devote our full attention to what we should be doing to cope with the situation. The technique called 'self-instructional training' can help in this situation."

Reappraisals: Stress-Busters

"Let's talk about stress-busters first. A key to mentally coping with stress is to become aware of the automatic thoughts that generate distress. Whenever you feel yourself becoming upset, the first thing you should tell yourself is: '*I* am creating this feeling by the way I'm thinking. How can I stop myself from being upset?' This statement, or one like it, will not only place things in proper perspective, but will also cause you to focus on your own stress-producing thoughts and on how you can substitute stress-reducing thoughts.

"As you go through the program, you will identify your particular hot thoughts and generate a set of alternative reappraisals or self-statements that you can use to counter the stress-producers. Starting next session, I'll also help you practice using these stress-busters in conjunction with your relaxation techniques to reduce emotional arousal. As you begin to apply your stress-busters out in the real world, you'll be rewarded with a reduction in stress. Because rewarding consequences strengthen behaviors that lead to them, the strength of the stress-busters will increase. You'll soon find that the new appraisals start to replace the old hot ones and become the newly dominant automatic thoughts that make you more stress-resilient. Combined with continued mastery of your relaxation skill, you will have increased ability to regulate your emotions and added a powerful weapon against stress in your life.

"Let's consider some examples of stress-buster statements that have proven useful to previous participants in this program. You'll find these in the handout I'll give you today. I want to emphasize again that each of you is a unique individual and will need to develop self-statements that work best for you. But these, along with the handout, should give you some useful leads. [Present these exemplars to the clients, either in hard copy or PowerPoint.]

1. "'I don't like this situation, but I can definitely stand it. No sense getting strung out.'
2. "'No sense blowing it out of proportion; it's not that big a thing.'

3. "'Unfortunately, people don't always behave like I want them to. That's the way it goes—no use getting upset.'
4. "'Other people's needs are as important to them as mine are to me.'
5. "'I don't have to be perfect. I can make mistakes, too. I don't have to please everyone.'
6. "'Okay, so I don't like this. It's not the end of the world.'
7. "'Don't catastrophize now. Put this in perspective.'
8. "'It would be nice if everything always went perfectly, but that's not the way life is.'
9. "'If I catastrophize about *this*, I'm bound to be upset.'
10. "'If I can change this situation, I should do so. Thinking about what I can do to handle this situation is better than getting upset. I may not like it, but I can definitely stand it.'
11. "'Keep cool. It's not that big a thing. Relax.'
12. "'Life is too short to let things like this make me miserable.'

"These examples should help you develop your own set of self-statements for coping with difficult situations. You will find that you can almost always short-circuit unpleasant emotions by placing things in a noncatastrophizing perspective.

"As you'll see when you read the handout on the mental control of stress, there are two ways to challenge stress-producing automatic thoughts. One way is to examine them logically and decide whether they are valid. Many of the stress-busters I just shared with you do that. The other way is to examine the evidence for and against your stress-producing automatic thoughts based on your own experience. For example, a person who thinks 'I'm a total failure' can challenge the thought by considering whether it is indeed the case that he or she has never succeeded at anything."

Self-Instructional Training: Performance-Enhancing Thoughts

"Unlike the stress-busters, self-instruction is not a way of attacking or replacing irrational beliefs. Instead, it can guide you through the encounter, reduce stress, and keep your attention on the task at hand. Intense emotions can disrupt performance because we become so bound up in self-defeating thoughts that we cannot devote our full attention to what we should be doing in order to cope. Psychologist Donald Meichenbaum (1985) developed a technique called 'self-instructional training' to help people talk more adaptively to themselves before, during, and after stressful situations. Here are some self-instructional self-statements that people have used to help them reduce stress and keep their minds on the task at hand:

Preparing for a Stressful Event

- " 'You can develop a plan to deal with this.'
- " 'Run through your mind and visualize how you want to respond.'
- " 'Concentrate on keeping your cool. You can handle this.'

Confronting the Stressful Event

- " 'Don't think about being upset, just focus on what you have to do.'
- " 'Don't get all bent out of shape; just do what has to be done.'
- " 'Relax and slow things down. You're in control. Take a deep breath.'
- " 'This upset is a cue for you to use your coping skills. Relax and think rationally.'
- " 'Don't try to eliminate stress. Just keep it manageable and focus on the present.'

"Behaviors that lead to positive outcomes become stronger and more efficient. When saying adaptive things to yourself helps you control your stress, the new thoughts are rewarded and strengthened. Use these statements in conjunction with your relaxation coping response. Together, they give you powerful weapons against negative emotions. You can help the strengthening process by internally rewarding yourself immediately after you use them effectively. Here are some examples of rewarding self-talks:

Following the Stressful Event

- " 'Way to go! You're in control.'
- " 'Good—you're handling the stress.
- " 'Beautiful—you did it!'
- " 'How can you handle it better next time? You can do an instant visualization replay.'

"Coping competently with life's stresses increases self-confidence and resiliency. By developing your coping abilities, you can gain increasing control over your emotional life.

"You'll find a more detailed discussion and more examples of self-guiding thoughts in the handout."

Homework Assignments

1. "Continue to practice the three-muscle-group relaxation technique once a day, and practice breathing during the day, pairing your cue word with exhalation. Also practice full body tension and relaxation as often as possible during the day. Again, don't forget to use your cue word with exhalation (Handout A-2). I'm giving you two additional assignments to help you develop your mental coping skills.

2. "One assignment is to read and use Handout A-3, Mental Control of Emotions and Stress. The handout contains much of what we talked about today, plus sets of stress-buster and performance-enhancing statements that you can use either as is or as a basis for making up your own. Our goal is for you to have a set of stress-reducing statements that you can use in situations that create stress in your life.

3. "That is where the second assignment comes in. I'm giving you a set of Stress and Coping Diary forms, Form A-1 [and/or Form A-2, Analyzing Thoughts and Feelings]. The forms ask you to describe a stressful situation and your emotional response to it; for example, feeling overburdened, anxious, or angry. You are also asked to identify the automatic hot thought that likely triggered the emotional response. Finally, at Step D (which stands for *dispute*), you're asked to think of what you could have said to yourself instead that would have countered the hot thought and reduced your emotional response. This could be a stress-buster or a self-instruction or perhaps one of each. [For clients using the Stress and Coping Diary:] You'll find the exercise on Item 8 of the diary. I'm also giving you a worksheet (Form A-3) that you can use to evaluate the evidence for and against your stress-producing hot thoughts. This exercise can help you formulate alternative thoughts that are more balanced.

"This exercise accomplishes two important things. First, it helps you analyze the connections between situations, your thoughts, and your emotions and it helps you identify the automatic thoughts that are hot ones for you. Doing this over time will also help you identify your 'hot-button' vulnerabilities that make certain situations particularly challenging. These could be issues involving fear of failure or disapproval, issues with trust or self-worth, feelings of being mistreated or attacked, worries about disapproval, and so forth.

"The second function of this exercise is to help you develop a set of rational thoughts that you can use to reappraise situations and reduce their capacity to produce stress responses. Hopefully, these will include some 'all-purpose' ones as well as some that help you handle recurring stressors of the same kind. We're going to use Step D from the exercise in Form A-2 to identify and refine the ones that are most likely to be useful for you as an individual. [Note: If you are using the Stress and Coping Diary instead of Form A-2, ask clients to focus on Items 7A and 7B, plus the hot buttons, Item 4.] I'd like you to fill out a copy of Form A-2 each day, choosing the most stressful event you've experienced. If none has occurred, choose a recent past event that was significant for you. Situations that push your buttons can be especially valuable. Put as much care and effort as you can into analyzing the thoughts involved. I want you to bring some usable ones with you for our next session. Use this Anti-Stress Log (Form A-4) to transfer the stress-producing and corresponding stress-reducing thoughts that you discover in these exercises. As this log is developed, it will help you identify your most critical hot thoughts and develop effective stress-reducing thoughts to counter and eventually replace them.

"Again, I'm reminding you that these are critical weeks for building your coping skills, so please make sure to apply yourself to the out-of-session assignments."

Distribute copies of Handout A-3 and Forms A-2, A-3, and A-4.

INDIVIDUAL ADMINISTRATION

Session 2 covers the same content as the group session. The difference, of course, is that you have the advantage of working with only one person and are able to personalize the steps of the session in a manner not possible in the group administration. You can also more closely monitor the client's progress and compliance with homework assignments—another important consideration.

Review Relaxation Training Progress

With individual clients, we begin by asking each client about the out-of-session relaxation training exercises, assessing his or her degree of compliance, and eliciting the client's experience and degree of satisfaction with the procedure. We ask the client to evaluate how useful the skill will be and explore any problems or issues that arise. The following discussion occurred with Harlan, the socially anxious client described in Chapter 4.

THERAPIST: I want to review your experiences doing the relaxation exercises. Think of a tension thermometer that goes from 0, totally relaxed, to 100, as tensed up as you could possibly get. How much tension did you experience when you tensed up, when you let the tension out halfway, and when you released it completely?

CLIENT: I'd say about 80 to start with, then 40 at the halfway point, and by the end of the week, I was down to probably 10—pretty deeply relaxed. The first time I did it, maybe 20 or 25.

THERAPIST: Great. As you were releasing the tension, were you able to detect different levels or degrees of tension?

CLIENT: Definitely, and more so as I practiced over time.

THERAPIST: Did you combine your cue word with the exhalation and tension release?

CLIENT: Yes, but I changed my cue word from *relax* to *calm* after about 3 days because it worked even better.

THERAPIST: Again, great. I want you to feel free to adapt everything we do to what works best for you. Did you imagine the wave of relaxation flowing through your muscles? If so, tell me what your wave is like.

CLIENT: Yes, I did, and that works, too. My wave is warm and light blue.

THERAPIST: How often did you practice your relaxation skill?

CLIENT: My Post-it reminders helped me, but I did miss a few practices. Once, I started after dinner and fell asleep. Another time, I was out late with friends and felt sedated by a few beers, so I went to bed. But I did practice the breathing paired with *calm* lots of times during the day, and it really helps at work when I start to get frazzled because of time pressures.

THERAPIST: One of the reasons we use the relaxation training is to help people increase their body awareness. Did you discover any places in your body where tension seems to pool?

CLIENT: I never realized how much tension I carry in my shoulders and neck.

THERAPIST: Fine. If that's a tension site for you, you can do some focused practice involving only those muscles. Find a muscular movement that allows you to tense the muscles, then concentrate on relaxing them with the cue word. Any concerns or issues about the relaxation?

CLIENT: No. I think this is going to work well for me.

THERAPIST: Have you applied it in any life situations?

CLIENT: Yes, the other day. Chelsea came over and I thought she might ask me about going out with her cousin. I started to tense up, then exhaled, relaxed, and used my cue word and had an immediate drop in tension. But it turned out to be a false alarm. She didn't mention her cousin. But it was neat to see I could actually use the relaxation and it worked.

THERAPIST: I'm very pleased with your progress, and I appreciate your conscientiousness and dedication to learning this skill. I think you're ready to go to an abbreviated exercise where you simply do a moderate generalized body tension that includes all of the muscle groups at once, then release the tension and do the cue-enhanced relaxation with exhalation. This one only takes 10–15 seconds, so you can get lots of practices in each day. Because the tension phase might look a little weird if done in public, I recommend that you do it when others are not observing.

Remember to practice the exhalation, accompanied by the word *calm* (or whatever other word the client has chosen), and the muscle relaxation in your daily life whenever you think of it. It takes a few seconds and you can have many practice trials during the day without going through the entire tension sequence. When you get good at this, you'll be surprised how effectively you can turn off physical stress reactions.

Noncompliance with Homework Assignments

If the client has not complied with the relaxation training assignment, you should thoroughly explore the reasons why that occurred. Is it a question of forgetfulness, poor time management, or a lack of credibility regarding the usefulness of relaxation? Questions like the following can elicit the information:

- "I'm wondering, what got in the way of your relaxation practice?"
- "You said you kept forgetting. I wonder, what could we do to set up reminders?"
- "I realize that you're so stretched already with your various responsibilities that it's one reason you're here. Having experienced how hard it is to find time for one more thing, can you think of a way to block in the 5–10 minutes it takes to do the exercise?"
- "I'm wondering if the rationale I gave you last week for the relaxation training made sense. Did some other strategy that we discussed, such as working on stress-producing thoughts, make more sense?"
- "Do you think that if you learn the relaxation, it would be helpful to you? People don't like to spend time on something they don't believe in. Or, they may feel that they tried something similar in the past and it didn't work for them. Because this is an important

part of the training program, I want to be sure you're on board with it. What do you think?"

Noncompliance at this stage is not a good sign, for it means that the client is already behind schedule if you are working within a time-limited format. It is important to explore the client's attitudes and expectations toward each training component. If the client holds a negative attitude or is dubious about any element of the program, the entire program may be compromised. A pattern of resistance and noncompliance will almost guarantee an unsuccessful outcome. It may be that the client wants some other approach to treatment, or believes that the origins of the stress-related problem resides in childhood or unconscious experiences that need to be worked through. An approach like this may seem superficial and representative of pop psychology. In such instances, a different treatment approach may be warranted. For example:

THERAPIST: I'm wondering if this program is what you hoped for or expected when you came to see me. People have expectations about the kind of approach that might best fit their needs. If that's the case and this program is not your cup of tea, we should certainly discuss it, for there's no sense spending our time and your money on something that does not live up to your hopes and expectations. Can we talk about that possibility?

CLIENT: I almost didn't come back today because I felt so guilty about not doing my relaxation exercises. I've tried to relax in the past, and it wasn't helpful in reducing my anxiety. I should have told you that last week. And when I came to see you, I actually did expect that we would be talking about the roots of my problem so I could get rid of it. I was in therapy like that about 5 years ago and we talked a lot about how my parents made me feel like a loser, but I had to stop because I moved here for a different job.

THERAPIST: Did that therapy help your anxiety?

CLIENT: Not really, but I understood more about myself. I think it would have helped if I could have gone for more than the 6 months I was in treatment.

THERAPIST: Tell me about your use of relaxation. How did you learn it?

CLIENT: I read in a magazine that deep breathing relaxes the body, so I tried it.

THERAPIST: How did it compare with the level of relaxation you experienced last week when we went through the exercise?

CLIENT: I got pretty relaxed by the end, but I'm not sure I could do that without your instructions.

THERAPIST: It could be that it didn't work because you didn't have enough training to master the skill. I don't think deep breathing alone would work, either. But I am confident that with practice, you could relax yourself to a level you experienced when I did it with you, or even beyond, and in a lot less time—perhaps one or two breaths. Now obviously I'm not going to force something on you that you don't want to do, but I really do believe that this could be useful to you if you give it a legitimate try. It's a core skill in this program. How about trying it on a daily basis for the coming week, following the instructions closely? I think you'll find that the level of relaxation you can attain to be much deeper than you get with deep breathing. If by next week you don't think you can quickly relax more deeply, then we can junk it. Does that sound reasonable? This program has helped so many people that I'd like you to give the relaxation and the mental skills we're going to talk about today a chance. They won't hurt you in any way, although they will require some time and effort on your part, but they might be helpful to you. If you decide that's not the case, I'll be happy to refer you to someone who does the kind of therapy you want, or we can move more in that direction. Does that sound reasonable?

Encouraging Problem Solving to Enhance Compliance

If a noncompliant client expresses confidence in the potential usefulness of the program and expresses no reservations about the components and their potential value, other factors may be at work. Perhaps the client is expecting something to be "done to" him or her and has not accepted personal responsibility for change, or perhaps is not yet committed to it.

"You tell me that you have a lot of stress in your life that you want to deal with more effectively. You indicate that the rationale for the program and the methods that we plan to use make sense and could be useful. You also found yourself able to get very relaxed when I did the relaxation exercise with you last week. And yet it's been a struggle for you to clear out space and time to do the practice needed to master one of the truly useful stress reduction skills. So there seem to be some barriers that we need to figure out and problem-solve, because the program can't work for you unless you are able to find a way to devote yourself to learning the coping skills. Both of us want you to profit from this training program, so we should work together to find a solution to this problem. I wonder if you have any thoughts about how we can make sure that you get the benefits of the program. For example, are there any times during the day when there are blocks of time that are completely in your control?"

Although, if needed, you can make suggestions couched in terms of what previous clients have found useful in overcoming this barrier, it's even better if the client comes up with a plan on his or her own. The client can then take personal credit for its success, thereby reinforcing a sense of personal resourcefulness. Be sure to positively reinforce such efforts.

CLIENT: I have an hour lunch break that I usually spend in my office. That's a time I could use to set 15 minutes aside to practice the relaxation. I could also do it before I go to bed. I just need to get this booked into my daily schedule. I know it would help me to learn this.

THERAPIST: I'm really pleased that you've come up with a training assignment plan that you think will work, for I'm going to give you some additional things to do for next week that involve the mental side of the coping equation. It's really important that you have some usable relaxation and mental coping skills by next week so we can move to the next phase, where you actually practice them to reduce stress. You didn't mention this as a possibility, but we could draw up a formal contract, signed by both of us, that specifies that you agree to do the training activities in the coming week. Contracts of this type are often useful in solidifying a commitment to change a behavior. What do you think?

CLIENT: Yeah, that might actually help, because I try to be a man of my word.

Relaxation Exercise

"Before we go on, I'd like to take you through a quick relaxation exercise like the one we did last week."

Take 5 minutes to go through the three-group-muscle relaxation routine with the client again. Observe the client and elicit feedback on how relaxed the client got this time through the procedure. Explore any relaxation issues, such as difficulties in relaxing certain muscle groups. If that occurs, instruct the client to focus special attention on those muscles during the out-of-session relaxation practice.

Mental Control of Emotions

With an individual client, you cover the same points as in the group administration but in a more interactive manner that is related to the client's own experiences. If the client has been completing the Stress and Coping Diary during the previous week, you will have the opportunity to review the entries and gain some advance knowledge of his or her stressors, emotional reactions, and coping strategies, as well as some indication of the client's ability to identify stress-evoking appraisals. Take a few minutes to go over the entries with the client. In the following instance, the therapist uses Harlan's Stress and Coping Diary responses to make the point that stress involves thoughts and physical responses.

THERAPIST: I can see by your diary entries that this has been a pretty stressful week for you. It seems that at least three things happened that triggered a lot of anxiety. Which one would you most like to talk about?

CLIENT: Last Wednesday's was the worst one. The company brought in a productivity expert and arranged individual interviews with her for all of the assistant managers, including me. When I got the e-mail announcement for my appointment, I really got uptight.

THERAPIST: Tell me about your uptightness.

CLIENT: The usual. My heart started to pound, my underarms got sweaty, and I got all tense. I had trouble concentrating on my work and was really worried.

THERAPIST: A pretty strong emotional reaction of anxiety. Let's take a look at Item 7, where you listed the following thoughts on your diary form: "She will have looked at my sales figures and will think I'm incompetent." "She'll see how nervous I am and think I'm hiding something, which will be mortifying." "She'll think I'm incompetent and recommend that I be demoted or fired, and I couldn't stand if that happened." Do you think those thoughts had anything to do with how anxious you got?

CLIENT: Who wouldn't get anxious under those circumstances?

THERAPIST: How soon were you aware of these thoughts?

CLIENT: I had the immediate physical reaction. The thoughts popped into my head at about the same time, and I kind of pinned them down for sure when I did the diary entry afterward.

THERAPIST: Okay. We've established in this entry, as in most of your other ones, that your thoughts about others evaluating you negatively are a big trigger for your stress responses—which brings us to the topic

I want to discuss today, namely the mind–body connection in stress. Then we'll look at this a bit more closely from the perspective of helping you reduce your anxiety.

The ABC Model of Emotions

Present the ABC model of emotions, relating it to the client's situation and reaction whenever possible. Questions like the following can help personalize the process, as in this discussion with Harlan.

THERAPIST: One thing you mentioned was that your anxiety occurred instantaneously, and then you became aware of the thoughts. This is very characteristic of why we call these *automatic* thoughts. Let's talk about these automatic thoughts and how they apply to your anxiety. Can you think of other times when a situation seemed to trigger a feeling instantaneously, before you could even think about it?

CLIENT: Lots of times when I'm put on the spot.

THERAPIST: We usually think of situations as directly triggering our emotions. Almost always, however, the situation triggers thoughts and *thoughts* trigger the emotion. For example, have you ever overreacted to a situation, then feel differently when you rethought the situation or understood it better? How about the interview situation?

CLIENT: Well, yeah—when I looked back at it, I realized that I blew things out of proportion when I thought I was going to fall apart in the interview and lose my job. It was true that I would probably have looked nervous during the interview, but as it turned out, I used my relaxation skill when the anxiety hit, and it calmed me down somewhat and the interview went okay. I didn't go in frazzled. I think it went pretty well.

THERAPIST: Good. I'm glad you thought to use your relaxation to calm down your anxiety. The more often you apply your relaxation skills in such situations, the better they will get. This example also shows how rethinking the situation influences how you feel. We all have "hot-button" situations to which we're especially emotionally responsive. Do you have a sense of what yours might be?

CLIENT: No question, feeling on the spot and being judged by other people makes me feel inadequate.

THERAPIST: So, it looks like we can link these hot-button situations to certain hot thoughts that run automatically and trigger your stress response.

CLIENT: I've noticed that when I do the daily diary, social situations where

I feel on the spot, where I don't want to be disapproved of by others, always seem to trigger these exaggerated thoughts.

THERAPIST: That's a great insight. Does this thought pattern seem to be one that you'd like to work on so that you can counter or replace it?

CLIENT: If I could do just that and actually believe the new thoughts, I think it would be great.

THERAPIST: Well, let's proceed in that direction. At this point, I want to summarize some key ideas in the training materials we'll be using for that purpose. I'm going to show them to you as we proceed, so that I can point out some pertinent sections. I'll want you to take them home, read them carefully, apply them to yourself, and begin to develop some alternate thoughts that would reduce your stress.

Have Handout A-3; Forms A-2, A-3, and A-4; Table B-1; and Figures B-1 and B-2 available to point out relevant sections and exercises. Do not give them to the client at this point because he or she is likely to start reading them.

Characteristics of Automatic Thoughts

THERAPIST: The first key idea relates to the nature of automatic thoughts. We've been talking about how easy it is to overreact emotionally to situations. We've also looked at some thoughts that tend to trigger your emotion and stress. We therapists use the term "catastrophizing" to describe the kind of thinking that leads to needless stress and emotional disturbance. Relatively minor frustrations, inconveniences, and concerns are mentally blown up so that they become, for the moment, catastrophes to which we emotionally react.

Now, let's apply this idea to our model of stress (showing the model in Figure B-1) and to how you thought about the upcoming interview with the productivity expert. In particular, let's look at the appraisal portion of the model. Note that it lists four different levels of appraisals that we can make: of the situational demands, of coping resources, of the consequences that could occur, and of the meaning of those consequences for our personal identity. Stress-producing appraisals can occur at any of those levels and may occur in all of them. In your interview situation, did you do any catastrophizing? How about demands?

CLIENT: I guess I saw it as a lot more threatening than it was. I kind of pictured a severe woman doing a third-degree on me about my performance. It turned out that she was friendly and pleasant and never mentioned any inadequacy in my performance. She was more interested in my ideas for increasing productivity.

THERAPIST: So in your mind you constructed a really threatening situation that turned out not to be the case. How about your own coping resources? Any catastrophizing there?

CLIENT: I was really worried that I couldn't keep composed and that I'd blow it. I could see myself looking so nervous that I would make a bad impression.

THERAPIST: And what about the consequences of not being able to perform?

CLIENT: I could see how I could make a terrible impression, look totally incompetent, and get demoted or even lose my job. I'd probably never be able to get a job this good.

THERAPIST: So you saw some pretty negative consequences. On a scale from zero, "of no concern" to 100, "the worst thing I could ever experience," where did those consequences fall?

CLIENT: In my mind at the time, probably at about 70.

THERAPIST: And in your mind, how likely were these terrible consequences to occur on a scale of zero percent to 100%.

CLIENT: I'd say about 80%.

THERAPIST: So in your mind at the time, you created consequences that were very bad and highly likely to occur. No wonder you got so anxious. Suppose you were saying those things to yourself right now. Let's try a little experiment. Could you think of some realistic things you could say instead?

CLIENT: (*pause*) Well, I guess I could say that I've never actually fallen apart in the way I imagined I might. I know my job and can explain it, and I actually do it at an okay level.

THERAPIST: And what about all the awful things that you imagined might happen? What's the evidence that they would actually occur?

CLIENT: Maybe the thought that she'd recommend that they fire me was less likely than I thought at the time. My boss hasn't criticized me for anything.

THERAPIST: Now, let's assume that you had said these current things to yourself when you got that appointment e-mail. First, you reported a score of 90 out of 100 for the terrible consequences you thought about. Would that score change?

CLIENT: Yeah, it would go down, maybe to 40 or so.

THERAPIST: Okay, that's a lot less severe. Now what about the score of 80% likelihood that these consequences would occur?

CLIENT: Maybe down to 25 or 30%.

THERAPIST: If those ideas are realistic and had passed through your head at the time, how would your anxiety have been affected?

CLIENT: It would have been much lower.

THERAPIST: I would think so, too. If we accept the notion that the intensity of an emotional response is linked directly to the intensity of the appraisal, then we see here an example of how catastrophizing—blowing things out of proportion—can create excessive stress. In reality, it was entirely reasonable for you or anyone else to get a bit concerned if they got an e-mail that suggested that an expert was going to evaluate them, but your automatic thoughts turned it into a far more threatening situation. So if you can learn to ferret out such thoughts and change some of your unrealistic appraisals, you can develop some mental coping skills. These skills parallel the physical skill you're learning in your breathing and relaxation training. The goal is for you to develop a set of explicit stress-reducing thoughts—stress-busters—that you can use when you get into evaluative situations and thereby reduce your anxiety. I'm going to get you started in this process by giving you some reading materials on the mental control of emotions and stress. But let's take a moment to preview one element of what you'll be reading.

Irrational Core Beliefs

Go over Table B-1, Some Core Beliefs That Cause Problems, with the client.

"Here's a list by psychologist Albert Ellis of widely held and usually unquestioned beliefs that can cause needless disturbance. We typically learn them from significant people in our past, such as parents and friends, and from our culture in general. Many of the automatic thoughts that flash through our heads in hot-button situations can be traced back to these beliefs. Let's take a look at each one and see if we can figure out which distressing emotions each one might trigger."

Guide the client through each irrational belief with leading questions if necessary. Finish by saying something like the following: "You've got some real good insights about how people can be indoctrinated into beliefs that create particular 'hot buttons,' or types of situations to which they are particularly vulnerable."

THERAPIST: As you learn more about your hot thoughts, you may find one or more of these core beliefs lurking in the background. But even now, looking at this list, do you see any of them that we should keep an eye out for?

CLIENT: They all look irrational to me. I don't think I believe any of them.

THERAPIST: You're right about that. They are quite extreme. And people can have basic beliefs that are less absolute than this version but that still produce automatic thoughts that are troublesome. Now, as I understand your hot-button issues, they involve concerns about other people's impressions of you, so that you experience social anxiety and tend to avoid evaluative situations. Am I understanding correctly?

CLIENT: That's true.

THERAPIST: So which of these would best fit that pattern?

CLIENT: This one is probably the closest. (*Points to "To be a worthwhile person, it is essential that one be loved and approved of by virtually everyone."*)

THERAPIST: Good analysis, Harlan. That would fit well with your earlier statement that feeling on the spot and being judged negatively by other people make you feel inadequate. Usually, what goes along with that is the second idea here: "In order to be worthwhile, one must be perfectly adequate, achieving, and competent in all possible respects." For many people with concerns about approval and disapproval, performing well is a must, whether that means socially or in any other area where people can get evaluated. What do you think?

CLIENT: The ideas seem so extreme, but I can see that if someone believes them, they could have the kind of anxiety I have.

THERAPIST: For now, let's just consider this as an initial hypothesis that we can follow up on. I introduce it now because I want to give you a bit of a head start for analyzing your automatic thoughts and coming up with some countering stress-reducing thoughts. But before we end, I'd like to share a master idea that underlies catastrophizing. Ellis suggested that almost all of these beliefs find expression in one master stress-producing statement that you'll read about in today's handout: "It's terrible, awful, and catastrophic when things (life, other people, the past, or me) are not (or are certain not to be) the way that I demand that they be, and I can't stand it when things are this way." I'd like you to really think hard about this statement or master core belief and how it might underlie your social anxiety. What do you demand of yourself in order to be worthwhile? To what kinds of situations do you respond with "awful" appraisals? And do you ever react as if it's so awful that you can't stand either the situation or falling short of your "should" or "oughts"?

Let me say one last thing as we finish up today. It is important to emphasize that the goal of what we're doing is *not* to deny or distort reality by turning negative appraisals into phony positive appraisals. *Rational thinking* is not the same thing as *rationalizing*. It is indeed the case that some events are, in fact, objectively difficult and demanding, and most people want to be liked by others and to view themselves as competent. So, don't beat yourself up for having typical human desires and preferences. Rather, the goal is to recognize that negative events and consequences fall along a scale from a bit negative to truly catastrophic. The tendency to overreact with thoughts like "It's awful!" and "I can't stand it!" results in an escalation of negative emotions. It is a question of putting events and consequences into perspective, based on the evidence, so as to reduce needless distress.

(*Show the client the portion of Handout A-3 entitled, Self-Instruction: Performance-Enhancing Thoughts.*) This handout also has material on another procedure called *self-instructional training*, another way of "talking to yourself" in a manner that reduces stress. Unlike the stress-busters, self-instruction is not a way of attacking or replacing irrational beliefs. Instead, this portion of the program can guide you through the encounter, reduce your stress, and keep your attention on the task at hand. Intense emotions can disrupt performance because we become so bound up in self-defeating thoughts that we cannot devote our full attention to what we should be doing in order to cope. Self-instructional training helps people talk to themselves before, during, and after stressful situations in ways that turn their attention to task-relevant aspects of the situation, direct their coping efforts, and develop a plan for reacting to the situation (such as telling themselves to stop and think before reacting to a hot situation). As you develop your stress-reducing self-talk, you may find these quite useful as well.

End-of-Session Summary and Homework Assignments

End the session by verbally summarizing the session and giving the client copies of Handout A-3 plus a set of daily Stress and Coping Diary forms (Form A-1) and also Forms A-2, A-3, and A-4 for self-monitoring and developing coping self-statements.

"As we end, let's summarize today's session. First, we reviewed your relaxation training and discussed how it's going. We also did another relaxation go-through. Then we talked a lot about how thoughts cause feelings, and how many of these thoughts are automatic ones that run underneath our usual awareness. They constitute our appraisals, how we interpret situations. We found that we could tie some of these ideas to the stress reactions you experienced before your interview with the productivity consultant. We focused a lot on a common form of thinking called *catastrophizing*, which can cause exaggerated stress responses, and we looked at some widely held beliefs that cause problems and underlie some of our troublesome automatic thoughts. Have I missed anything, or do you have any comments or questions?

"If not, let me tell you about your homework assignments for next week. I want you to continue your relaxation training, taking care to associate exhalation and your cue word *calm* with tension release. By next week, you should have a pretty good relaxation coping skill under your belt that can tone down the physical part of the stress response. Is that okay with you?

"This week's other assignments are going to building up your mental coping responses. I want you to read this handout (Handout A-3), Mental Control of Emotions and Stress; fill out this form (A-2), Analyzing Thoughts and Feelings; and also fill out Challenging and Replacing Stress-Producing Thoughts: Where's the Evidence? (Form A-3). [If the diary is being used]: Keep completing your Stress and Coping Diary (Form A-1). In the diary, Items 4 and 7, in particular, get at hot-button situations, hot automatic thoughts, and ask you to come up with stress-reducing thoughts. These materials will help you zero in on stress-producing automatic thoughts and begin to replace them with stress-reducing ones. You'll be developing a list of your own personalized stress-busters. You should also choose some from the section titled, "Self-Instructions" in Handout A-3 that you can use to tell yourself what to do before, during, and after stressful situations to cope more effectively. Transfer the stress-producing and corresponding stress-reducing thoughts that you discover when filling out the two forms, Analyzing Thoughts and Feelings and Challenging and Replacing Stress-Producing Thoughts, to this Anti-Stress Log (Form A-4). As this log is developed, it will help you identify your most critical hot thoughts and create stress-reducing thoughts to counter and eventually replace them.

"Using these materials, I'd like you to come up with some new anti-stress statements for this Anti-Stress Log that we can examine next week and that you can use in reducing your emotional arousal. It's important that you do these exercises because next week, we're going to explore how you can use them to control your stress response. Be sure to keep all of the exercise materials you complete, for we'll be using them later on."

[Show the client Figure B-1 for the session wrap-up.]

"We've covered a lot today, and I know that the handouts I'm sending home with you will help you digest it. But as we end, let's put every-thing in context so you can see where we're going. This graphic (Figure B-2) shows the stress model and the procedures we've introduced thus far. As you can see, we're focusing on building your coping skills to handle the portions inside the bracket—that is, inside you. The relax-ation coping skills you're learning are directed at giving you control over the physiological part of the stress response. To address the mental appraisal portion and build mental coping skills, we're challenging and replacing your irrational self-talk with stress-reducing self-talk. This approach is called *cognitive restructuring*. We're using self-instructional training so you can learn to inwardly talk your way through stressful situations and keep focused on the task at hand. As we proceed, we're going to put the mental and physical coping skills together into what we call an *integrated coping response*, which we plug into the breathing cycle. Then in our final sessions, we'll introduce additional stress-reduction techniques that you can use to develop your coping skills still further.

"Does this all make sense? Do you have any questions or concerns? If not, we'll continue next week with some practice in actually applying the physical and mental coping skills."

CHAPTER 6

Session 3: Induced Affect Reduction Using Relaxation and the Integrated Coping Response

ABOUT SESSION 3

By this third session, clients should have mastered the relaxation and breath training sufficiently to use it as an active coping skill to reduce arousal. The IA technique will be used twice in this session. Although cognitive skills were introduced in Session 2, only exceptional clients are well-enough developed to reduce arousal with the same level of success as with relaxation. Therefore, in Session 3, clients use relaxation alone to counter arousal under conditions of IA in an initial trial. We then do a second IA trial to introduce the integrated coping response. Clients are instructed to insert a self-statement of their choosing, selected from their Anti-Stress Log, into the inhalation phase and to apply relaxation upon exhalation. The effects of relaxation should continue to facilitate arousal reduction even if the cognitive coping skill is not yet well established.

OVERVIEW

Training Objectives

1. Monitor clients' progress in acquiring relaxation and cognitive coping skills.
2. Apply IA to clients, with relaxation alone to dampen arousal.
3. Introduce and practice the integrated coping response.

4. Continue work on clients' development of stress-reducing self-statements.
5. Instruct clients in how to construct an Anti-Stress Log and coping cards.

Session Outline

- Assignments check-up
  - Review breath and relaxation progress
  - Review the Analyzing Thoughts and Feelings form (or diary equivalent)
- First IA administration
  - IA rationale
  - Initial relaxation phase
  - Arousal phase
  - Affect reduction phase using relaxation
  - Discussion phase
- Second induction using integrated coping response
  - Initial relaxation phase and arousal phase
  - Affect reduction phase using integrated coping response
  - Discussion phase
- Continuation of cognitive skills training
  - Anti-Stress Log and coping cards
- Homework assignments and handouts

Materials Needed

- Subjective Units of Discomfort Scale (SUDS) (Figure B-4)
- Anti-Stress Log: Stress-Reducing Self-Statements (Form A-4)
- Analyzing Thoughts and Feelings (Form A-2)
- Stress and Coping Diary (Form A-1) copies

Homework Assignments

- Practice daily abbreviated breathing and relaxation practice (Handout A-2).
- Develop Anti-Stress Log (Form A-4) and coping cards (in Handout A-3).

GROUP ADMINISTRATION

Assignments Check-Up

Review Breath and Relaxation Progress

Check on how relaxation practice is going. Reinforce those who have practiced regularly and ask if anyone has been applying it in daily life.

Group members are likely to report that they have applied the relaxation skill with positive effects. Reinforce such accomplishments and use them as instances of positive modeling and encouragement for other participants. Emphasize the importance of continuing to practice in order to fully master this skill and to also enjoy the experience of relaxation. In a group administration, not much can be done for those who are not complying with relaxation training except to encourage them to do so in order to experience its benefits. They can still experience the IA portion, being instructed to use abdominal breathing to reduce arousal, since the arousal level induced in this session is not excessive. Typically, clients who have not been highly motivated enough to do the exercises drop out by this session. We typically experience an attrition rate of 10–15%.

Occasionally, clients will maintain that although the stress they experience is excessive and aversive, they fear that if they are not stressed, they will not have the necessary motivation to perform. For example, test-anxious students sometimes say that they need their anxiety to motivate them to study or to perform well on tests; they've always experienced it before and during tests and have done fairly well. In such cases, it can be useful to differentiate between a positive motivation to succeed and a negative fear of failure. These are two distinct motivational systems (Atkinson, 1964) that have different results on behavior. Fear of failure is not only aversive, but it also can have negative effects on performance (Sarason, 1984). In contrast, positive motivation to achieve enhances performance. Most people have varying levels of both motives. Reducing a dominant fear of failure can free positive motivation to drive the behavior with effects that are likely to be more enjoyable and positive.

Sometimes clients do not comply with the relaxation training because they believe they do not experience high physiological arousal. Two factors may be involved in such reports. First, some people carry around a high level of baseline tension that is normal for them. Once they start practicing relaxation, however, it is not uncommon for such clients to report, "I never realized how tense I was all the time." When clients deny or minimize the intensity of their arousal responses, ask them to test it out by doing some relaxation training.

People can clearly differ in the relative extent to which they experience the somatic and cognitive components of anxiety (Sarason, 1984; Smith, Smoll, Cumming, & Grossbard, 2006). Among the anxiety disorders, both cognitive and somatic components are observed to varying degrees. Generalized anxiety disorder is characterized by a particularly strong worry component (Borkovec et al., 2004), whereas panic disorder has a particularly strong physiological component (Craske & Barlow, 2014). Therefore, a client who does not comply with relaxation training because of low somatic involvement may nonetheless profit from the cognitive coping skills training. Conversely, clients who do not develop highly effective cognitive coping self-statements may still be able to use relaxation as an effective emotion regulation strategy.

Feedback data from clients on the CASMT components show individual differences in the perceived helpfulness of the relaxation and cognitive skills components (Smith et al., 2011). Some find the relaxation skills more useful, others the cognitive coping skills, but most find both helpful. Again, it is useful to frame the coping skills program as a buffet from which one can choose the most helpful items.

Review Analyzing Thoughts and Feelings Form

Ask clients about the stress-producing and stress-reducing statements that they discovered when they did the Analyzing Thoughts and Feelings (Form A-2) exercise or the daily Stress and Coping Diary (Form A-1). As per the trainer's request, participants should have brought their written materials with them, particularly their Anti-Stress Log (Form A-4). Check to see if anyone had difficulty doing this or understanding what they were to look for in relation to the Mental Control of Emotions and Stress (Handout A-3).

Next, discuss specific self-statements that participants developed. For example:

"I'd like everybody to profit by being part of this group. You've all been working, I hope, on stress-busters and self-instructional statements that you think would counteract the hot thoughts that trigger distress. I asked you to bring some along with you today. Hopefully, you've started your Anti-Stress Log. Or, you may have your Analyzing Thoughts and Feelings form with you, so you could look at your D statements. What I'd like to do now is go around the group and ask you to share some of the self-statements you've developed, if you are willing to do so. It may be that someone didn't think of one that you did, and your self-statement could be exceedingly useful for him or her as well. It may also be possible to consider some variations that would make it even more of a stress-buster. With your permission, I may make some suggestions if I think of something that might be helpful. I don't want anyone to feel on the spot or to worry that he or she will be negatively evaluated. We're all in this together, and these groups work best when the members are supporting one another. We should also remember that this is something new for you, and I guarantee you'll get even better at this with practice.

"Is someone willing to go first? Others should feel free to share similar self-statements that you've developed and to write down ones offered by others that you think might be useful for yourself. So, let's view this as a stress-buster problem-solving exercise."

Depending on how active the group is, devote perhaps 5–10 minutes to this discussion, reinforcing members for their contributions and inviting others to share similar self-statements. At this point, the majority of the self-statements will likely be anti-catastrophizing ones, although groups vary. Some of the self-statements may need shortening so they can fit better into the inhalation phase of the integrated coping response. For example, "Even if I do poorly on this test, I'll probably still be able to go to medical school" might be shortened to "It's not the end of the world." Feel free to take notes of promising self-statements and encourage other group members to consider their potential usefulness. For example, at one session, a collegiate golfer who experienced severe performance anxiety because she considered herself a total failure when she underperformed, came up with this self-statement: "Golfing is what I do; it's not who I am." This statement was derived from challenges to the core irrational idea that unless one is totally achieving, one cannot be a worthwhile person. By the end of training, she reported that the anti-stress self-statement served as the stimulus for a major reappraisal of her internalized conditions of worth. She later added another statement: "Success is giving my best effort. No one can do more." This reduced outcome-oriented pressure is tied to the personal meaning of consequences, the fourth type of appraisal in the stress model. Her disclosure stimulated a group discussion of irrational ideas that link self-worth to success, social approval, and related conditions of worth.

"I hope this has been helpful in giving you some additional ideas and self-statements. Now, I'd like you to choose two moderately stressful situations you've experienced recently or in the past, and for each one, I'd like you to write down one or two stress-reducing statements that you think would have been helpful. I don't want you to choose a traumatic event that could trigger an intense response at this point in your training. I'll ask you to imagine these situations and then practice your coping skills to reduce the emotion."

In choosing situations to imagine, clients can select ones that elicit different emotions, such as anxiety and anger, to broaden their anti-stress arsenal. They should also focus on recurring stressful situations that they will be encountering repeatedly in the future and that are particularly important for them to master. Examples might be speech or academic test situations for performance anxiety, social-evaluative situations to learn to reduce social anxiety, or interactions with challenging people who tend to induce anger.

First IA Administration

This will be the participants' first exposure to IA. You can expect some anxiety in clients about letting out potentially overwhelming feelings or about reacting so strongly that they might embarrass themselves in the group setting. Trainers often have similar reservations about eliciting strong emotional responses. To date, hundreds of individuals (including people with psychotic disorders) have experienced the IA procedure in both clinical and research settings without untoward effects. One reason is that even intense affect can be brought under control with relaxation instructions or abdominal breathing, particularly if the client is already trained in relaxation skills.

In group administrations, it is unusual to get high levels of affective arousal, at least in initial IA administrations. Evaluative concerns tend to dampen overt emotional expression. Also, we ask participants to choose a moderately stressful event, and not a traumatic event, in this session. We want the participants to feel sufficient emotional arousal to experience the efficacy of their coping skills. Moreover, we do not do IA until participants have had several weeks of training in relaxation and we are confident that they can use it to reduce arousal. If a group member is having difficulty "getting down," we administer relaxation instructions to the entire group

IA Rationale

"You've been working on your relaxation skills for 2 weeks and we're ready to put them to work. We know that any skill is best learned when you can practice it in the kinds of situations where you'll actually use it. If you want to get good at tennis, you have to learn not only how to swing the racquet, but also you need to go out on the court and try the skill. The same is true for stress management skills. If we're to practice applying your stress management skills to reduce or control feelings, we have to get the feelings into the room. So today we are going to use a method called *induced affect* (the word *affect* means emotion) that will allow you to practice coping with stress. We will do this twice. I'll ask you to imagine two stressful situations that you choose, let emotional arousal develop, and then use your coping skills to shut it down. Now, if you've been practicing your relaxation, you'll be good enough at it by now to turn off or greatly reduce any emotion you experience in this procedure. Don't be afraid to let yourself get into the scene and experience your feelings. You should also have some anti-stress self-statements on hand that you can use for the second induced affect practice. By the end of both exercises, you'll be relaxed and calm again.

"Because stress responses are unpleasant, you may be a bit apprehensive about experiencing them here. A common reaction to uncomfortable feelings is to avoid or suppress them, but if you're to practice your coping skills in this controlled and safe environment, it's important that you allow the process to take place so you can demonstrate for yourself how these skills work.

"I'd like you to do this with your eyes closed so you can concentrate on your inner experiences. Here's what we're going to do. I'm going to help you get relaxed. Then I'm going to ask you to imagine the first situation you chose. I will try to help you experience the stressful feelings. As I said, it's important that you let this happen and try not to avoid experiencing the feelings. You're safe here because, as you'll see, you've learned stress-reducing skills. Then, I'm going to have you demonstrate to yourself how quickly you can control those feelings using your relaxation skill. The whole procedure, including the relaxation phases, will take less than 10 minutes. Of course, I should emphasize that your willingness to do these procedures is completely voluntary, and you can decline to do so. If you decide that this approach is not for you, you can just sit back and relax or imagine pleasant scenes. Or, if you wish, you can quietly leave at any time." [The latter rarely occurs, as almost all participants do the IA procedure.]

Initial Relaxation Phase

In this initial IA administration, start with a brief generalized breathing relaxation induction based on the training exercise:

"To begin, let's practice our relaxation. Just settle back and begin focusing on your breathing. Feel the cool air as it enters your nostrils and the warmer air as it leaves your body. Breathe without any effort down into your stomach. Each time you exhale, let your body relax more deeply. Feel the muscles in your body just . . . let . . . go as you let the chair support you completely. Just focus on that deepening sense of relaxation as your body reacts automatically to your effortless breathing out. Use your personal cue word—for example, *relax* or *calm*—each time you exhale. If anything comes to mind, just focus your attention back on your breathing.

[After 6–10 breaths:] "Now as you breathe comfortably into your stomach, imagine a pleasant wave of relaxation that flows down your body, beginning at the top of your head. It's as if your skin is transparent and you can look right through it at the muscles, like you can in one of those plastic anatomy figures. Each time you exhale, picture that wave wash down over the muscles and see them relax even more deeply, like rubber bands becoming limp and loose. . . . That's good. . . . Let that wave of relaxation move right down your body with each out-breath, relaxing you ever more deeply. Enjoy the sensations of relaxation as your body sinks more deeply into your chair."

Arousal Phase

When the participants are relaxed, begin the IA phase, using the group protocol that follows.

"Now, I would like you to think of the first stressful situation that you recently experienced. Try to recreate that situation in your mind as vividly as you can. [Pause for 10 seconds.] Let all of your senses be engaged. . . . What are you seeing? . . . What do you hear? . . . What are you doing? . . . Are there any odors present? . . . Feel any touch sensations that were present. Try to reexperience the situation as if it were occurring at this very moment. [Pause for 10 seconds.]

"Now I want you to shut out the outside world except for my voice and focus your attention inwardly . . . deep down inside yourself where you have your feelings. . . . Be very receptive to any feelings or thoughts that might come to you. . . . As you focus your attention inwardly and imagine that situation . . . notice any feelings that are beginning to emerge and allow them to grow stronger. . . . They may be rather vague feelings, but as you concentrate on them, allow them to begin to emerge and grow stronger. . . . That will occur automatically as you focus your attention more closely on them. . . . That's good. Let the feelings come from deep inside you . . . deep inside yourself where all your feelings and thoughts begin. Stay with the feelings that begin to emerge, and allow them to begin to grow stronger. . . . As you focus on these feelings, the feelings from deep inside yourself, allow yourself to feel these feelings, your own feelings . . . and let the feelings grow stronger. . . . Let the feelings come from deep inside yourself, and as they grow stronger, let them come to the surface. . . . Let the feelings grow and any thoughts or images merge with them. . . . Feel the feelings and allow them to grow stronger. Allow yourself to feel the feelings . . . let them come out. . . . Keep focusing on your feelings and let them come to the surface. Let the feelings come from deep inside you, and as they grow, and become more intense, let them come to the surface. Feel the feelings . . . feel the feelings . . . that's good. . . . Stay with your feelings . . . allow yourself to feel your feelings . . . your own feelings. Let the feelings become stronger and stronger . . . let them build . . . let them grow. These are your own feelings. Stay with your feelings . . . feel the feelings.

"You may find that as you focus on the feelings, they start to spread from one part of your body to others. The spreading feelings may increase body tension, your heart may beat faster, your stomach may have certain sensations. Your breathing may become faster and shallower, and it may move up into your chest. I can see these reactions in many of you. They're perfectly normal and appropriate to this situation. Whatever sensations you have as the feelings grow, focus on them and let them grow even more. Don't be afraid to do so, because you're going to turn them off presently. Your feelings . . . stay with them . . . allow them to come from deep inside yourself . . . stay with them . . . and let any thoughts or images merge with them and let them come to the surface. . . . Stay with them . . . your feelings . . . coming out now."

Watch for any physical signs of affect from the clients, including faster breathing, swallowing, muscle twitches, etc., and verbally reinforce them.

"That's right, that's good. Get into that feeling and let yourself really experience it. Let it out. Feel the feeling grow and spread through your body. Don't be afraid of it, for in a little while, you'll find that you can control even a strong feeling with your relaxation skill.

"Let the feelings come out and grow stronger and stronger . . . more and more powerful . . . more and more intense. Coming out now, coming to the surface from deep inside you . . . your own feelings . . . feel your feelings . . . concentrate on your feelings . . . and as they come to the surface, allow them to continue to grow more and more intense . . . and stay with them. Let the feelings begin to spread through your body . . . as the feelings come from deep inside . . . to the surface. . . . As you allow them to grow more and more powerful, let them spread into the muscles of your body . . . feel the feelings and let them grow . . . your own feelings As the feelings come out now, feel them spread into the muscles of your body . . . and feel the feelings. Let the feelings come to the surface . . . and feel the feelings getting stronger and stronger, more and more intense. . . . Feel the feelings . . . allow them to come out . . . allow yourself to feel these powerful feelings. Let them spread across your body . . . into your muscles . . . feel the feelings and let them come out."

Keep reminding participants to experience themselves in the situation. Also, ask them to focus on any thoughts, images, or memories that might come to mind. During the induction phase, these cognitions can intensify the affective response. This focus also helps clients (1) gain insight into the specific cognitions that are involved in their stress responses and (2) direct the development of their stress-reducing self-statements.

"As you experience that situation and focus on the feelings, see if any thoughts or images come to mind that seem related to the feeling. If so, say those thoughts to yourself, or focus on the images, and notice what effect they have on the feelings. The feelings bring up the thoughts, and the thoughts bring up the feelings.

"Let the feelings from deep inside spread across your body . . . feelings from deep inside . . . let them spread into your muscles. . . . Perhaps you can feel those feelings in your neck . . . around your eyes . . . very distinct sensations getting stronger and stronger in these muscles as you feel the feelings. Feel the feelings in your face and neck . . . feeling these very powerful feelings. Now feel the feelings in your hands and fingers . . . in all the muscles of your arms . . . feel the feelings . . . and let them come to the surface. . . . Allow yourself to feel these feelings, your own feelings . . . building . . . moving to all parts of your body. . . . Feel them in all the muscles of your body. Let the feelings grow . . . make the feelings build . . . increasing in intensity . . . getting stronger and stronger. . . . Let the feelings come to the surface . . . feel the feelings. . . ." [Allow the induction to go for about 5–7 minutes.]

Affect Reduction Phase Using Relaxation

"Now, while continuing to see and feel yourself in the situation, I want you to experience how you can turn off that feeling with the coping skills you're learning. While continuing to imagine that situation, I'd like you to take a series of soft, easy breaths into your stomach. As you slowly exhale, tell yourself to *relax* and just let the feeling melt away. Breathe without any effort down into your stomach. Each time you exhale, let your body relax more deeply. Feel the muscles in your body just . . . let . . . go as you let the chair support you completely. Just focus on that deepening sense of relaxation as your body reacts automatically to your effortless breathing in and out. Use your personal cue word—for example, *relax* or *calm*—each time you exhale. Concentrate in particular on the sensations as you control the feelings you just had. Now as you breathe comfortably into your stomach, imagine a pleasant wave of relaxation that flows down your body, beginning at the top of your head. Each time you exhale, picture that wave wash down over the muscles and see them relax even more deeply, like rubber bands becoming limp and loose. . . . That's good . . . just let that wave of relaxation move right down your body with each outbreath, relaxing you ever more deeply. Enjoy the sensations of relaxation as your body sinks more deeply into your chair.

"Is everybody relaxed? If not, please raise your index finger so I can see it and we'll do a little more relaxation to help you get yourself back down. If you're already completely relaxed, just enjoy the relaxed state if I continue the relaxation a little longer so that everyone is relaxed."

Continue relaxation until all clients look relaxed.

"Now, I'm going to count down from 5 to 1. As I do so, I'd like you to bring your focus back to this room. Open your eyes when I get to 3 or 2 and at 1 become fully alert. Stretch a bit to get comfortable, if you wish."

Discussion Phase

Following the initial induction, some time should be devoted to a discussion of participants' experiences during the IA exposure. Start the discussion by acknowledging that no two people had exactly the same experience because they imagined situations that differed in important ways. These differences include how stressful the situations were, the different emotions experienced, and the different emotional intensities. Group members also have varying levels of relaxation skills. Continue along the following lines.

"Despite the differences, I'd like to tap into what your experiences were like in the hope that there are some common experiences.

- "I'm wondering in particular if you were able to get relaxed at the beginning? At the end?
- "How many of you were you able to experience a level of emotion that you would regard as at least moderate in intensity?
- "How quickly were you able to get into the maximum level of intensity? [If needed, explain that the IA protocol is group-oriented and may not be of optimal length for people who react very quickly or slowly.]
- "How close did you come to an emotional response like the one you'd expect in the actual situation? Did anyone experience an even stronger one?
- "Did focusing on the thoughts that accompanied the emotion increase the emotion? Did my asking you to catastrophize about the situation have any effect?
- "Were you able to shut down the emotional arousal with your relaxation? How many breaths did it take? How did you feel about your ability to get back down? If you were able to experience that actual situation tomorrow, how do you think you would react?
- "Have I missed anything that is relevant to your experience?"

Reinforce and encourage any positive reactions, any slight success. Be accepting of any feedback you might receive, even negative feedback. In a group, there may be one or more individuals who did not experience affect because the IA procedure was too short or who had difficulty bringing down the affect, perhaps because they haven't practiced their relaxation enough. In general, however, you should expect that the experience was as intended. In the event that a client reports difficulty imagining the scene, feeling arousal, or reducing the arousal, suggest that he or she practice visualizing the scene at home, using relaxation to reduce any arousal that might occur.

Second Induction Using the Integrated Coping Response

"Now I want to do a second induction exercise to introduce you to the use of what we call the *integrated coping response,* which combines your mental and physical coping responses into a double-barreled mind–body stress reducer. You've just used the physical relaxation skill with your cue word as you exhaled to reduce emotional arousal. Now, we're going to add a stress-reducing statement as you inhale along with using your cue word to relax as you exhale. This practice creates a mind–body coping response tied into the breath cycle.

"This time, I want you to imagine the second stressful situation you selected and to use the stress-reducing statement you think will be effective. This could come from the Analyzing Thoughts and Feelings Form (A-2) [or Form A-1, Stress and Coping Diary] you did on that particular day, or from your Anti-Stress Log (Form A-4) or coping cards. You may refer to those materials at this point if you have them with you and wish to do so. Please write down or commit to memory the stress-reducing statement you're going to use. Let me show you how this works." [Show graphic of the integrated coping response (Figure B-3).]

Initial Relaxation and Arousal Phases

Do a brief relaxation induction to establish a low baseline level of arousal. When the participants seem relaxed, repeat the IA procedure as in the first induction. Then administer the arousal reduction phase, this time adding the self-statement into the inhalation phase.

Affect Reduction Phase Using the Integrated Coping Response

"Okay, were now ready to turn it off, as before. But this time, as you inhale, I want you to say your stress-reducing statement to yourself. At the top of your inhalation, you can add the word *so* or *and* and then your cue word, such as *relax*, as you exhale. Go ahead and do that now, and see how many breaths it takes you to get calm and relaxed. If you have more than one stress-reducing self-statement that applies to this situation, use the others as well to see how they work for you."

Stay largely silent, but if any participants seem to be having difficulty in reducing their affect, administer verbal relaxation instructions until all participants seem comfortable and without distress.

Discussion Phase

When all the participants look relaxed, ask them about their experiences. Tell them that a major goal of the stress management program is to help them develop an effective integrated coping response, with a variety of stress-reducing self-statements that they can tailor to the particular situation. Some of these can be all-purpose anti-catastrophizers that are widely applicable. Others will be stress-busters and self-instructions that are tailored to particular emotions and situations. Clients should leave the program armed with an array of coping responses that they can modify, add to, and refine in the future. From this point on, in coping skills rehearsals using IA, make use of the integrated coping response.

Tell clients that, beginning with the next session, you are going to expand the stress-management buffet by teaching them other stress reduction strategies that research has shown to be effective.

Continuation of Cognitive Skills Training

In groups, ask one or more participants to describe a stressful situation from their homework and the stress-producing and stress-reducing statements they discovered. When they get stuck on justifying one of their stress-producing statements, use questions to help them learn to question the underlying belief: "Yes, but *why* should you always succeed or do things perfectly?" If they use a stress-reducing statement that is not optimal or doesn't work, analyze with them why it didn't work (e.g., statement was too global; statement didn't address a more fundamental, stress-producing belief). Engage the group members to formulate a more effective one. Search for any unspoken "buts." Ask if they have been using any of the stress-reducing statements in the Mental Control of Emotions and Stress handout (Handout A-3) in their daily lives and reinforce such attempts. Encourage them to use both reappraisals and self-instructional statements.

Tell them that they need to *practice* these cognitive methods in order to learn how to do them successfully. Like any new skill, these new methods feel hard and awkward at first. Participants will make mistakes, but with practice, the coping responses will become much easier and clients will be successful more often—much like learning to ride a bike or how to skate.

Anti-Stress Log and Coping Cards

Encourage clients to continue to work on their Anti-Stress Log (Form A-4) and to transfer the content to coping cards as described in Handout A-3, Mental Control of Emotions and Stress. Explain that the log is an aid for recording their characteristic stress-producing cognitions and the stress-reducing alternatives.

Remind clients to continue recording in the Anti-Stress Log those stressful situations along with their self-statements and to try various stress-reducing statements if the first one doesn't work. Have them use the materials in Handout A-3, Mental Control of Emotions and Stress, and Form A-2, Analyzing Thoughts and Feelings, as the basis for their cognitive restructuring and self-instructional training. Our experience and the results of outcome studies (e.g., Smith & Nye, 1989; Jacobs et al., 2013) indicate that in a group setting, people can use these materials very effectively on their own by adopting some of the adaptive self-statements listed in the handout.

Forewarn participants that their initial attempts to use stress-reducing self-statements may not work well initially but *will get more effective over time*:

"The thought patterns you've developed, including your beliefs and self-statements, are a product of many years of learning and use, so they aren't displaced easily or quickly. But the main purpose of what we're doing now is to help you examine your thought patterns and begin to challenge and replace some of the self-statements that cause unnecessary stress with new ones that are more useful for you. Maybe when you begin the process, your new self-statements won't be as successful as you'd like. But with practice and use, the new self-statements will be strengthened because they reduce or prevent negative feelings and, with use, will replace the old ones.

"For example, one person put himself through hell by being a total perfectionist. If everything wasn't done perfectly, he beat himself over the head with statements like, 'That should be done *right*' (by which he meant *perfectly*), 'I screwed it up,' and 'I'm a failure.' Once he began to challenge those statements, he saw that he applied a much higher standard to himself than he did to other people. He could be compassionate toward and understanding of them, but not himself. He agreed that a more reasoned self-statement, such as, 'I am, and will always be, an imperfect human being who makes mistakes. All I can do is my best, and that's good enough.' As he applied this self-statement in situations where he agonized about his imperfect performance, he began to feel a reduction in his anxiety and upset with himself. He found that his new attitude and standards took a lot of the self-imposed pressure off him. Eventually, they replaced his old stress-producing thoughts because they led to a rewarding outcome."

Homework Assignments

Abbreviated Relaxation

Remind participants to continue daily relaxation practice at home, adopting this regimen:

1. In the muscle relaxation exercise, they can move to tensing and relaxing all the muscle groups at once and slowly releasing the tension, combining exhalation with the cue word (e.g., *relax, calm*).
2. Practice the yoga breathing exercise described in Step 4 of the muscle relaxation exercise by itself, again remembering to pair the cue word with the slow exhalation. Do three repetitions of this exercise three times a day, or more often if possible.
3. Concentrate on using abdominal breathing and the paired cue word numerous times each day to help maintain a comfortable and relaxed state, but especially in any stressful situation that occurs.

Cognitive Skills Development

Have the clients use the Stress and Coping Diary (Form A-1) and/or Analyzing Thoughts and Feelings (Form A-2) to develop material to list on the Anti-Stress Log (Form A-4) and the coping cards. Provide clients with several copies of the Anti-Stress Log form.

INDIVIDUAL ADMINISTRATION

Individual administration follows basically the same protocol as above, except that it is tailored to the client. It is particularly helpful to have information from the Stress and Coping Diary (Form A-1) to review before the session and with the client. The diary data will provide information about the situations the client has encountered, the resulting emotions and their impact, the coping strategies employed, and the cognitions (both stress-producing and stress-reducing) reported by the client. This information will provide fertile material for optimizing the session for the client and for evaluating the client's psychological mindedness and progress in skills development.

Working with an individual rather than a group allows you to tailor the IA phase to the client. Occasionally, you can ask the client what he or she is feeling and what thoughts or images come to mind. You can use this information not only to increase affect elicitation (e.g., "Okay, just focus on that feeling in your stomach . . . let that feeling of pressure become even stronger . . . and just focus on that idea that you're going to screw up"), but it also can also be a very effective diagnostic technique, since intense affect frequently elicits or makes more accessible stress-related self-statements, images, and memories. To illustrate the collaborative assessment and IA procedures with individual clients, we present two cases. The first describes the first induction with Harlan, the socially anxious client from previous chapters. The second is with Susan, a woman with a severe approach–avoidance conflict involving a desire for closeness and a fear of intimacy.

ASSIGNMENTS CHECK-UP

Review Breath and Relaxation and Analyzing Thoughts and Feelings

Review the client's progress practicing relaxation. Also review the client's entries on Form A-2, Analyzing Thoughts and Feelings; Form A-3, Challenging and Replacing Stress-Producing Thoughts: Where's the Evidence?; Items 4 and 7 of the Stress and Coping Diary (Form A-1); and/or the clients Anti-Stress Log (Form A-4).

It is important to identify any personal and environmental barriers to regular practice that might be holdovers from previous discussion in Session 2, or any new ones. Some clients maintain that their lives are so demanding and stressful that they don't have time or opportunity to practice. To deal with this excuse, suggest that they block out a defined time period each day to ensure that practice occurs. Also, probe to see if they simply do not believe that relaxation will be helpful to them.

A useful framework for understanding noncompliance is the transtheoretical model advanced by Prochaska and DiClemente (1984). The hierarchical model identifies six stages of change. The first is *precontemplation*, in which the existence of a problem is either unrecognized or denied. In the *contemplation* stage, a problem is acknowledged, but the client is not ready to complete the steps necessary to deal with it. In the *preparation* stage, the problem is acknowledged, and although the client has decided to take action, the active process of changing behavior has not begun, or the client is not fully committed to doing what is necessary to deal with the problem. Clients at this stage, though participating in a program such as CASMT, may fail to commit themselves to homework assignments, or they may show uneven compliance with the program. In the *action* stage, the client is committed and actively involved in behavior change efforts both within and outside of the treatment context. Once coping skills are learned, the *maintenance* stage becomes a critical focus for continued compliance with the program and improvement of coping skills, as the client proceeds toward the final stage of *termination,* in which the skills have become ingrained and are sufficiently under personal control that stress management is permanently improved.

Most clients who seek out stress management training are at least at the precontemplation stage, acknowledging that life stress is having a negative impact on them and that it is worthwhile to consider a stress reduction program. From the first session on, we make it very clear that in order for the program to be helpful to them, they will need to take personal responsibility for doing what is required to learn the coping skills taught in the program. The initial goal is to move such clients from precontemplation and preparation into the action stage, where they are committing themselves to attending sessions and doing the out-of-session training assignments. Early failures to comply with homework assignments should be explored and dealt with promptly and assertively by the therapist, for these failures are an opportunity to move clients in the pre-action phase into the action stage where they can help themselves develop stress resilience.

During the maintenance phase, a critical issue is the possibility that the client will lapse into ineffective ways of coping, particularly if situations are encountered that overpower the coping skills that he or she has learned. Clients must be prepared for the inevitable setbacks that will occur so that *lapses* (i.e., single episodes in which self-regulation failures occur) do not become *relapses,* defined as a sharp reduction in coping efficacy accompanied by a regression to previous maladaptive behaviors. When relapse occurs, attempts at coping may be abandoned because of a dramatic reduction in coping self-efficacy, and the client may backslide into experiential avoidance and maladaptive coping patterns. In substance abuse problems, for which the relapse prevention model was originally proposed (Marlatt & Gordon, 1985), the tendency to become discouraged by lapses was termed the "abstinence violation effect," and this construct has been applied to many forms of psychopathology and is now seen as relevant to the maintenance of gains in any behavior change program.

*   *   *

The following material picks up with the case of Harlan, the socially anxious client from previous chapters. In this session, Harlan reported that his 20th high school reunion was in 2 weeks. His social anxiety had prevented him from attending previous reunions, but he was considering going to this one and it was causing him considerable anxiety. On the one hand, he was interested in seeing some of his former male classmates, but he was also curious to see if any of the women in his class were unattached. He reasoned that because he had high school experiences in common with them, it would be easier to converse with a female classmate than with a woman he did not know. Significantly, he also saw the reunion as an opportunity to "test my wings" and try out his stress management skills. Additionally, information from his more than 20 daily Stress and Coping Diary entries revealed a strong tendency to use social avoidance as a coping skill in evaluative situations. He regretted his avoidance of the blind date opportunity several weeks earlier and realized the limitations on his professional and social life that his avoidance was creating. This reunion was an opportunity to counter that tendency.

The therapist commended Harlan's willingness to confront his anxiety about the reunion. In examining the coping diary entry for the day he decided to attend the reunion, Harlan and the therapist found that his stress-producing self-statements included "I won't be able to carry on a good conversation"; "Other people will have been more successful than me"; and "I'll look nervous and they'll find me boring." Harlan and the therapist examined the stress-reducing statements as well, deciding that the following provided a valid reappraisal of the potential pros and cons of attending: "I have little to lose and much to possibly gain if I reconnect with people I like"; "It's possible I could meet a nice woman who's also looking for a relationship, and I'll meet no one by staying home"; and "I'm perfectly able to carry my end of a conversation."

Harlan's First IA Administration

In individual administrations, where the absence of group-based inhibitions typically results in stronger emotional responses to IA, no client is ever allowed to leave the session in a high state of distress, even if the session needs to be extended for that client to employ an additional relaxation induction. A similar approach occurs in prolonged exposure treatment for PTSD, where clients are encouraged to experience intense affective responses elicited by imaginal reexperiencing of traumatic events. In such exposure sessions, the affective response can be controlled with relaxation if habituation does not occur (Foa & Jaycox, 1999).

THERAPIST: Harlan, last week I told you that in today's session, we'd begin applying your coping skills so you could practice them to reduce emotional arousal. If you're agreeable, I'd like to propose that we use this reunion situation to get you into some emotional arousal. It's also an opportunity to actually prepare for being in that situation. Most importantly, it'll allow you to demonstrate to yourself that you can handle your anxiety better than in the past.

HARLAN: Well, might as well jump into the pool.

THERAPIST: First, I'm going to get you relaxed. Then, I'm going to ask you to imagine being at the reunion and help you immerse yourself into the scene. I'll help you get into the feelings, encouraging you to fully experience your feelings, and then we'll use your relaxation skill to turn off the arousal as quickly as you can.

As we go through this exercise, I'm going to check in with you from time to time on your level of relaxation versus discomfort using this scale. (*Shows a copy of the SUDS in Appendix B, Figure B-4.*) As you can see, the scale goes from 0, none; to 30, mild; to 50, moderate; to 7, severe; to 100, unbearable, worst imaginable. We call these 100-point readings the Subjective Units of Discomfort Scale, or SUDS (*pronounces* suds). So, if I ask you for a SUDS reading, I'm asking where you are at the moment on this scale. Is that clear?

Initial Relaxation Phase

The therapist administers cue-enhanced muscle relaxation as in the group protocol, reminding the client to use his or her subvocal cue word, such as *relax*, with each exhalation. The following is an abbreviated transcript of the IA administration. An actual rehearsal trial may take 10–15 minutes to elicit and then reduce the arousal.

THERAPIST: Just settle back and begin focusing on your breathing. Feel the cool air as it enters your nostrils and the warmer air as it leaves your body. Breathe without any effort down into your stomach. Each time you exhale, let your body relax more deeply. Feel the muscles in your body just . . . let . . . go as you let the chair support you completely. Just focus on that deepening sense of relaxation as your body reacts automatically to your effortless breathing out. Use your word *relax* each time you exhale. If anything comes to mind, just focus your attention back on your breathing.

[After 6–10 breaths:] "Now, as you breathe comfortably into your stomach, imagine a pleasant wave of relaxation that flows down your body beginning at the top of your head. It's as if your skin is transparent and you can look right through it at the muscles, like you can in one of those plastic anatomy figures. Each time you exhale, picture that wave wash down over the muscles and see them relax even more deeply, like rubber bands becoming limp and loose. . . . That's good . . . let that wave of relaxation move right down your body with each outbreath, relaxing you ever more deeply. . . . Now, what reading would you give on the stress thermometer that goes from 0 to 100?

HARLAN: I'd say about a 10, though it goes higher when I think about what's going to happen.

Arousal Phase

THERAPIST: OK, let's go to the reunion. Please describe the scene you're imagining.

HARLAN: I'm walking into the country club lobby. There are some men and women milling around; I recognize one guy, but not the others. Most of the people are already in the ballroom.

THERAPIST: Please describe how the people are dressed. (*Client does so.*) What do you hear?

HARLAN: People are talking and laughing. I hear glasses clinking. Lots of people have drinks, and everyone seems involved in conversations— except me.

THERAPIST: Can you smell anything?

HARLAN: Yes, some food.

THERAPIST: How do you feel? What's your SUDS reading, from 0 to 100?

HARLAN: I'm feeling tense thinking about it. It's about 40. One of the women looks over at me, and it goes up to 50.

THERAPIST: Okay, turn your attention down inside and focus on the feeling. Feel those sensations in your body. And as you focus on the feeling, it will begin to grow, just automatically. Just let that happen. The feeling is going to get bigger and bigger, more and more intense. Just let it loose. (*Harlan begins to grimace.*) That's good, just letting it grow, bigger and bigger, more and more intense. It's your feeling, and it's getting bigger and more intense as you focus on it. That's good, that's fine. Just let it come. (*Continues encouragement, suggestion, and reinforcement of affective expression.*) Tell me about the feeling and what's happening in your body.

HARLAN: My stomach is all knotted up, and I'm cold and tense all over. My heart is pounding.

THERAPIST: What's your stress reading on the 0 to 100 SUDS scale?

HARLAN: About 60.

THERAPIST: That's good, just keep feeling what's happening in your stomach, your muscles . . . feel your heart beating harder and faster. Do any thoughts accompany your body's reaction?

HARLAN: I'm thinking that this could be a disaster. I'm so strung out that I'll look like a stammering, sweating basket case. Everyone will focus on me and say, "Where'd that guy come from?" I feel like turning around and leaving.

THERAPIST: Feel that sense of being strung out, the sense that you're looking weird, like a basket case. Feel that. (*Harlan appears tense and agitated, with fast, shallow breathing and clear muscle tension.*) That's good. You're doing great. Your stress reading now?

HARLAN: High—about 70 or 75.

This rating would be considered a relatively fast emotional reaction by the client. We strive for a maximum SUDS reading of 60–70 on the first administration to increase the likelihood of successful self-administered relaxation by the client. The therapist therefore stops the induction at this point.

Arousal Reduction Using Relaxation

THERAPIST: With all this anxiety, you have the natural tendency to escape or avoid the feelings. But rather than turning around and leaving, you're going to turn down that feeling. It's your mind and your body, and you have some new tools to control them and deal with emotions, even those as intense as what you're experiencing right now. Let me show you how much control you have. Keeping that scene in mind, I want you to focus on your breathing and relax your body using your cue word *relax* each time you exhale. With each breath, you just breathe out that tension and watch those feelings in your stomach, heart, and muscles begin to fade away. Just letting go . . . more and more relaxed. With each breath, you become calmer and more relaxed. That's good, just letting go, letting that wave of relaxation spread through your body and replace the tension. (*Observes Harlan's "coming down" to a relaxed state.*) What's your SUDS reading now?

HARLAN: Pretty relaxed. Probably back to a 10.

Discussion Phase

THERAPIST: I'm interested in what this experience was like for you.

HARLAN: Well, I got into it pretty quickly, and by the end, I was more

stressed than I would have been in the actual situation. What surprised me was how quickly my relaxation brought it down.

THERAPIST: How many breaths did it take?

HARLAN: Only the first five or six to get me to 20 or so, which I can easily
tolerate.

THERAPIST: Needless to say, I'm very pleased with how you've applied
yourself to learn relaxation. With continued practice and application
in stressful settings, you can do even better. It will be interesting to
see how it works for you at the reunion. Remember, all it takes is a
breath and your cue word when you want to use it.

Harlan's Second IA Administration

In the second administration of Session 3, the therapist shows Harlan the
integrated coping response schematic (Figure B-3), pointing out how the
integrated coping response is created by adding a stress-reducing statement during inhalation.

In Harlan's second IA administration, he and the therapist decided
that because of the salience and impending nature of the reunion, they
would use another reunion scene, this one involving his approaching an
attractive former classmate who was, like himself, unaccompanied. Harlan worried that she would find him nervous and boring if he couldn't
create an interesting conversation.

Harlan was asked to think of a potentially useful self-statement that
would apply to this stressful situation. Harlan decided on the statement,
"I only need to carry my half of the conversation." He used this statement
during the inhalation phase of the breath cycle.

The subsequent induction resulted in a reported SUDS reading of
75. The integrated coping response reduced it to 30 in fewer than 10
breaths. Harlan was somewhat surprised and quite pleased with his success in reducing the moderately uncomfortable arousal. He decided that
if he could control anxiety at that level in an actual conversation with a
woman, he would be capable of functioning well in that type of situation.
The therapist congratulated Harlan on his success, attributed it to the
work he had done in learning progressive relaxation, and assured him
that his coping skills would increase with further practice and application.

*   *   *

To illustrate another use of the integrated coping response, we
present a second condensed IA administration with a different client,
Susan.

Susan's Second IA Administration

Background

Susan sought treatment initially because of work-related stress. She also complained of loneliness stemming from relationship problems with men. Susan had a number of borderline personality disorder characteristics, including emotional dysregulation, interpersonal issues, and a history of difficult intimate relationships. She described a series of failed heterosexual relationships, some of which she terminated because of malevolent attributions—what she viewed as insincere behaviors (e.g., "I doubted that he really cared about me"). In other instances, she saw herself as rejected and abandoned.

Susan had a childhood history of father-related sexual abuse and reported generalized difficulty with trust and intimacy; at the same time, she greatly desired closer relationships. This approach–avoidance conflict involving desired intimacy was the focus of a treatment plan that began with the use of CASMT to deal with her emotional dysregulation and distress intolerance. Later, other components of dialectical behavior therapy (Linehan, 1993, 2015) were introduced.

In previous sessions and in homework assignments, Susan was trained in relaxation and developed some potentially adaptive statements. She faithfully did her training assignments. The therapist began IA once he believed that Susan's coping responses were sufficiently well developed to control the emotional arousal elicited by the procedure.

The first induction involved a conflict with a female coworker with whom the client had recurring problems. In order to deflect blame for her own sloppy performance, the woman had lied so that Susan was unjustly suspected of the error. The initial IA administration elicited strong anger that Susan was able to control after an extended application of her relaxation skill together with a brief relaxation protocol administered by the therapist.

Selecting the Second IA Situation and Coping Statement

After a discussion of the incident and the success Susan had enjoyed in reducing her strong arousal, the therapist identified a second incident that he considered to be highly salient in her life.

THERAPIST: In looking over the data from your Stress and Coping Diary, it looks like you've been really stressed this week, starting last Tuesday. You mentioned that you went out with Kevin again. How did that go?

SUSAN: We get on really well, and I find him very attractive. I could get serious about him. But when he said he's developing feelings for me, I started having mixed feelings. I now remember I couldn't sleep for a long time that night. Actually, just remembering what Kevin said that evening is making me feel confused and conflicted.

THERAPIST: Confused and conflicted?

SUSAN: On the one hand, I was excited that he was feeling like I'm starting to feel, and I'd love to get close to him. But it also scared me a bit. It was like alarm bells went off. I began wondering if I could trust him. Does he really care? That feeling is scary for me, and I know it makes me want to pull back to feel safer.

THERAPIST: Let's take a closer look at that feeling and try a bit of practice in handling that feeling with the skills you've learned. To get ready, can you choose a self-statement or two from your alternative thoughts list or your coping cards, or perhaps think of one right now, that could counter that scared feeling that you have about trusting Kevin? Let's take a look at your diary entry for that date and see how you responded to Item 8, which asks what you could have told yourself instead that would have helped allay that fear of letting yourself get close to Kevin. Do you remember the ones you put in your diary after that date?

SUSAN: (*long pause*) I can think of two that I have on my coping cards. One is "What's past is past, and not the present or future." The other is that "I need to take the risk, or I'll never get what I want."

(When the client puts forth a potential stress-reducing self-statement, it is important for the therapist to establish that it is credible and potentially useful to that client. If this is not the case, the therapist and client should formulate one that meets those conditions and maximizes the efficacy of the integrated coping response.)

THERAPIST: What do you think of the validity of those ideas?

SUSAN: Well, I can accept them as true, but I can't buy into them completely. They could be wrong in this case.

THERAPIST: That's true. And if you think that Kevin is just like your father and other men who've used you, and you think that it's certain that you'll be exploited once again, it's likely that you'll avoid getting close, either by withdrawing from the relationship or doing something to provoke his withdrawing. Does that seem like a reasonable hypothesis, or am I misreading the situation?

SUSAN: Yes, I can see how that happens.

THERAPIST: But let's examine the evidence. If that's not true and you can replace the idea that the worst is sure to happen, then there's a good chance that you can face and overcome the fear, let yourself get closer, and maybe get the kind of relationship you want. To explore that notion further, let's start with a question: What percentage of men are totally insincere and only want to use women for their own ends and then dump them? Think of all the men–women relationships you've seen or heard about in your lifetime.

SUSAN: Well, maybe 30% of them. But there's a lot higher percentage in those I've gotten involved with.

THERAPIST: Okay, so if 30% are heels that you'd want no part of, what about the other 70%? Given all of the evidence you have so far about Kevin, which group is he more likely to be in?

SUSAN: We'll, I've not caught him in any lies and he's been gentle and seems sincere. But he could be fooling me.

THERAPIST: True, but how likely is that? What's the evidence? If you had to make a general bet, where would you put your money?

SUSAN: I'd guess that he's in the 70% group.

THERAPIST: Given the analysis that you've just done, where are you now in relation to Kevin's trustworthiness compared to the thoughts the other night that triggered your fear of letting him get close?

SUSAN: It seems less risky now.

THERAPIST: And how does that less risky feeling square with the two stress-reducing self-statements you came up with, which I thought were very good ones, by the way?

SUSAN: I'll need to work on really believing them, but I think they'd work.

THERAPIST: Well, we've talked about one goal of the program is to make you a better personal scientist. One of the things scientists do is conduct experiments to see if their theories are supported by the evidence. That method applies here in two ways. First, you looked at the evidence that favors or does not favor Kevin's sincerity, and you came up with two self-statements that you hypothesized would be stress reducers. So we're ready to do an experiment to see how well those self-statements work for you. I'd like to do another emotion exercise in which you use those self-statements in conjunction with your breathing and relaxation to form a combined mind–body coping response. We call it an *integrated coping response* because it combines both a mental and a physical stress reduction response in a double-barreled fashion. This time, you will again use your cue words *relax* and *relaxation* while you exhale, but we're also going to have you say one of the stress reducers to yourself while you inhale. Here's a picture of what it looks like. (*Shows Susan the integrated coping response schematic [Figure B-3].*) Okay, now I'd like you keep those new self-statements in mind. Why don't you sit back in your chair and we'll get you relaxed. And then I'll help you get in touch with that feeling. OK? (*Susan nods.*)

Arousal Phase

THERAPIST: Let's return to last Tuesday when Kevin told you he has feelings for you. Describe the situation as closely as you can, and hear and see him as he said it.

SUSAN: (*Describes the scene in detail as the therapist explores all sensory modalities—e.g., "He said it in a very soft and gentle voice. I was so scared that I just hugged him harder and didn't say anything. I hope he didn't notice how tense my body was. I was afraid I'd start shaking."*)

THERAPIST: As you relive that scene, can you feel any of that alarm bell reaction down inside you?

SUSAN: (*Nods.*)

THERAPIST: Holding that scene in mind, I'd like you to turn your attention down deep inside, and I want you to focus on that alarm bell feeling. . . . As you do so, the feeling will start to grow a bit stronger in your awareness . . . and it'll become bigger automatically as you focus your attention on it and it becomes the center of attention. Just let that feeling grow and as you focus on it, it gets stronger—just automatically—because it's at the center of your attention. . . . Just let it grow, stronger and stronger. . . . It's getting bigger and bigger. (*Susan begins to show signs of arousal.*) That's good, that's fine, just let it grow, stronger and stronger. . . . You're doing great . . . just let it come and grow, because you're going to show yourself how you can turn it off. . . . But for now, let it spread through your body and get stronger . . . like a tiny flame that gets bigger and bigger until it's a blaze. Pay attention to how it grows . . . to what's happening deep inside. Let it grow . . . getting stronger and stronger . . . bigger and bigger . . . stronger and stronger. Just feel that . . . that's good.

SUSAN: (*Becomes more aroused, begins to cry.*)

THERAPIST: Tell me about the feeling.

SUSAN: I feel scared and alone. It's like an icy hand in my stomach and chest. I want to run away from it.

THERAPIST: Focus on that feeling in your stomach and chest. . . . That feeling is spreading like an icy grip and getting even stronger. . . . What thoughts are you having about that feeling?

SUSAN: I hate it . . . I want to get away from it . . .

THERAPIST: . . . and you want to run from it. . . . Feel that desire to run from it.

SUSAN: Like I usually do. . . .

THERAPIST: But this time, you're going to face it down. Focus down inside . . . let it come . . . feel the feelings and let them come. Feel the feelings and let them come . . . feel the feelings and let them grow . . . feel the feelings and let them bubble up like a fountain, let them grow . . . just let them grow. That's good, stronger and stronger . . . stronger and stronger. Those feelings come from deep inside and spread throughout your body. . . . The feelings come from deep inside and spread throughout your body . . . growing more and more . . . more and more . . . stronger and stronger . . . just let them grow . . . feel the feelings . . . feel the feelings deep inside . . . that's good . . . let them come . . . feel the feelings deep inside. Do any thoughts come to mind?

SUSAN: I'm so scared about letting myself get hurt again. If I open myself to Kevin, I'm scared he'll play me for a while, get the sex he wants, and then dump me or hurt me like the others have.

THERAPIST: It's a scary thing to think about letting yourself get close and being so vulnerable to getting hurt. Feel that scary feeling.

SUSAN: I also wonder if anyone could really love me. I feel defective, ruined. . . . I hate being alone, but I couldn't stand going through the thought of being unlovable and waiting for the axe to fall. Even my father treated me like a sex object.

THERAPIST: Let that feeling of being vulnerable, that scary feeling, get even stronger. Look at it, see what it's like. It's so scary to put yourself out there, to open yourself to Kevin and take the chance he'll use you or find that you're not what he wants, that you are defective. Feel that feeling of being somehow defective, ruined. It's so hard to trust, given what you've been through in the past. Feel that feeling . . . feel it.

SUSAN: (*sobbing*) But I can't stand the feeling. I hate it. I want to run away.

Arousal Reduction Using the Integrated Coping Response

THERAPIST: Okay, we're going to talk about this experience and what it means for you. But for now, let's practice turning that feeling off with the skills you've learned, instead of running away from it. I'd like you to keep that scene and how you feel in your mind while you breathe down into your stomach and relax. Just letting go of all that tension, and each time you exhale, letting those muscles relax. That's good, just letting go. . . . It's your body and you can control it. Your muscles becoming limp and loose and relaxed. The inside of your body becoming calm and relaxed as the tension drains away, flowing out through your fingers and toes. . . . And now we're going to put one of those self-statements you chose together with your relaxation as you breathe. So, as you inhale into your stomach, say one of those stress-buster ideas to yourself. Then, at the top of your breath, say "so" and then a long, slow "relax" as you exhale. Do that with each breath and see how you can turn off that feeling. Show yourself that it's *your* mind and *your* body and you can have greater control over the feelings that block you from getting the intimacy you want in your life. Try out the other self-statement by itself as well.

SUSAN: (*Takes a series of breaths that move gradually from her chest down to her abdomen and exhibits a decrease in arousal.*)

Discussion Phase

SUSAN: It worked. Even though the scary feeling was really strong, I was able to get it back down.

A discussion of the feelings she experienced and their relevance to her life followed. The discussion centered on the conflict between her desire for and fear of intimacy and her vulnerability to being hurt or exploited. They discussed how, as closeness begins to develop, she experiences increasing anxiety that causes her to conceive of relationship events as "trust tests." Her fear makes her hypervigilant to signs of disapproval or rejection or to indications of trustworthiness. She reduces the anxiety caused by increased intimacy by either pulling away or behaving in a distrustful or hostile manner that drives the other away. The loss of the relationship reinforces her belief that it is safer to keep people at arm's length, and reinforces her avoidance. At the same time, it frustrates her desire for a close relationship.

THERAPIST: I think this has been a good session, and I hope you do, too. We've covered some important ground, and you've seen some relations between your needs, your feelings, and how you cope with them. As we work more on practicing your coping skills and as you apply them outside of our sessions in your life, you'll be in a position to risk intimacy on a more rational basis. You can use the same integrated coping response on those feelings if they come up in a relationship. You learned early in life that closeness led to exploitation and hurt, and that was repeated and reinforced in other relationships. But, as your self-statement says, that need not be the case in the present or the future. As you begin to master that fear of being hurt again, you won't need to run away from closeness or do things that drive the other person away. Instead, you can let your desire for a close intimate relationship be the dominant motive in how you relate. If you can decrease your fear of being hurt again, you'll reduce a big barrier to getting the closeness you desire. If you agree that this is important to you, we'll do more work on this conflict as we work together.

SUSAN: I'm realizing how important this distrust of others is in my life.

As practitioners of dialectical behavior therapy can attest, this type of conflict is a challenging one to work with in therapy, and the therapist can expect that as intimacy begins to develop in the therapeutic relationship, the client's fear of vulnerability may be triggered. Should that occur, the therapist may choose to use IA to bring the fear component to the fore and assist the client in applying stress management coping skills. Clearly, individual administration allows a therapist to personalize the intervention to focus on specific issues and to tailor the coping responses, particularly the cognitive ones, to the client's needs.

Generally, we have found that the use of two distinct situations as the basis for rehearsal is preferable because if the client successfully applied relaxation to reduce arousal, it may be difficult to repeat the induction a second time using the same situation and achieve the same level of arousal. However, a therapist may decide to repeat the situation involved in the first IA trial if there is a strong affective load or a particularly salient situation that might profit from the application of the integrated coping response in the second IA administration.

By Session 4, the client may be able to use coping self-statements alone to reduce arousal. The therapist may choose to take that route if there is a desire to focus on cognitive control of stress and the client seems particularly attuned to the cognitive interventions. We ask clients to continue to practice the integrated coping response through the remainder of the program because although we have found variability in cognitive restructuring skills, we are confident that relaxation will be successful in dampening arousal. In one sense, we take advantage of the confounding of thought and relaxation, for even if most of the arousal reduction is carried by the relaxation component, it reinforces the notion that controlling thoughts can have salutary effects as well.

Homework Assignments

The out-of-session assignment is the same as for the group administration. Clients can now use the abbreviated muscle relaxation exercise:

tensing all muscle groups at once and slowly relaxing, using their cue word with exhalation. They should also practice the yoga breathing exercise using the cue word on exhalation—three repetitions three times a day, or more if possible. Use the Stress and Coping Diary (Form A-1), Analyzing Thoughts and Feelings (Form A-2), and Form A-3 (Challenging and Replacing Stress-Producing Thoughts: What's the Evidence?) to develop self-statements to list on the Anti-Stress Log (Form A-4) and on their coping cards.

POTENTIAL TREATMENT ISSUES

Potential issues and problems that might emerge during this phase of CASMT center around two issues: (1) the ability of the client (and therapist) to tolerate strong affect, and (2) difficulties in creating cognitions that can counteract and eventually replace maladaptive appraisals and irrational core beliefs.

Client Unwillingness or Inability to Experience Affect

The ability of the client to experience affect during IA is a key factor in the rehearsal of coping skills as well as in the identification of automatic thoughts, intermediate beliefs, and core beliefs. One of the virtues of IA lies in its potential value for countering emotional avoidance. However, there are a number of reasons why clients may inhibit affective display. In group administrations, social factors, including fear of embarrassment or fear of potentially negative reactions from other group members can have an inhibitory influence. This is especially the case with clients whose issues involve social anxiety. As one client confided, "I don't want to make a fool of myself by becoming unglued." The same can occur in individual sessions, where clients may be concerned about a negative evaluation by the therapist if they appear weak or psychologically disturbed. Clients have expressed concerns that they may cry or "break down" if they let their emotions out. Others may be ashamed of emotions they find unacceptable, particularly "unjustified" anger. One deeply religious client who had lost both his spouse and his business was deeply ashamed of his unexpressed anger toward a God who had placed him in very difficult life circumstances. Some clients have a fear that if they "let themselves go," their emotional response may become uncontrollable. One client confided to his therapist that he was concerned that "I won't be able to get the toothpaste back into the tube."

　　Like other psychological interventions, the relationship between therapist and client is of paramount importance. It is important to nurture a trusting and supportive atmosphere, assuring clients that any distress that they experience will be reduced by their own coping skills, and with the assistance of the therapist if necessary. One useful analogy is to compare the process with learning a physical skill, as in the following:

> "We're working together because you experience unwanted stress reactions in your daily life. If you want to learn to reduce those emotional responses out there, it's a good idea to practice doing so in here, where you can strengthen your coping skills. Mastering any skill requires that you practice it, particularly under conditions that are similar to where it will be applied. You can read all you want about how to swim, but if you're going to learn to swim, you eventually need to get into the pool. That's why I'm asking you to invest in experiencing the stress response here so you can practice controlling it. Succeeding here will give you more confidence in your ability to do it out there in your daily life. This procedure is all about empowering you. One additional benefit is that when you're emotionally aroused, you may become more aware of the stress-producing automatic thoughts related to the emotion. This is the first step in eventually replacing them with stress-reducing thoughts."

It is not necessary that clients experience intense affect in the rehearsal of coping skills. As noted above, in this session we prefer a moderate level of intensity (60–70 SUDS) so that the client enjoys initial in-session success. Very rarely, however, one will encounter a client who claims to be unable to experience any arousal under IA. If the treatment is time-limited and the problem continues, the therapist can switch from IA to covert rehearsal, in which the client imagines successfully applying relaxation and adaptive self-statements, as is done in stress inoculation training (Meichenbaum, 1985) and occasionally in cognitive therapy (J. S. Beck, 2011). Covert rehearsal can be an efficacious approach to rehearsing coping skills. Though in need of replication, one study that compared the approaches to coping skills rehearsal suggested that, as Bandura's (1997) self-efficacy theory would predict, successful rehearsal in reducing high emotional arousal creates stronger coping self-efficacy (Smith & Nye, 1989).

Therapist Reluctance to Induce Strong Affect

Therapists can feel initial uneasiness about arousing intense affect in clients, whether doing exposure treatments or IA. They should be reassured that the benefits of such treatments justify the use of these efficacious methods. High-intensity emotional reactions are readily brought under control, particularly if the client has already learned the relaxation coping skill.

When using IA, a client should never be allowed to leave the session in an agitated or anxious state, even if the session needs to be extended by administering relaxation instructions until the client is calmed down. Once arousal is contained, the client's discomfort should be acknowledged and his or her courage in responding emotionally should be positively reinforced. The occasion should also be used to demonstrate to the client the power that using relaxation (even if therapist-administered) can have in managing arousal. It should be emphasized to clients that with time, practice, and application in stressful situations, their coping skills will become increasingly effective.

Cognitive Skill Development Issues

Cognitive therapists posit three layers of dysfunctional cognitions: automatic thoughts, intermediate beliefs (e.g., attitudes, rules, assumptions), and core beliefs (A. Beck, 1976; J. S. Beck, 2011). At the situational level, automatic thoughts influenced by underlying intermediate and core beliefs constitute appraisals and generate emotional responses. Cognitive restructuring can target any of these levels. In rational–emotive therapy (Ellis, 1962; Ellis & Harper, 1961), the focus is primarily on core beliefs, whereas in cognitive therapy, the focus typically proceeds from chronically accessible automatic thoughts to the less accessible intermediate and core beliefs. Nonetheless, many clients have almost immediate insight into underlying core beliefs. Our cognitive restructuring approach is to focus on all levels and provide examples of stress-reducing appraisals that can apply to any of them. Subsequently, clients can develop adaptive self-statements that address all three levels. For example, Harlan quickly seized upon the core belief, "In order to be a worthwhile person, I must be approved of by virtually everyone and succeed in everything." To the extent that access to intermediate and core irrational beliefs becomes available, many clients can quickly see their self-defeating qualities and begin to counter them with new self-statements that short-circuit the automatic thoughts that elicit their stress responses.

Cognitive restructuring requires an analytic mode of thinking, and clients differ in their conceptual abilities and psychological mindedness. Some clients have difficulty identifying automatic thoughts or challenging them. In instances where clients struggle to identify intervening thoughts and continue to view their stress responses as being directly triggered by the situation, several measures may be used. First, as is suggested in the protocol described in Chapter 5 and in Handout A-3 on mental control of stress, one can work back from the emotion and ask what specific thought would be required to generate that emotion in that situation. Another approach is to report thoughts that have been identified by other clients in similar situations and ask if they might possibly apply to the client. Finally, if cognitive restructuring seems beyond the client's capabilities in a time-limited treatment, self-statements derived from self-instructional training can be applied effectively by most clients, and there is much empirical evidence to support their efficacy (Meichenbaum, 1985). Indeed, we encourage our clients to develop Anti-Stress Logs and coping cards that contain self-statements derived from both cognitive restructuring and self-instructional training.

CHAPTER 7

Session 4: Induced Affect Skills Rehearsal and Introduction to Meditation and Mindfulness

ABOUT SESSION 4

Session 4 includes two more IA trials to practice using the integrated coping response. Additionally, this session includes an introduction and application of a simple breath-focused meditation technique, the Benson relaxation response technique (Benson, 1975; Benson & Proctor, 2010). It is easy to learn and serves both as a stress reduction measure in its own right and as an introduction to other mindfulness techniques that are presented in Session 5. The efficacy of meditation as a self-administered stress management coping skill is well established (Alidino, 2015; Edenfield & Saeed, 2012).

OVERVIEW

Training Objectives

1. Monitor progress in acquiring relaxation and cognitive coping skills.
2. Apply IA with the integrated coping response.
3. Continue work on the development of stress-reducing self-statements.

Session Outline

- Assignments check-up
  - Review relaxation.
  - Review development of stress-reducing statements.

- First IA with the integrated coping response
- Second IA with the integrated coping response
- Introduction to the Benson meditation technique
  - Practice Benson meditation technique.
- Homework assignments

Materials Needed

- Benson Meditation Technique (Handout A-4)
- Anti-Stress Log (Form A-4).
- Analyzing Thoughts and Feeling (Form A-2)
- Stress and Coping Diary (Form A-1)

Homework Assignments

- Practice abbreviated (whole-body tension) relaxation and breathing–cue word pairing.
- Practice Benson meditation technique daily.
- Use diary and/or Analyzing Thoughts and Feelings to develop the Anti-Stress Log and coping cards.
- Apply relaxation and integrated coping response in stressful situations when opportunities occur.

GROUP ADMINISTRATION

Assignments Check-Up

Review Relaxation

Check with each client about relaxation practice. Ask how real-world use of the breathing and relaxation skills is going and how it is working for them. Describe how they can use relaxation when they are experiencing stress, rather than only as a once-a-day exercise.

"Practicing the relaxation once a day for 10 minutes does not automatically cause people to feel more relaxed during the whole day. However, using the technique with a few breath cycles periodically during the day can help you maintain a more relaxed state throughout your day. The beauty of this technique is that you can do it hundreds of times a day, if you wish. After all, we take, on average, about 15 breaths per minute, so you can imagine how many opportunities you would have to increase your feelings of well-being. Additionally, by practicing, you will learn how to feel deeply relaxed fairly quickly so that you can use it when you really need it. It can be used before, during, and after stressful events.

"Specifically, you can use your relaxation skills to reduce stress when *preparing* for a stressful incident. Sometimes, you may be waiting for an event that you know will be challenging, and you may feel tense just waiting for it—waiting to take an exam, waiting to get a performance evaluation from your boss, dealing with a difficult coworker, or having to confront a problem occurring in a close relationship. Often, there is a period of time before the event when you are just waiting or preparing. Relaxing and breathing deeply and slowly can reduce the amount of tension you feel during this stressful waiting period, so that you will be able to handle the situation more effectively. The yoga breath (*demonstrates short inhalations and slow release at exhalation*) that you do last in your relaxation practice can work very quickly. You can also prepare by rehearsing remaining calm during the event and rehearsing what you are going to say and do.

"You'll especially want to use your skills *during* a stressful event. By using your cue word, paired with exhalation, you should be able to relax yourself with one or two abdominal breaths without interfering with ongoing activity. That's why we work so hard to combine exhalation, relaxation, and the cue word with one another: so your self-command will automatically increase your relaxation. There is also a technique called *differential relaxation* that you can use while you are going through a stressful situation. What this means is that you can concentrate on relaxing just the muscles that you don't actually need to handle the situation. For example, when you drive in heavy traffic, you may notice your hands clenching the steering wheel, your shoulders hunching up, and your forehead furrowing (*demonstrates in extremis*). Now, you can't sit back and tense and release all your muscles while driving down the highway. But you *can* concentrate on relaxing your fists, shoulders, and forehead, for you don't need them tensed in order to drive. This focused relaxation will reduce your overall stress level, making you better able to cope with the situation. Relaxing your body in the dentist's chair or when undergoing a painful procedure actually reduces pain sensations, in part by directing your attention away from the body sensations. You can 'untense' your hands and legs while talking with your boss, or relax your body while expressing a grievance (*demonstrates relaxing most of the body while sitting upright and talking*). Some of your relaxation practice should be done while standing upright, as you will be in some stressful situations in that position.

"Finally, you can use your relaxation *after* a stressful incident. You may be sitting there stewing about how upset or angry or tense you feel about the situation now that it is over. You could keep yourself worked up for hours afterward. This is an ideal time to plug in your relaxation skills to 'come down' emotionally."

Review Development of Stress-Reducing Statements

Check in individually with all participants about the stressful situations they have experienced and their homework of recording the stress-producing self-statements and the stress-reducing self-statements that seem to work for them. Especially focus on the stress-reducing statements they have been discovering.

It is important to help clients find the self-statements that work best for them. As noted earlier, there are two classes of self-statements in the Mental Control of Emotions and Stress handout. One set derives from cognitive restructuring and the other from Meichenbaum's (1985) self-instructional training. The latter are generally more useful for children and people who are not psychologically minded enough to analyze their self-statements using cognitive restructuring. Self-instructions that direct attention and guide behavior are very useful in task performance.

Explore some stressful situation(s) in detail. You might want to focus on emotions such as anger, worry, or depression (which lends itself more to the cognitive coping skills than to relaxation). If you want to make sure one of these topic areas is addressed, ask for a sample situation from the participants. Similarly, you might want to address issues that have been neglected so far, such as perfectionism, fear of assertion, test anxiety, or some other topic important to this group.

Help clients through trouble spots and objections, search for "buts," and help them find alternative stress-reducing self-statements. Encourage any efforts and all little successes. If someone expresses discouragement or skepticism, remind him or her that this is a complex skill that takes time and practice to learn.

"In order to practice and strengthen your coping skills, we are going to do a few run-throughs of imagining the stressful situations again. As before, I'll help you get into the feelings that arise in you, and then we'll practice turning them off by using the combination of a stress-reducing thought and the relaxation response, or what we call the *integrated coping response*. Again, let yourself really get into the feeling so that it is as intense as possible. I'm sure you'll be pleased with your ability to turn it off using your coping skills. Take a minute to think of the stressful situation you're each going to practice, and the self-statements from your Anti-Stress Log that would be the best stress-busters or self-instructions."

First IA with the Integrated Coping Response

As in Session 3, ask if everyone has a recent stressful situation in mind, or one from the past that is particularly troublesome and elicits strong affect. Ask them to close their eyes and vividly imagine themselves in the situation. Administer the IA procedure, repeatedly suggesting that they feel the feelings start to grow stronger and stronger, and reinforcing signs of affect, as in Session 3 (takes about 5 minutes). Then ask them to turn off the arousal by using their integrated coping response.

"Now, I want you to continue to think about that situation, but say to yourself one of your stress-reducing self-statements as you inhale. Then as you exhale, relax. . . . That's good, keep doing this with each breath. You might try more than one of your stress-busters or self-instructional statements for variety and to see which one works best."

Stay largely silent, just reminding clients occasionally to keep thinking of the stress-reducing cognitions while in the situation (about 5 minutes). If any participants seem to be having difficulty in reducing their affect, administer relaxation instructions. Then, lead the clients in a discussion of the IA practice, especially the feelings they experienced and the effect of the self-statements and relaxation on the feelings. Reinforce and encourage them in every way you can.

Second IA with the Integrated Coping Response

Ask participants to choose another situation (or the same situation as in the first induction if they want more practice on it). After they choose the self-statement that applies best and is most likely to be useful, repeat the IA procedure (5 minutes), followed by discussion. In the discussion, ask participants to share how successful they were in reducing the affect. Also ask them to share the stress-reducing statements they used and to report how well they worked. Encourage participants to write down self-statements shared by others that they might find useful.

Introduction to the Benson Meditation Technique

"Now that you've had experience using the integrated coping response, we are going to start adding to your stress management techniques. Today, we're going to do some meditation.

"Have you ever had the experience of feeling physically relaxed but being unable to get to sleep because of thoughts racing through your mind? If so, you've experienced the difference between body relaxation and mental relaxation—that is, relaxation of the mind. Today I want to take you through a meditation technique that produces both physical and mental relaxation. This simple but powerful technique was developed by Dr. Herbert Benson of Harvard Medical School. Benson was a pioneer in researching the ancient practice of meditation. A fixture in Eastern cultures, meditation is a technique that's been practiced for thousands of years as a way to gain inner peace. Using sophisticated physiological measures, Benson studied what happens to the body when people meditate. Soon he ran out of expert meditators in the Boston area, so he decided to train volunteers to meditate so he could study them as they gained expertise. When he did, he found that ordinary people could learn a simple, breath-related technique rapidly and when he measured their physiology, he discovered that it had rather profound effects on their minds and bodies. He found evidence for a mental and physical state that was the exact opposite of the fight-or-flight stress response. While meditating, his subjects showed a sharp drop in their metabolism and in oxygen consumption, greater than occurs during sleep, even though the subjects were in a state of relaxed wakefulness. Heart rate, muscle tension, and breathing decreased as well. Brain wave activity also changed. In later research Benson termed this meditative state the 'relaxation response' and published a book with the same title that became a runaway best seller. Today, there is a surge of interest in meditation because of its stress- reducing properties as well as other positive psychological and physical effects.

"Surveying the many meditation techniques that exist, Benson found that they had four important components in common.

"Number one is a quiet environment: Ideally, you should choose a quiet, calm environment with as few distractions as possible. The quiet environment makes it easier to eliminate distractions.

"Second is a comfortable position: A comfortable posture is important so that there is no undue muscular tension. We favor, as did Benson, an upright sitting position with eyes closed, like we'll do today. Some practitioners use the cross-legged 'lotus' position of the yogi, but only use that position if you have flexible knees and find it comfortable. If you do this meditation lying down, there is a tendency to fall asleep—which, by the way, is one reason it's also been used successfully in the treatment of insomnia. You should be comfortable and relaxed.

"The third component is a mental device to direct your attention inwardly as you concentrate on the normal process of breathing. To shift the mind from logical, externally oriented thought, many forms of meditation use a sound, word, or phrase repeated silently or aloud; or fixed gazing at an object. In Eastern meditation practices, this is sometimes called a *mantra*. Benson's mental device is either a word, like your relaxation cue word, a short phrase that denotes peace and tranquility, or simply the word *one*. Think your cue word or *one* to yourself each time you exhale. Since a major difficulty in the elicitation of the relaxation response is 'mind wandering,' the repetition of the focus word or phrase is a way to help focus the mind.

"The final component of meditation is perhaps the most important. Benson, referred to it as a 'passive attitude.' When distracting thoughts occur, as they are sure to do, they are to be disregarded by saying 'Oh, well' to yourself and redirecting your attention to the repetition of the breath and the focus word. Do not worry about distracting thoughts or dwell on their content. Don't attempt to actively suppress or control them. Instead, adopt a 'Let it happen' or 'Oh, well' attitude."

Practice of the Benson Meditation Technique

"Today, I'm going to teach you Benson's simple technique, which you'll find easy to learn because of the abdominal breathing you've been doing. Put anything you're holding on the floor and sit comfortably in your chair with your feet on the floor and your hands in your lap. Think of a focus word that you'd like to try.

"Close your eyes and relax your muscles, starting from your head and proceeding down to your feet. [Wait 15 seconds.] Now, breathe slowly and peacefully down into your stomach, so your belly rises and falls while your chest stays still. Observe as much detail about your breath as you can. Feel the coolness of the air as it enters your nostrils and flows down your throat and into your lungs. Feel your diaphragm rise and fall effortlessly as you breathe in and out. Feel the warmth of the air as it exits your body when you exhale.

"When your breathing becomes soft and steady, each time you exhale, say the focus word or *one* silently to yourself, slowly throughout the exhalation. Let your body sink down further into the chair with each breath. If fleeting thoughts, sounds, and other sensations come into your mind, just say, 'Oh, well' to yourself and bring your attention back to your breath and the word *one*.

"I'm going to let you go with that for a few minutes. Just let that peaceful state of mind and body develop at its own pace. Let time stand still."

Allow the meditation exercise to proceed for 8–10 minutes, then softly intrude:

"Okay, just keep your eyes peacefully closed. Scan your body and mind to see what the body–mind relaxation state is like. Now I'm going to count backwards from 5 to 1. With each count, let your attention return more fully to the room, and at the count of 1, open your eyes."

Ask members to report on their experience. Were they able to get physically relaxed? Did they become mentally as well as physically relaxed? What did saying the focus word or *one* do for them? Did anyone have thoughts, feelings, or sensations come into their mind? Were they able to put them aside by thinking "Oh, well" and returning their attention to their breathing and focus word? Was it difficult to put aside the cares of the day and immerse themselves in the here and now? Was it stressful? Overall, did they like the experience?

Reassure participants that difficulty in staying focused on their breathing is normal. Some people get anxious because they're not "doing something," which points to the frenetic pace and the many "shoulds" that are part of modern life. Reassure them that as they practice, they will learn to attain a deep state of mental and physical relaxation.

"The experiences that accompany this meditation vary among individuals. A majority of people feels a sense of calm and relaxation, like some of you reported. Other descriptions involve feelings of pleasure, refreshment, and well-being. Some report a clearing of the mind and a relaxed mental state, even though thoughts come and go as they meditate. Many people report that after meditating, they feel a sense of physical rejuvenation and an increase in their energy later on, as if the body has recovered some of its resources while idling in neutral gear. Still others report little change at first, but more of these experiences as they practice it over time. Regardless of the subjective feelings, there is objective evidence of the physiological changes that accompany meditation. Research by Benson and others shows that after about a month of meditation for 12–15 minutes a day, its effects become more stable during daily life. For example, meditators have lower average blood pressure all through the day—before, during, and after meditation. After about 8 weeks of daily practice, genetic analysis shows stress-decreasing and health-enhancing changes in gene expression. The book *Relaxation Revolution*, by Benson and his coauthor William Proctor [2010], cited in today's handout, describes many scientific studies on the health-promoting benefits of the relaxation response."

Ask participants to describe any differences they experienced between the muscle relaxation exercise and the meditation. Then provide this rationale:

"Both the quick muscle relaxation and meditation approaches like the Benson technique have their places in stress management, but the places and uses are different. Meditation is a general mind–body relax-ation technique that is used as an overall stress reducer. The meditative relaxation response is good for cancelling out the effects of stress. Obvi-ously, you can't say 'Time out!' in a stressful situation and sit down to meditate for 10 minutes.

"That's where the breathing and muscle relaxation technique that you've learned earlier comes in handy. You can instantly relax yourself while remaining fully present and functioning in the stressful situa-tion. In any breathing cycle, you can also combine the relaxation with a stress-reducing or self-instructional statement that will help keep you on task. So each of these has its specific contribution to the general goal of stress reduction.

"I might note one other use for this technique. As I mentioned ear-lier, it can be very helpful for insomnia. Here's one way to use it if you're having trouble getting to sleep: First, do a whole body tense-and-release sequence and take some relaxation breaths with your cue word to get physically relaxed. Then apply the meditation technique in this fashion: As you inhale into your abdomen, imagine your inhalation 'sucking' all thoughts out of your mind. Hold your breath for 5 seconds. Then, as you exhale slowly, say 'sleep' or 'down' or some other word that denotes going into a state of sleep to yourself. Stretch out the word for the length of the slow exhalation. The combination of physical relax-ation and the quieting of the mind helps put one to sleep."

Homework Assignments

1. Instruct participants to continue to practice general muscle relax-ation using deep breathing and their integrated coping response in daily stress situations. By this time, clients have often discovered particular bodily hot spots that hold tension, so they can use their tense–relax proce-dure to focus on those specific muscle groups (e.g., shoulders, neck mus-cles). People who suffer from tension headaches often find that focusing relaxation on the forehead (frontalis muscle) and neck muscles is helpful.

2. At least once a day, they can practice the integrated coping response to imagined stressful events. The procedure is to (a) think of a recent, recurring, or anticipated stressful event; (b) choose a stress-reducing thought that would apply to the event; (c) imagine the event as vividly as possible, allowing the associated emotion to occur; and (d) utilize the integrated coping response to shut down the arousal. This pro-cedure is a good way of preparing for anticipated stressors.

3. Clients should continue to complete the Anti-Stress Log (Form A-4) of stress-producing automatic thoughts and situations and alternative

stress-reducing statements. They should try using the alternative statements after a stressful event. Particularly useful are self-instructions in which clients tell themselves how to behave effectively (e.g., "Breathe and relax and focus on what you have to do"; "Blowing up won't help—pause, keep your cool, and hear him out"). The stress-reducing self-statements from the Anti-Stress Log should be transferred to coping cards to which clients can refer frequently to help establish the reappraisals and self-instructions.

4. Clients should practice the Benson technique 12–15 minutes per day, following the procedure just described in the preceding material, and using the guidelines in the Benson meditation handout (Handout A-4).

End the session by telling participants that you hope they are pleased with their progress in developing coping responses. Emphasize that whatever they've accomplished to this point is due to their commitment and effort. This acknowledgment helps to facilitate self-efficacy and to encourage learned resourcefulness. It is important that positive change be attributed to clients' own efforts.

INDIVIDUAL ADMINISTRATION

Individual administration follows the group format closely, with two skills rehearsal trials using IA and the introduction to Benson meditation. Again, however, the individualized format allows for a more personalized administration and more feedback and participation by the client. If the Stress and Coping Diary was used, the therapist and client will have a week's worth of data to examine, including the situations encountered, the emotions experienced, the stress-enhancing and stress-reducing cognitions produced by the client, and the coping strategies employed, together with their perceived effectiveness.

Eliciting Associated Cognitions and Feelings with IA

As discussed in Chapter 1, network models such as the CAPS (Mischel & Shoda, 1995) describe the facilitating and inhibitory associative links that form among system elements such as construals, affects, expectancies, goals and values, and self-regulatory behaviors, both cognitive and behavioral. Entering the system at the level of affect can be a "royal road" to discovering important links that appear during IA as thoughts, feelings, images, and behavioral predispositions. This process is illustrated in the following transcript from a Session 4 IA transcript. The transcript has been altered in some respects to preserve anonymity. It is derived from an IA audio recording used to train therapists in the technique.

The client was a college football quarterback at a major university. As a freshman, he was called into action when the starting and backup quarterbacks were lost for the season with injuries. Unexpectedly rushed into a pressure situation, he was referred by the team physician because performance anxiety was having major negative effects on his athletic performance, academic functioning, and physical well-being. Embarrassed and frustrated with his poor performance, his confidence at a low ebb, and feeling he was letting his team down, the athlete was reportedly withdrawing from relationships with teammates and his girlfriend, was sleeping poorly, and was losing weight. Bouts of pregame vomiting were sapping his strength on game days. In the past month, a poor performance had cost his team an important game. Before his exposure to this stressful situation, however, the athlete had exhibited good adjustment and therefore received a formal diagnosis of adjustment disorder.

Though extremely talented, the athlete was exhibiting a variety of stress-related dysfunctional behaviors. He reported that his concentration was adversely affected by intrusive and worrisome thoughts and vivid images of past mistakes. This disruption in his concentration was reminiscent of the perceptual narrowing and poor external cue utilization that occur under stressful conditions as described by Easterbrook (1959) and Nideffer and Sharpe (1987). The athlete described his experience as "tunnel vision . . . as if I'm looking downfield through a cardboard toilet paper roll." This constricted perspective caused him to lock onto a particular receiver or area of the field, and thereby to fail to process other relevant cues such as alternate receivers or defensive players who were closing on the play. It also allowed defensive backs to "read his eyes" to detect the targeted receiver and converge on the pass. A series of interceptions that cost his team two early-season games, critical comments about his performance in local newspaper articles, and some booing by home fans who wanted him replaced as the starting quarterback only served to increase his anxiety.

At a physical level, the coach reported that this quarterback's "million-dollar arm" sometimes disappeared because muscle tension disrupted his natural fluid motion, resulting in some erratic passes. He had also become tentative and hesitant with his throws. To everyone's frustration, the athlete performed well during practice, but "seized up" on game day. The coach summarized the situation by saying "I've got a Wednesday All-American who can't perform on Saturday." The coach correctly pointed out that because of the athlete's exceptional talent, this was the first time in his athletic career that the young man had experienced adversity and failure, and he was not equipped to handle it.

The athlete was intelligent, highly motivated, psychologically minded, and committed to doing whatever it took to reduce his performance anxiety. He devoted himself to completing out-of-session assignments and developing cognitive and somatic coping skills, which he found immediately helpful. Because of time pressures to reduce his anxiety as early in the season as possible, the athlete was seen twice a week. He viewed development of the "mental side of the game" as a key to attaining his goal of a future professional career. By the time he reached the IA rehearsal phase of the program, he had a well-developed repertoire of coping skills to be rehearsed under conditions of high affective arousal. He had done well in Session 3 in reducing arousal, first using relaxation alone and then the integrated coping response.

The athlete appeared for the fourth session expressing satisfaction with his ability to handle game-related stress the previous Saturday.

THERAPIST: So you were fairly satisfied with the way things went Saturday?

CLIENT: Yeah, things went pretty well. You know, I started to get really tense Friday when we were going over the game plan. When I first noticed it, I told myself, "Okay, now that's the signal to start coping." I could tell that I was, you know, starting to say something to myself like "My God, what if I screw up and blow the game for us again?" So I attacked that idea with the idea that if I gave it everything I had and made a mistake, well, tough shit. You know, there will be 100 other college quarterbacks and most of the pros screwing up at times, too. You know, even though they are doing their best. Who am I supposed to be, God? I also reminded myself that I have enough talent to do well at this level if I stop locking up with worry and just let it rip. And it worked. It was really neat. It was nice not feeling like a basket case before the game.

THERAPIST: Well that sounds great. You are plugging in a good and effective internal sentence to deal with that idea, "What if I screw up?" So, today, let's build on what you've learned so far. You know the importance of practice in football better than I do. In the same manner, the best way to keep building your coping skills is to practice and rehearse them like we've been doing. So let's do some more work today. Again, we're going to work on putting together the anti-stress sentences, the relaxation, and the breathing into what we call the *integrated coping response*. Okay?

CLIENT: Yeah, okay.

THERAPIST: Let's pick out a really tough situation to practice on. Think of a really bad one.

CLIENT: Okay, that one happened 2 weeks ago, and it's about as bad as you can get.

THERAPIST: Okay, well let's use that one to get those feelings going. Now before we do, let's think about what would be the best anti-stress sentences for you in that particular situation. We talked about a number of possible ways of handling that kind of situation.

CLIENT: Yeah, uh, I don't know . . . the one I like best went something like, "Okay, just concentrate on what you have to do and let's go kick some ass."

THERAPIST: It's important to choose one that's really personal and effective. So let's use that one when you're ready to turn off the stress. It's equivalent to "You don't have to stress yourself. Let's just concentrate on the present and what you have to do now, and let's go kick some ass." Can we shorten that a bit so you can say the key idea to yourself while you inhale?

CLIENT: Okay. (*pause*) How about "I have what it takes so just focus and relax."

THERAPIST: Lean back then and close your eyes. And now just take a deep breath and relax. [When the client appears relaxed after five to seven breaths:] That's it. Now, like before, I'll describe the scene and you just visualize it and imagine it as vividly as you possibly can. Okay? Just try to see everything that's going on in that situation, to hear it, to smell it if that's the case. Just try to get into that as if it were happening right now. It's late in the fourth quarter and you're trailing by 5 points, and the reason you're trailing by 5 points is because you haven't been having a good day. In fact, you've thrown three interceptions and you've lost a fumble near the goal line that probably cost a touchdown. So now you're behind and this is the last time you have the ball. You're driving. It's a forth and five at about the 30-yard line and in front of you, you can see the scoreboard and the time is running down. There's 29 seconds left in the game, and as you look at the scoreboard, you can see the time running down: 28 . . . 27 . . . 26 seconds. . . . You're out of time-outs. Now, what are the things that stand out as you think about that scene, as you imagine it?

CLIENT: Well, I can see the crowd, I can hear everyone roaring, and as we move up to the line, they get quiet. And everybody, the crowd, our guys on the sideline, coaches, everybody's watching me. I can see the TV camera in the end zone pointed at me with the red light on.

THERAPIST: And now you're walking up to the line, you call the signal in the huddle. . . . And you get under center and then what happens?

CLIENT: Well, just as I put my, put my hands under the center's butt, they,

they roll up their zone so that my primary receiver's going to get double coverage, and I don't recognize the damn defense. I don't have a clue which of my secondary receivers is gonna get open. It looks like their corner may be coming on the blitz, and the back, who's supposed to move over to block him, is going in motion, so he won't be in position if the blitz happens. Their middle linebacker shouts, "You're toast!"

THERAPIST: Okay, fine. I want you to hold that scene now in your imagination. You're in that situation. It's really a tight situation, and I want you to focus your attention down inside, okay, down inside where there's a feeling, and as you focus on that feeling, that feeling's going to grow. That feeling's growing; it's getting stronger and stronger. Focus your attention on that feeling. It's getting bigger and bigger. Now just let that feeling grow. As you focus on it, it will grow kind of automatically. Just turn it loose. You can feel it grow. (*Client begins to show signs of arousal, and thoracic breathing begins to occur.*) That's fine, that's good. You're really getting into it. Just let that feeling grow. Just let it grow. It'll do it all by itself and get stronger and stronger. Just feel what's happening inside. You can feel it more and more. It's getting very, very strong now. That's good, that's good. Just let it grow, that's fine. That's right. Just let that feeling grow. Just let that feeling grow. Let it come out now. It's okay. Just let the feeling get stronger and stronger. That's good. Just letting that feeling grow. That's good. Just letting that feeling grow. It's getting stronger and stronger. It started out as a flickering flame of a candle and now it's growing, growing, growing into a huge blaze inside your body. You can feel it spreading throughout your body. Your whole body is having that feeling. Letting that feeling grow, stronger and stronger now. That's good. That's good. Just letting that feeling grow. That's good. That's really good. You can feel that feeling in your body. Feel that feeling in your body. That's good. The feeling growing stronger and stronger. That's good. It's getting stronger and stronger. You can really feel that feeling. Feeling that feeling. It's just growing and growing and you're going to continue to let it grow. It's going to get stronger and stronger. You can let it become as strong as it can possibly become because you know you're going to be able to turn it off when you want. So just let that feeling grow. Just feel that feeling all through your body. That's good. Just letting it grow. Just letting it grow. Getting stronger and stronger and bigger and bigger. Bigger and bigger. Spreading, spreading through your body. How do you feel? (*Client is showing increased respiration, hand-clenching, facial grimacing.*)

CLIENT: I'm . . . I'm really . . . I'm really getting strung out.

THERAPIST: Okay, what do you feel in your body?

CLIENT: Well, mainly, mainly right . . . right here in my stomach, but my, muscles . . . my muscles are getting tight all over and my . . . my heart's pounding.

THERAPIST: Okay, fine. Well concentrate on those feelings in your stomach. Kind of a churning feeling in your stomach, it's getting stronger and stronger. That starts to grow. As you focus on that part of the feeling, it gets stronger and stronger. That's good. That's fine. Just let that feeling grow. Just let it grow. It'll do it all by itself . . . and it's getting stronger and strong. That's good. You're doing really great. Just letting it grow. And those muscles . . . kind of like rubber bands just tightening up. You can feel those feelings in your body. And your heart, you can feel the feeling in your heart as it pounds faster and faster. Feel that feeling, feel that feeling. It's growing. It's getting stronger and stronger. You can let it get as strong as it can become. That's good. That's fine. That's really great. Just letting it grow. Okay. That's fine. You tell me, what are you thinking about now? What comes to mind?

CLIENT: Well . . . well, I feel like it's . . . like it's my fault that, that we're behind and like I've, I've just, I just got to come . . . come through. That everybody will say that I'm a goddam choker if I . . . if I screw up again. Just a hell of a lot of pressure.

THERAPIST: Okay, I want you to focus on that pressure, that feeling of pressure, that feeling of pressure is growing, continues to grow and get stronger and stronger. Focus on every aspect of that feeling of pressure in your body and your mind. That's good. Just letting that pressure grow. It's a feeling of pressure. You feel like it's your fault that you're behind. You're feeling that you've just got to come through, a lot of pressure. You don't want to be called a choker; you don't want to feel like a choker. You don't want to screw up again. All of those feelings. Part of that pressure. The pressure just growing, growing, getting stronger and stronger. Just stronger and stronger. Stronger and stronger. That's good. That's fine. Okay. Doing great. Just letting that feeling of pressure grow. Just letting that feeling of pressure grow. You're in that stadium. There are 60 thousand people watching you. You're up to the line. You don't recognize the defense. The clock is running down. You can see it in front of you . . . 20 . . . 19 . . . 18 seconds. And that pressure, that pressure, just building and building and getting stronger and stronger. Feel that pressure, just feel it, feel it. That's good. That old familiar feeling of pressure. Okay, that's good. That's good. Just letting it grow.

Okay. Now I want you to focus very carefully on what's going to happen to your body next because now we're ready to turn off those feelings. Okay? Remember now, as you inhale deeply, say the "Let's kick ass" anti-stress statement to yourself, then as you get to the top of the inhalation, you say "so . . ." and then a long, slow *"relaaaaaax"* as you exhale. Okay, now go ahead; see how quickly you can control that pressure feeling. That's good, just plugging in the sentences and the relaxation.

CLIENT: [after 10 seconds:] Hey, that's all right.

THERAPIST: You're down already?

CLIENT: Yeah, it only took me two or three breaths to get back down. And I really got into it this time. I think I was really more strung out than I would be in the real situation. Putting the sentence and the relaxation together like that really worked.

THERAPIST: It seemed like you got into the feeling really quickly. More so than you have in the past.

CLIENT: Yeah.

THERAPIST: I guess just thinking about it got it going, and maybe also the fact that you know from your past experience in here that you can control it made it easier to let it grow.

CLIENT: Yeah.

THERAPIST: Nonetheless, it took guts to let the feelings get that intense. Okay.

CLIENT: Well, this was a chance to see just how good I've gotten at controlling the stress. No way I could have done this a few weeks ago without falling apart. I think I'm going to be able to carry this out onto the field. We'll find out soon. This game Saturday is a biggie.

THERAPIST: Well, I saw some real mental toughness in what you were able to do today. Let me ask you something else. Did anything else come to mind while you were in the feeling? Did you become aware of any specific sentences that you were saying to yourself while you were getting really upset in the situation?

CLIENT: Umm, like, yeah, like . . . like "God, what if I screw up again?!"

THERAPIST: So that, just thinking about that is enough to really get the feeling going. What if, what if, what *if*.

CLIENT: Yeah, yeah, *what if* I throw one more interception. *What if* we lose because of me. It's fourth down and my last shot.

THERAPIST: Yeah. The problem is that thoughts like that interfere with what you're trying to do. It doesn't work to just try to drive them out of your head. The harder you try to suppress them, the stronger they become—like, if I tell you not to think of a blue elephant. What does work is to counter them with thoughts that help you get to your goal.

CLIENT: You know, there was something else. I had an image of my dad pop up out of nowhere. Before he died, he used to come to every game, from grade school to college. He had really high expectations for me and would get on me pretty good if I screwed up. Thank God he hasn't seen what's happened this season. Had he been at the game, it would have made the pressure even worse.

THERAPIST: What did your dad look like in your image?

CLIENT: He was frowning, looked very worried.

THERAPIST: How did you deal with that image?

CLIENT: It was there for just an instant and then it was gone, so I went back to the game situation.

This case provides an example of how high levels of affect can activate other elements of the personality system, such as associated thoughts and images. The appearance of his father's image is clearly something that should be and was explored during later discussions with this athlete. It served as a catalyst to deal with the fact that his father's unrelenting expectations were still influencing him. His father had been an excellent athlete whose athletic career was cut short by a catastrophic knee injury. As his son began to exhibit exceptional athletic talent, the father became increasingly involved in his athletic life and began to define his own worth in terms of his son's success. "He lived through me, and I felt I had to succeed for him as well as myself. It was never an option to fail."

To counter the conditions of worth he had internalized, the athlete worked on the development of some adaptive self-statements that focused on maximum effort rather than outcomes. To assist in this process, the therapist provided the athlete with a book written by the revered UCLA basketball coach John Wooden (Wooden & Jamison, 2010). It was important for this athlete to internalize the definition of success offered by Wooden: "Success is peace of mind which is a direct result of self-satisfaction in knowing that you did your best to become the best that you are capable of becoming. . . . No one can do more" (p. 32). Focusing on effort and preparation rather than defining success solely in terms of outcomes helped this young athlete alleviate the self-imposed "shoulds" and "musts" that created his anxiety. Conferences with his coach helped to reinforce this mindset.

The athlete responded well to the intervention. He and his coach reported an increase in composure during games and increased resilience, defined as an ability to bounce back from a poor play. His performance improved markedly, as shown in the performance grades made by the coaching staff based on studying the films of practice sessions and games. During the remainder of the season, the quarterback reported decreased anxiety and greater enjoyment of competition, performed closer to his potential, and led his team to a successful season.

POTENTIAL TREATMENT ISSUES

Meditation-Related Issues

Although most people are able to engage in meditation in a manner that relaxes and refreshes them, the practice may pose challenges and potential difficulties that vary from person to person. Some people (particularly those who are chronically sleep-deprived because of stress or poor sleep hygiene) report falling asleep during the procedure. It is useful to normalize this experience and to reframe it as an indication of how relaxing the technique is, and to tell clients that during meditation, many people show brain waves associated with sleep even if they feel awake (Pagano, Rose, Stivers, & Warrenburg, 1976). We encourage clients to meditate sitting up rather than lying down. A few clients have found that keeping their eyes open prevents falling asleep.

Intrusive thoughts and feelings are a common challenge during meditation, particularly during initial sessions. Some clients say that they are unable to quiet the mind and keep out thoughts, or that feelings make it impossible to stay focused on breathing and their focus word. Clients may therefore believe that they are doing it "wrong." They should be reminded that the key is to stop resisting thoughts and trying to make them go away, for thinking is a natural activity of the mind and thoughts are therefore a part of meditation. When we stop resisting what is naturally happening (e.g., with the "Oh, well" response suggested by Benson and Proctor [2010]), we experience calmness and peace. Redirecting attention back to breathing and *one* or the chosen focus word deflects attention away from thoughts and feelings, without trying to suppress them, and thereby fosters a feeling of inner calm.

A third issue for some clients is restlessness. Cut off from external stimuli, they feel fidgety and anxious. They begin to think of all the things they could or should be doing instead of "just sitting and breathing." This common experience can be reframed as showing how conditioned we are to frenetic activity in a chaotic world; we feel we should always be "doing something." We can feel restless as the body unwinds from its high baseline of activity and tension. It takes time for the body to settle down and feel at rest, and so it is best to continue meditating. Instead of stopping the meditation practice, suggest to clients that they give themselves permission to take time out for meditation. Remind clients that the key to achieving a state of deep relaxation is to stop resisting feelings and be present instead to "what is," even if its restlessness. Thoughts, emotions, external stimuli, and bodily sensations come and go continuously in the natural flow of life. Left to themselves, these sensations will ebb and flow. The goal of these meditations is not to have special or mystical experiences, but to become more at ease with *whatever arises*. By meditating regularly, ease in meditation will grow and translate into greater ease in living—the ability to flow with whatever life brings.

"I Tried It and It Didn't Work"

A statement from a client that a coping strategy didn't work can be disconcerting to a therapist. In such instances, a therapist might well apply his or her own integrated coping response, counter any defensive attributions, and deal with the situation as an opportunity to promote the personal scientist and the learned resourcefulness concepts that are integral to CASMT.

A useful approach is to engage the client in a collaborative functional analysis of the two main elements of the statement: "it" and "didn't work." Focus on antecedents, coping behaviors, and consequences. Questions like the following can facilitate this process:

- "Obviously, we'd both prefer that it did work for you. It's been said, however, that we often can learn more when things don't work out. [Avoid the word *failure* because it may reinforce a pejorative interpretation already being made by the client.] If we can find out what went wrong, then we can use that information to create something that is more effective. How about putting our heads together and analyzing what happened?"
- "Can you describe the situation in detail?"
- "What stood out in that situation that made it stressful?"
- "Can you recall what you told yourself about the situation—that is, what automatic thoughts might have come up?"
- "So, what exactly did you do to cope with this situation?"
- "You say you tried your integrated coping response. What exactly was the self-statement you used and how did you apply the relaxation?"
- "In what way did it not work?"
- "What would you estimate your SUDS ratings were before and after your coping response? How would you have known if the coping response *did* work?"
- "What did you conclude from this experience?" (Is the client

thinking things such as "It will never work"; "This program is useless"; "This is hopeless"; "I'm a failure doing this"?)

The client's responses can provide useful information for both the therapist and the client. What exactly did the client do, when, and in response to which type of situation? Was the situation so demanding that it overpowered the client's developing skills, or is it reasonable to assume that it should have been dealt with more effectively? If the latter, an analysis of the "it" portion of the proposition is in order. Was the coping response appropriate to the situation? Was the cognitive element appropriate? Was it derived from cognitive restructuring or self-instructional training? Has the client mastered relaxation to the extent that it can be used effectively to reduce arousal? If in-session observations suggest that relaxation has been mastered to a reasonable degree, what needs to be done to foster generalization to *in vivo* situations?

On the "doesn't work" side of the proposition, the client's expectations and standards of success should be explored. Is the client applying unrealistic standards or expectations to either the intervention or to him- or herself? This type of situation can be a golden opportunity to access core beliefs about success and conditions of worth that can be the focus of cognitive intervention. For example, if the client reports a decrease in SUDS readings after coping, but defines "working" as reaching a score of zero, such an expectation clearly reflects unrealistic standards.

The therapist should also focus on the attributions the client is making in regard to the perceived failure to cope successfully. Is the lack of perceived success being attributed to the treatment, to inadequacy on the part of the client, or both? Are the coping skills inadequately developed? Does this one event mean the client is a failure? If so, is the cognitive error of overgeneralization characteristic of the client in other domains as well?

Whatever the case, it is well to reemphasize several points that were made in in Session 1's orientation to the program. First, learning to coping with stress is not an instantaneous process. It involves unlearning well-established mental and physical stress responses and ineffective coping strategies while acquiring new, more effective stress management skills. The unlearning–relearning process takes time, practice, and application, so that it is not unusual to experience some challenges. In fact, failures are virtually certain to happen from time to time. Just as an athlete working with a coach can learn as much or more from errors as from correct performances, so can the stress management client working with the therapist. At this point, clients are in the early learning stage of skill development, discerning what works best for them and how and when to apply the skills. Clients can also be told that when people learn physical skills, their performance improves not in a smooth pattern of improved performance, but in fits and starts, with periods (plateaus) of no improvement during which the skills are being consolidated as new brain circuits are strengthened. The same pattern occurs with psychological skills. Moreover, every individual is different and confronts unique situations. What works in one situation and with one client may not work as well for another. Therefore, it would be a huge mistake to despair and abandon the process of learning coping skills. The goal is progress, not perfection, and the path is crooked rather than straight. The important thing is to have faith in oneself and in the scientifically supported coping skills from which to choose.

Finally, reemphasize to the client that the goal of this program is not to eliminate stressful experiences from daily life. That would be impossible. The goal is to increase the client's coping resources so that stressful situations can be more successfully managed and his or her quality of life enhanced. As Meichenbaum (1985) noted, an important goal of coping skills training is to "encourage clients to view stressful situations as problems-to-be-solved rather than as personal threats. The goal is to make clients better problem solvers to deal with future stressful events as they occur" (p. 30).

As therapists, we would like to see our therapeutic efforts and techniques bear immediate and lasting fruit. However, it is important to frame treatment as a place where the client has the license to fail and is expected to do so from time to time. By inoculating the client to setbacks and ineffective coping episodes, the therapist is establishing the realistic expectations that underlie relapse prevention.

CHAPTER 8

Session 5: Integrated Coping Response Practice, Acceptance, and Cognitive Defusion Training

ABOUT SESSION 5

Session 5 continues the use of IA to rehearse somatic and cognitive coping skills, and also introduces participants to a mindfulness meditation technique, acceptance as an aspect of mindfulness, and a series of mindfulness exercises designed to promote defusion. *Fusion* is when we mistake our thoughts for reality; *defusion* is the process of separating ourselves from our thoughts and seeing thoughts for what they are: mental events that may or may not represent reality (Hayes et al., 2012). Within the conceptual framework underlying CASMT, defusion can be regarded as an additional cognitive coping skill.

OVERVIEW

Training Objectives

1. Continue self-regulation training using the integrated coping response under IA.
2. Introduce mindfulness and acceptance as a new coping approach and conduct acceptance exercises.

Session Outline

- Assignments check-up
- IA with the integrated coping response

- Introduction to acceptance techniques
  - Monitoring and Labeling Thoughts
  - White-Room Meditation
  - Letting Go of Thoughts
- Homework assignments

Materials Needed

- Mindfulness, Acceptance, and Defusion (Handout A-5)
- Stress and Coping Diary (Form A-1) or Forms A-2 (Analyzing Thoughts and Feelings) and A-3 (Challenging and Replacing Stress-Producing Thoughts)
- Anti-Stress Log (Form A-4)

Homework Assignments

- Continue to practice the integrated coping response during imagined stressful encounters and in real-life situations.
- Practice the mindfulness meditation, acceptance, and defusion techniques described in Handout A-5.

GROUP ADMINISTRATION

Assignments Check–Up

Clients were given an unusually large number of assignments to do during the preceding week, including (1) practicing general relaxation in their life situations; (2) covertly rehearsing the integrated coping response in relation to imagined stressful situations; (3) continuing to work on developing stress-reducing self-statements, using their Anti-Stress Log and coping cards; and (4) practicing the Benson meditation technique daily. Begin the session by asking clients about each of these assignments. Ask them how the meditation practice went, how they experienced it, and any difficulties they may have encountered. Ask them to compare the two relaxation methods they've learned: the muscle relaxation exercise and the Benson meditation technique. Ask about their experience using the integrated coping response in life situations during the week. Encourage continued practice and application to increase their effectiveness.

"I know I gave you a lot to do last week. We're down to our last two sessions, and we're going to use them to build on the skills you've already learned and to add some new techniques to your stress management toolbox. The goal is for you to leave the program with skills that scientific studies have shown to be effective and with materials that will enable you to continue to develop your skills. We want you to have a variety of skills from which to choose, because people differ in the skills they find most useful. Different situations can demand different approaches, and coping flexibility is very useful.

"Today, we're going to do a session like last week's so you can practice shutting off emotional arousal that you create by imagining stressful situations and letting me help you get into the feelings Then, we're going to build on the meditation procedure I taught you last week. I'm going to teach you some techniques you can use when you need to gain some distance from disturbing thoughts and feelings. These techniques come in handy if you get a bit overwhelmed and you find it hard to make use of your integrated coping response. However, these mindfulness techniques are effective in their own right, and some people adopt them as primary rather than as fallback skills. Again, the guideline is, use whatever works best for *you*. The only way to know, however, is to give each of them a chance."

IA with the Integrated Coping Response

Ask participants to choose one stressful event and one or two self-statements from their Anti-Stress Log. Then ask them to vividly imagine the situation and conduct an IA session of 5–8 minutes' duration, as in previous sessions. Try to elicit a high level of arousal, and then instruct the participants to shut it off using their self-statements combined with relaxation (i.e., the integrated coping response). Briefly discuss how the process went, how successful they were in reducing their arousal, and how many breaths it took. Reinforce favorable reports and attribute their success to their work developing their coping skills.

Introduction to Acceptance Techniques

The following discussion links the CASMT model and the previous discussion of automatic thoughts to a new set of strategies based on mindfulness and acceptance models.

"If you've got a handle on the integrated coping response and have been successful in identifying and changing stress-producing self-statements, you are more capable than before these sessions began of preventing or controlling your stress responses. You've already seen that improvement in the exercises we've done with the emotion-induction procedure. Today, I want to introduce you to some new tools you can use in situations where you can't change the situation or short-circuit the emotion but must tolerate negative thoughts, sensations, and emotions. There are times when the best strategy is to distance yourself psychologically from such inner experiences. As a group, these are termed 'mindfulness and acceptance strategies,' some of which build upon the meditation technique you've been practicing.

"Scientists who study physical pain make an important distinction between *pain* and *suffering*. They say that there are two aspects to our experience of pain. One is the basic sensation from pain receptors that are sent into the spinal cord and up to the brain. The sensations alone constitute *pain*, but when they're fused with the appraisal of how much they hurt and the consequent negative emotional reaction, they create *suffering*. The more negatively people appraise the sensations and catastrophize about them, the more those people suffer.

"Studies have compared champion marathon runners with novices on how they handle the discomfort of exertion as the race progresses. As discomfort begins, both the novices and the champions often distract themselves by focusing their attention outside of their bodies, studying trees, watching clouds in the sky, counting their steps, and so on. Eventually, however, the discomfort becomes too much to ignore. When that happens, the novices continue to try distraction, but it no longer works, and they hit what is called 'the wall.' But the experts shift to a new mode, focusing on and accepting the sensations of their physical discomfort in a detached, nonjudgmental manner. They are better able to tolerate the discomfort and even use it to pace themselves during the late portions of the marathon. Lots of research has shown that people can learn to uncouple pain sensations from negative appraisals and thereby increase their pain tolerance, sometimes even doubling the amount of pain they can tolerate. It's the meaning that counts.

"You can apply that same principle to yourself. Recall that one aspect of automatic thoughts is that they're so overlearned, they seem true and real. So if you have the thought, 'I'm a failure,' you take it to mean that you are, in reality, a failure. In our previous work, however, we've seen how such thoughts can be detected and challenged. Their believability is reduced and we can distance ourselves from them.

"There are other ways to achieve distance from negative thoughts and feelings without changing them. We can learn to regard negative whisperings in the mind not as reflections of reality but as what they are, 'just thoughts': mental events that come and go. We can let them go in one ear and out the other without getting caught up in their negative effects. It's a little like disregarding unacceptable advice given by a misinformed but well-meaning friend or relative. We can politely take in what he or she says without buying in to the idea and acting on it. The advice goes in one ear and out the other.

"When feelings are too intense to control, we can accept the sensory, 'gut' aspects of them without judging them, without getting swept away by negative thoughts and meanings. This distancing approach is called *acceptance*. Acceptance involves allowing the presence of stressful thoughts and feelings and waiting for them to pass, rather than trying to control or resist them. Now, this may sound completely incompatible with the active emotion control skills you've been learning in this program, but in reality, they complement one another, proving that there's more than one way to get something done. Now, acceptance, as we'll be using the term, does not mean that you do nothing in the face of stressful situations and simply give up and suffer. Nor does it mean seeking out stressful situations so you can have lots of negative emotions. The form of acceptance I'm going to teach you is a special kind that is based on the mindfulness meditation you've been doing. Instead of avoiding negative thoughts and feelings, you can learn to accept their temporary presence without negative evaluation and by so doing, become more emotionally free and less constricted.

"Mindful acceptance leads to a coping skill called *defusion*, in which thoughts are detached from their ordinary emotional consequences. Defusion involves recognizing that your thoughts are not facts and that the content of your thoughts is not necessarily the same as reality. The only reality a thought has is as a mental event. In this way, all thoughts are the same. Acceptance and defusion do not involve confronting, disputing, or changing the thoughts. Nor do they mean avoiding or suppressing thoughts—which, by the way, doesn't work very well. Mindful acceptance simply changes your relationship to your thoughts so that you can detach from them and see them for what they are: temporary experiences in your stream of consciousness. In that manner, you can treat negative thoughts in the same way that premier marathoners learn to tolerate their painful sensations by stepping back from them and from the catastrophic appraisals that usually accompany pain.

"Language plays a role in this new response pattern. Much of our thinking involves language that is loaded with meaning from our personal experiences. For example, a child who is rejected and degraded by her parents can come to believe that she is 'unlovable.' The emotionally loaded word becomes fused with her sense of self. When that word appears in a thought about herself, it can trigger a cascade of negative thoughts and emotions, and those thoughts are likely to be accepted as reality. But what if those thought are stripped of their meaning? Let's see what happens with a 1-minute exercise."

The following exercise is based on a finding by Edward Tichener (1916) that if a word is repeated around 50 times, it begins to lose its meaning and becomes more of a sound than a concept. ACT therapists use this exercise to demonstrate defusion, often using the word *milk*, but more emotionally loaded concepts can be used as well (Hayes et al., 2012).

"In a moment, I'd like you to say the words *not okay* out loud. First, I'd like you to apply the words to yourself; think of some important way in which you're not okay, in which you fall short of the person you'd like to be. Does that idea bring up some feeling? Try to make the feeling as real as possible. [Pause briefly.] Now rate how intense the feeling is on a 1–10 scale.

"Now, we're going to say the words out loud repeatedly. Say them loudly and with me until I tell you to stop. Ready? 'Not okay,' 'Not okay.' [Initially, speak once per second for 60 seconds, with the interval decreasing over time until the words are being said in rapid succession.]

[When finished:] "What do you notice now about those words? What happened as you kept repeating them? Do they have the same loaded meaning as before? Rate how intense the previous feeling is right now on the same 1–10 scale."

Clients typically report that the words became "just sounds" largely devoid of the meaning they'd had originally, and their emotion ratings are correspondingly lower.

"This little demonstration shows us that when words are stripped of their emotional meaning, they lose their capacity to distress us. The first step in defusion is becoming aware of what's going on in your mind. Normally, what goes on in the mind 'just is,' operating in the background like a radio playing in the next room, with little awareness on your part. But, as we've seen in our previous work identifying automatic thoughts, we can tune into the mind's productions and become more aware of them. Now, we're going to build on the meditation technique I taught you last session and use it to show how you can become more aware of your thoughts and begin to view them from a distance rather than being immersed in them.

"When we did the meditation technique and when your practiced it during the week, did any thoughts, feelings, or sensations come into your mind as you concentrated on your breathing and the focus word? If not, you are truly a unique person, because virtually everybody reports that happening—even highly experienced meditators. No matter how hard we try to stay with the breath, thoughts keep showing up. You may have found yourself doing a lot of 'Oh, well'-ing, which is one acceptance technique that works. Today, we're going to use the intruding thoughts to practice some other techniques for acknowledging those thoughts while staying with our breathing during meditation. We're going to do a form of mindfulness meditation in which we focus on our breath without using the Benson technique focus word. I'm going to interrupt occasionally to allow you to experience different ways of watching and distancing yourself from your thoughts. When I do, keep your eyes closed and try to maintain your meditative state; then *go with* the experience I suggest to see how it feels to you. In this area, different things work best for different folks. What all the experiences I suggest have in common is that they do not involve changing your thoughts or even judging them, but simply accepting them as some of the more than 50,000 thoughts that will come and go through your mind today.

"Let's begin. Sit up straight in your chair, close your eyes and get comfortable, and relax. Focus on your breathing as you breathe down into your stomach, effortlessly. . . . Feel the sensation of the cool air passing into your nostrils and down your throat, and the warmth of the air that you exhale. Each time you exhale, let your body relax even more." [Allow 3 minutes, then speak in a soft voice during the next exercise.]

Monitoring and Labeling Thoughts

"You may already have had some thoughts pass through your mind. When the next one appears, I'd like you to briefly note whether the thought is positive, neutral, or negative. Say to yourself, 'Now my mind is having a positive thought,' or 'Now my mind is having a neutral thought,' or 'Now my mind is having a negative thought.' Then return to concentrating on your breathing and inner sensations until the next thought appears. Do the same thing again, simply labeling the thought as positive, neutral, or negative." [Allow 2 minutes, then move to the next exercise.]

White-Room Meditation

"Now we're going to get in touch with how thoughts come and go. I want you to picture your mind as an all-white room with nothing in it. You are in the room, and you can be wherever you want to be, on either side or even on the ceiling, so you can observe what's going on. The room has two open doors, one to the left and one to the right. Imagine your thoughts are like misty clouds floating in from the door to your left and exiting through the door to your right. Allow each thought to have a brief moment in your awareness as it passes through the room and disappears through the door before the next one floats in. Your only role is to observe how thoughts come and go." [Allow 3 minutes.]

Letting Go of Thoughts

"You can be a passive, accepting observer of your thoughts with no need to respond to them as they come and go by themselves. Continue this breathing meditation as I take you through a few strategies of letting go of thoughts and gaining some distance from them that people have found useful. [Allow 30 seconds.]

"As you continue to meditate, imagine you're sitting in a forest on the bank of a beautiful mountain stream with crystal-clear water. To your right is a bend in the stream. When a thought arrives, imagine that it becomes a bright autumn leaf that slowly floats down from the trees above and lightly lands in the stream. The leaf is caught up by the current and is swept away around the bend, where it disappears from view. As each thought arrives, let this process repeat itself. [Allow 2 minutes.]

"Now imagine you're driving down a long stretch of highway. At various points there are billboards to your right. When a thought occurs, imagine that it attaches itself to the next billboard ahead that disappears from sight as you pass it. As the next thought appears, let a new billboard pop up ahead and see the thought attach to it before you pass by. Each thought becomes a message on a billboard that you drive past. [Allow 2 minutes.]

"Now, imagine you are holding a big bunch of helium balloons. As each thought occurs, it appears on the backside of the balloon that turns in the wind to face you. Say to yourself, 'My mind put a thought on the balloon.' Then let the string slip through your fingers and watch the balloon float away on the breeze into the sky until it disappears. Repeat with each thought. [Allow 2 minutes.]

"Here's a final 'letting go' technique. This one is physical. Continue meditation with the breath as before, but place your hand at your side with the palm facing up. When a thought comes into your mind, imagine that it floats down into the palm of your hand. Feel the texture, weight, and temperature of the thought. Then slowly rotate your hand so that the thought drops out of your hand and out of sight. Return your palm upward to receive the next thought. [Allow 2 minutes.]

"This physical 'letting go' technique can be used anywhere, but here is a less conspicuous version. Your hand is palm-up in your lap. As a thought lands in your palm bend the fingers slightly to contain it, then let your fingers open slowly and jiggle them to release the thought. Many people report that letting thoughts go physically in this fashion makes the process seem more real and believable.

"Now let's finish with a few more minutes of uninterrupted meditation. When thoughts arrive, use any or all of the techniques you've just done to distance yourself from them." [Allow 3 minutes, after which count down from 5 to 1 to end the meditation and return attention to the room.]

Ask clients to discuss their experiences during the meditation. Ask them if any of the techniques helped them create distance from their thoughts. Look for individual differences in effectiveness to stress the "different strokes for different folks" theme. The goal in the training is to help clients fill a strategy toolbox with methods that work for them. Emphasize that nothing done in the sessions is going to make them masters of the coping strategies. They will need to practice and actively apply the coping skills that work best for them in their daily lives. They are investing their time and effort in developing skills that can benefit them for the rest of their lives. Emphasize also that a given technique may not work on all occasions and in all situations. It is important for clients to have a flexible array of stress management tools and to try them out in the real-life situations. This is how they can learn which work best in which situations.

"As an example of how different approaches can have similar effects, consider the two approaches we have been teaching you—the integrated coping response and meditation. Although the active integrated coping response may seem the opposite of the mindfulness techniques, research has shown that both approaches are effective. When active coping skills programs are successful, people say it's because they gained greater control over their thoughts and feelings and so could actively reduce their stress. When mindfulness and acceptance-based programs are successful, people say it's because they stopped avoiding and trying to control their negative thoughts and feelings and learned to accept and tolerate them in a nonjudgmental way. However, if you can learn to prevent stress responses with active coping skills, there's less to tolerate. When active skills don't work, mindfulness methods are a good alternative. Sometimes, especially in situations where you are overmatched, it's not about how to win the war; it's about how to step away from the battle and make it a smaller part of your life. That's what acceptance and defusion can do for you. Importantly, all these approaches are antidotes to suppressing thoughts and feeling, which is not a good strategy because it bottles up feelings and has negative effects in the long run.

"As a personal scientist, gather the information you need, use the resource materials we give you, and feel free to create your own combinations. For example, one could combine muscle relaxation with defusion techniques if that worked better than combining relaxation with stress-reducing statements."

End the session with a question and discussion period, time permitting. Ask clients if there are any elements of the program that are unclear to them and if they have any thoughts about the potential usefulness of the training elements for themselves.

Homework Assignments

1. Clients should continue to practice the integrated coping response during imagined stressful encounters and in real-life situations.
2. Give out the Mindfulness, Acceptance, and Defusion handout (Handout A-5) and ask the clients to practice the mindfulness and defusion techniques described therein.
3. Give out another Anti-Stress Log (Form A-4), to which they can add new or revised stress-reducing self-statements, and recommend that they also update their coping cards, if appropriate.

INDIVIDUAL ADMINISTRATION

Assignments Check-Up

Individual administration involves the same protocol as for groups, with the advantage of being able to discuss the Stress and Coping Diary results for the week and to get a personal report on the out-of-session assignments and how they were experienced by the client. Of particular interest is the extent to which the client utilized the integrated coping response *in vivo* and in the imaginal assignment that was given.

Review in Vivo Stress Management Experiences

THERAPIST: I saw on your diary form for Wednesday that you used both relaxation and rethinking the situation to deal with an anger-inducing situation at home. Were those used as parts of an integrated coping response? (*Client nods affirmatively.*) Can you tell me about it?

CLIENT: Well, Tom [her husband] came home an hour late from work without telling me he was going to work late, so the dinner I prepared sat on the stove for an hour. This has happened before and I've gotten really mad the last few times and we had a fight.

THERAPIST: And you reacted differently this time?

CLIENT: Yes. I recognized that this was a hot-button situation that I tend to catastrophize about [note adoption of this program term], so when I started to steam about it, I told myself, "I'm getting pissed. That's a signal to control myself." In the end, I was able to stop it and stay pretty calm.

THERAPIST: Great job of picking up what was happening and developing a plan to deal with it. What specifically did you do?

CLIENT: I told myself that this was a chance to practice my skills. So as I inhaled, I said several things to myself, and as I exhaled, I said, "So . . . *relax.*"

THERAPIST: What were the self-statements you plugged in as you inhaled?

CLIENT: One was "I may not like this, but I can definitely stand it." Another was "He's working hard for us and probably forgot." The one that was new was, "He's a fallible human being like me." I got that one off the self-statement handout.

THERAPIST: What would you have said in the past?

CLIENT: Something like, "That selfish bastard! He's so god-damned inconsiderate! This really pisses me off! I can't stand being treated like this!"

THERAPIST: I can see how thoughts like that could cook up some real rage. But this time, you rethought the situation. Are you pleased with what you were able to do?

CLIENT: Really pleased. The last time this happened, I blew up at him when he came through the door and said some things I really regretted. We had a terrible argument. This time, with my anger controlled, I calmly said, "I'm sorry you're late. I've been waiting with dinner." He apologized and said he was working so intently he lost track of time. I then said, "I understand completely and appreciate how hard you work. But it would be great if you could call me so I can time dinner and make sure it's fresh when you get home." He agreed, apologized again, and we had a nice dinner.

I was really ticked off, and I was able to calm down. I think it's helped to practice using self-statements and relaxation to control emotions in our meetings, even though they are usually intense. They're often more intense than the anger I felt in the situation at home, which made it easier to handle.

THERAPIST: We think that's one of the advantages in practicing these skills to reduce the very real emotions that clients experience in sessions. We've worked mainly with anxiety, but anxiety and anger both involve bodily arousal, so we get some transfer there, even though somewhat different self-statements are needed to get at the blaming aspect of anger. Do you have any sense of which part of the integrated coping response was more effective, the self-statements or the relaxation?

CLIENT: I'm not really sure. I think maybe the relaxation was more effective in the short term, but the self-statements put the situation in a different perspective that I was able to maintain, so the anger didn't come up again.

THERAPIST: I'm pleased to see how well you were able to control the anger. You've worked hard on your thinking and relaxation skills, and you can expect that they'll increase in their effectiveness as you apply them repeatedly in your life.

Several elements of this report are noteworthy. First, the client quickly identified the situation as a hot-button one and immediately used a self-instructional self-statement to prepare to cope with it adaptively. This reflects progress in the personal scientist goal of linking antecedents, responses, and consequences. The situation and her developing anger were signals to engage a coping response. She then applied a series of reappraisals to counter some of her more typical, catastrophizing, anger-inducing self-statements. Because the components of the integrated coping response are temporarily conflated, it is often difficult to determine their relative contributions. However, the pattern described above by the client is not unusual. Relaxation can quickly reduce arousal, but reframing the situation with adaptive reappraisals often has more enduring effects.

Review Meditation Practice

Discuss with the client how he or she experienced the meditation practice. Consider any difficulties the client may be experiencing. Common problems such as intrusive thoughts are a perfect *entre* to the later discussion on mindfulness and defusion in this session.

THERAPIST: Were you able to practice the meditation procedure?

CLIENT: Yes, I did it almost every day, but I had some problems and am not sure it works for me. Or maybe I'm not doing it right.

THERAPIST: Tell me what you've experienced.

CLIENT: I get pretty relaxed because of the breathing we've been doing already. Once I even fell asleep. What I have trouble doing is keeping my mind clear. Even when I'm using the word *one*, and especially when I'm doing the second kind with breathing alone, I can't clear my mind. All sorts of thoughts pop into my head, usually about things I should be doing. Once, the image of my mother, who died last year, appeared from nowhere and I became sad. I try, but I can't make them go away. They make me fidgety and nervous. I must be doing something wrong. The other thing that happens is that I get more anxious because I should be doing something instead of wasting time.

THERAPIST: Let me reassure you that your experiences are not at all uncommon. The thoughts that pop into your mind are normal. All meditators experience them, even highly experienced ones. Thoughts are a natural product of the mind, and they're also part of meditation. You're not doing anything wrong. In fact, if you noticed your mind drifting, you're doing the exercise correctly. It isn't the thoughts that are important, but how you relate to them. When intruding thoughts occur, there is no need to fight them off. There is a lot of scientific evidence that trying to suppress thoughts actually intensifies them. Here's a common demonstration: Try as hard as you can *not* to imagine a pink element . . . [wait 5–10 seconds]. Couldn't do it, could you? I have yet to meet anyone who can. I certainly can't. So, in response to thoughts or feelings that come up, simply continue meditating, being aware of the restlessness as you return to the breath.

As for the restlessness and anxiety that come up, it's a perfect example of how difficult it is for us to do nothing. We live frenetic lives that keep us in perpetual motion. Moreover, our environment is filled with vivid media images through the Internet, smartphones, videogames, and hundreds of cable TV channels. With all that stimulation as the new normal, it can be challenging to withdraw into ourselves even briefly. Restlessness can occur as the body and mind unwind in meditation. It takes time to settle down and feel at rest.

One of the things meditation does is to take us from a future-oriented to-do list where we live in our heads into a present focus on the body and the senses, where we are attuned to present experience as it occurs, without evaluation or judgment. This mode of being allows us to connect and experience being alive—and these sensations can provide inner peace. This is what the term *mindfulness* refers to: paying attention to immediate experience in a nonjudgmental manner.

Finally, we see in your concern about doing something wrong the core idea that we've talked about in past sessions that in order to feel worthwhile, you need to do everything right. That automatic thought rears its head in many places. I bring it up now only to increase your awareness of its pervasiveness. So, the bottom line is that you've done nothing wrong and that with continued meditation practice, you'll more easily be able to slip into a present-focused consciousness.

Review the distinction between meditation and the quick muscle relaxation technique in terms of cognitive and somatic relaxation and the benefits to be derived from each method, as illustrated next.

"We'll talk more today about how meditation opens up a number of new techniques for dealing with thoughts and feelings. For now, however, I want to be sure that we're clear about the relation between the muscle relaxation training we started out with and meditation. How do you understand that relationship and how they are best used?"

If the client correctly discriminates between them, verbally reinforce this understanding. If not, reiterate the differences.

"Both muscle relaxation and meditation produce physical relaxation, but meditation also can create a relaxation of the mind. That's why we include meditation in this treatment. You can decide which of the two meditation techniques in the handout works best for you in this regard: the Benson technique with the focus word or the mindfulness technique we will try today, in which we focus on the breath only, without a focus word.

"Another difference is that the muscle relaxation technique is designed to be used quickly in stressful situations to prevent or reduce arousal. By now, one or two breaths may be all it takes to relax. Meditation is a more general stress reduction technique in that you can't usually meditate in a stressful situation, or use it as part of the integrated coping response. I should add, however, that the calm state one develops through repeated meditation practice can be carried anywhere in your life and used as a stress reducer."

As in the group administration, discuss with the client how the meditation practice went and how it was experienced by the client. Make the distinction between meditation and the quick muscle relaxation technique in terms of cognitive and somatic relaxation and the benefits to be derived from each method.

Individual administration also allows the therapist to select, in collaboration with the client, a situation on which to focus the IA portion of the session. Again, the therapist can discuss the details of the self-statements chosen and the client's experiences during IA.

IA with the Integrated Coping Response

In this session, only one IA administration occurs so as to have time for defusion training. Ask the client to choose one stressful event and one or two self-statements from his or her Anti-Stress Log. Then ask the client to vividly imagine the situation and conduct an IA session of 5–8 minutes, as in previous sessions. Try to elicit a high level of arousal and then instruct the client to shut it off using his or her self-statement combined with relaxation (i.e., the integrated coping response). Briefly discuss how the process went, how successful the client was in reducing the arousal, and how many breaths it took. Again, the therapist can discuss the details of the self-statements chosen and the client's experiences during IA.

Introduction to Acceptance Techniques

The introduction of the acceptance and defusion methods represents a change of orientation from active coping as represented in the integrated coping response. The orientation described in the group administration section of this chapter (pp. 237–238) can be used with individual clients, as well as tailored to the client's personal concerns and proclivities identified in the Stress and Coping Diary forms. As an example, consider this orientation to acceptance and defusion for a client whose coping has been characterized by emotional avoidance.

THERAPIST: We're working together because you wanted to learn to deal more effectively with the stress in your life. One of the things that we found from your Stress and Coping Diary entries was a tendency to use the coping strategy of avoidance to deal both with threatening situations and with unpleasant feelings such as anxiety, sadness, and anger. Am I understanding that correctly?

CLIENT: Yes. In my family, we were taught that showing feelings is childish and weak, so I never learned how to deal with my feelings. I just pushed them down and didn't express them even when I felt them. I also learned to avoid situations that could make me feel bad. I worked hard in school so that I wouldn't fail and feel worthless. I looked like a rock from the outside because I never let my insecurities and fears show. I lived in a protective shell.

THERAPIST: What are the benefits of that way of coping?

CLIENT: Some degree of safety from distressing feelings. People also think I'm strong and mature.

THERAPIST: And what are the costs?

CLIENT: I've bottled up my feelings, missed out on lots of things that could have been great, including some romantic relationships. Worst of all, I've felt like a phony, showing a false face to the world. And in the end, I couldn't really escape being stressed. I realized that the costs outweighed the benefits, so I finally decided that I needed to be able to deal with my feelings in a better way.

THERAPIST: And where are things at this point?

CLIENT: I have a ways to go, but I've learned in our sessions that I can let out feelings, although that induction procedure terrified me at first. But the skills I've learned have actually worked. That has been really cool, my being able to use my self-statements and also relax away the emotions.

THERAPIST: I'm pleased that your skills are working for you, and I anticipate that they'll be even more effective as you get more experience in using them. But I want you to have a flexible array of scientifically proven coping skills when we finish. Therefore, I want to introduce you to a different approach to coping that also could work for you, especially in situations where you are forced to tolerate stress responses that you can't otherwise control. And, best of all, this approach is the exact opposite of the avoidance strategies that were so costly for you over the years.

(As in the group format): The new coping strategy is called *acceptance*. In your Stress and Coping Diary, it's one of the coping strategies, and it says, "Acceptance involves simply allowing the presence of stressful thoughts and feelings and waiting for them to pass, rather than trying to control them." Now, this may sound completely incompatible with the active emotion control skills you've been learning in this program, but in reality, they complement one another, proving that there's more than one way to get something done. Now, acceptance, as we'll be using the term, does not mean that you do nothing in the face of stressful situations and simply give up and suffer. Nor does it mean seeking out stressful situations so you can have lots of negative emotions. The form of acceptance I'm going to teach you is a special kind that is based on the mindfulness meditation you've been doing. During meditation, you gain the ability to focus in a nonjudgmental and accepting manner on ordinarily disturbing mental thoughts and images. That perspective can lead to what is called *defusion*. Defusion involves realizing that thoughts are not facts and that the content of thoughts is not the same as reality. The only reality a thought has is as a mental event. In this way, all thoughts are the same. This perspective strips thoughts of their capacity to spiral into negative streams that trigger distress. Instead of avoiding negative thoughts and feelings, you can learn to accept their temporary presence without negative evaluation, and by so doing, become more emotionally free and less constricted.

Today, with your permission, I would like to teach you some specific acceptance and defusion techniques that can help you distance yourself mentally from these events. But before we begin, do you have any questions or concerns?

If not, let me elaborate a bit on these ideas and tell you what we know scientifically about mindfulness and acceptance. Scientists who study physical pain make an important distinction between *pain* and *suffering*. They say that there are two aspects to our experience of pain. One involves the basic sensations from pain receptors that are sent into the spinal cord and brain. The other is the brain's appraisal of those sensations and the resulting emotions. The sensations alone are painful, but when they're fused with the appraisal of how much they hurt and the negative emotional reaction, they create suffering. The more negatively people appraise the sensations and the more they catastrophize about them, and the more they suffer.

Studies have compared champion marathon runners with novices on how they handle the discomfort of exertion as the race progresses. As discomfort begins, both the novices and the champions often distract themselves by focusing their attention outside of their bodies, studying trees, watching clouds in the sky, counting their steps, and so on. Eventually, however, the discomfort becomes too much to ignore. When that happens, the novices continue to try distraction, but it no longer works and they hit what is called "the wall." But the experts shift to a new mode, focusing on and accepting their sensations of physical discomfort in a detached, nonjudgmental manner. They are better able to tolerate the discomfort and even use it to pace themselves during the late portions of the marathon. Lots of research has shown that people can learn to uncouple pain sensations from negative appraisals and thereby increase their pain tolerance, sometimes even doubling the amount of pain they can tolerate. It's the meaning that counts.

Today, then, we're going to use the intruding thoughts that happen during meditation to practice some techniques for acknowledging thoughts while staying with your breathing. We're going to do a mindfulness meditation technique that is similar in many ways to the Benson technique, except that you focus only on your breath without using the focus word (such as *one*). I'm going to interrupt the process occasionally to allow you to experience different ways of watching and distancing yourself from your thoughts. When I do, keep your eyes closed and try to maintain your meditative state, *going with* the experience I suggest to see how it feels to you. In this area, different things work best for different folks. What all the experiences I suggest will have in common is that you should not try to change the thoughts or even judge them, but simply accept them as some of the more than 50,000 thoughts that will come and go through your mind today.

Let's begin. Sit up straight in your chair, close your eyes and get comfortable, and relax. Focus on your breathing as you breathe down into your stomach, effortlessly. . . . Feel the sensations of the cool air passing into your nostrils and down your throat and the warmth of the air that you exhale. Each time you exhale, let your body relax even more.

During the defusion exercises, the therapist can check in with the client on his or her experiences. Do the same three exercises as with groups: (1) Monitoring and Labeling Thoughts, (2) White-Room Meditation, and (3) Letting Go of Thoughts. Discuss the client's experiences during these exercises, and then restate the rationale for their inclusion in the treatment.

"These techniques come in handy if you get a bit overwhelmed and it's hard to use your integrated coping response. However, these mindfulness techniques are effective in their own right, and some people adopt them as primary rather than as fallback skills. Again, the guideline is, use whatever works best for you. The only way to know, however, is to give each of them a chance.

"To build on what we did today, I have a new handout for you that deals with mindfulness, acceptance, and defusion. It provides guidelines on how you can practice these methods of dealing with negative feelings and intrusive thoughts."

Homework Assignments

The out-of-session assignments are the same as for the group protocol. Present a brief introduction and the rationale for each one.

1. The client should continue to practice the integrated coping response during imagined stressful encounters and in real-life situations. Imaginal rehearsal can be done on a daily basis.
2. Give the client the Mindfulness, Acceptance, and Defusion handout (Handout A-5) and ask him or her to practice the mindfulness and defusion techniques described therein, preferably on a daily basis.
3. The client should update the Anti-Stress Log and coping cards.

POTENTIAL TREATMENT ISSUE

Control-Based Coping and Mindfulness/Acceptance: Contradictory or Complementary?

It is understandable that some clients view the active integrated coping response and the acceptance and defusion techniques as incompatible. We take pains to present them as alternative strategies ("more than one way to get something done") and to encourage clients to learn and apply both sets of skills in their appropriate contexts. We regard acceptance as a coping strategy in its own right. As pointed out by Hayes et al. (2014), "Acceptance is not passive tolerance or resignation but an *intentional behavior* that alters the function of inner experiences from events to be avoided to a focus of interest, curiosity, and observation" (p. 185; emphasis added). Acceptance represents a *volitional cognitive shift* from the content of the thought to the process of thinking it.

One analogy that might be helpful to clients in how and when to use the various coping strategies is to liken negative thoughts and feelings to a headache. If one has a headache that reacts positively to taking an aspirin, little is to be gained by adopting an acceptance strategy. However, if the headache is a severe one that does not react positively to a medication, then acceptance-based techniques can be an effective strategy to lessen the suffering (negative affect) component of the pain by distancing oneself psychologically from the aversive internal stimuli (McCracken & Vowles, 2014). The same is true of aversive thoughts and affective responses. Thus, the inclusion of mindfulness and acceptance helps expand clients' coping repertoire in a manner that can enhance the ability to respond effectively to the many varieties of stressors they are likely to encounter in their lives.

CHAPTER 9

Session 6: Coping Skills Rehearsal and Additional Cognitive-Behavioral Strategies

ABOUT SESSION 6

The last session of CASMT includes a final IA rehearsal using the integrated coping response, plus a second induction in which mindful acceptance and defusion are practiced in the presence of arousal. We teach a simple distraction technique as an additional coping strategy and add a cautionary note on the use of emotional suppression and avoidance. We also provide brief instruction in how to self-administer desensitization and covert rehearsal techniques as additional posttreatment training methods that can further enhance coping resources.

Finally, a brief relapse prevention element is presented to prepare participants to deal with unsuccessful coping episodes. It can be anticipated that no matter how well they have learned the targeted coping skills, there will be instances in which clients either apply them ineffectively or are overwhelmed by stressful situations. We want to be sure that occasional lapses in coping success do not cause participants to suffer an inappropriate decrease in self-efficacy or to abandon the coping strategies they have learned in the program.

OVERVIEW

Training Objectives

1. Final administrations of IA to rehearse the integrated coping response and practice defusion under IA.

2. Describe additional self-directed procedures, including distraction, self-desensitization, and covert rehearsal based on stress inoculation training.
3. Provide relapse prevention tips.

Session Outline

- Assignments check-up
  - Discussion of clients' stress and coping experiences
- Program summary and orientation to Session 6
- IA with the integrated coping response (as in Session 5)
- Rehearsal of acceptance techniques under IA
  - Discussion of acceptance rehearsal
- Distraction: The 5-4-3-2-1 technique
  - Caution: Avoidance and suppression as maladaptive coping strategies
- Self-desensitization and mental rehearsal
- Relapse prevention
- Final comments

Materials Needed

1. Self-Desensitization and Mental Rehearsal (Handout A-6)
2. Self-desensitization anxiety and anger stimulus hierarchies (Table B-2)

GROUP ADMINISTRATION

Assignments Check-Up

Discussion of Clients' Stress and Coping Experiences

Check with the group on how their attempts to use their skills in real life have been working. Again, reinforce successful attempts and efforts. Emphasize that not everything they try will be immediately successful, and that strategies that work on one occasion may be less effective on another.

Program Summary and Orientation to Session 6

"In the preceding five sessions and in the weeks between sessions, you've been exposed to a program of coping skills training designed to increase your ability to manage stress in your lives. You've learned an integrated coping response containing statements and muscle relaxation tied into your breath cycle. You've learned how to analyze and change self-defeating thoughts that cause distress, and how to talk to yourself to focus attention on the task at hand to keep stress under control. You have developed an Anti-Stress Log of stress-reducing statements to use before, during, and after stressful situations. You've practiced reducing the emotional arousal that I've helped you experience during our sessions, and the success that you've experienced should give you confidence in your ability to control the mind–body stress response. In the last two sessions you learned some meditation, mindfulness, and acceptance techniques, such as defusion, that can be used to psychologically distance yourself from distressing thoughts, feelings, and body sensations.

"Every strategy and skill we've covered is supported by research. That same research, plus our own experience, tells us that different people favor different techniques over others. You probably already have favorites. However, I want to stress how important it is to have a set of skills that you can apply flexibly in different situations. For example, if you're too stressed to use the integrated coping response skills, the best strategy may be nonjudgmental acceptance of your temporary thoughts and feelings.

"Today, for a final time, we're going to start by practicing the integrated coping response to reduce emotional arousal that I'll help you get into. We'll also try out some the acceptance techniques that you learned in the last session. Then, I'm going to introduce you to some additional stress management techniques. All of these will be covered in greater detail in the handouts I'll give you. You can practice them on your own and use them in your lives. Scientific studies show that people can learn to apply these techniques on the basis of self-help written materials. We want your learning of stress management techniques to continue after you leave this program so that you can expand your personal coping resources."

IA with the Integrated Coping Response (as in Session 5)

Ask clients to select a stressful situation and a stress-reducing statement. Then, using the IA procedure as in Sessions 3 through 5, have clients practice their integrated coping response. Afterward, discuss briefly how it went for them. Encourage clients to continue their search for self-statements that are best suited to them and to the situations they encounter, for both are highly personal.

Rehearsal of Acceptance Techniques under IA

In a second IA administration, we provide practice of how to use mindfulness and acceptance to let go of stress-related cognitions and emotions during induced affect.

"Now, I want to use this emotion-arousing technique to let you apply the acceptance and thought-distancing strategies we discussed last session. I hope you practiced these during the week. Recall that both approaches involve becoming aware of thoughts and regarding them as temporary products of your mind rather than as reality. We tried some distancing techniques in that last session. In one, you imagined the thoughts as leaves falling into a stream and floating away. In another, you imagined the thoughts falling into the palm of your hand and then being released by turning your hand over or opening your fingers. Do you remember those?

"Now, for just a few minutes, I'd like you to return to the stressful scene you just imagined for the integrated coping response. Once again imagine it as vividly as you can and get in touch with the feeling you experienced. Once again, just focus on that feeling and let it begin to grow stronger. That's good . . . just let it get bigger and bigger, more and more intense. Let that feeling grow again all by itself as you let it become more intense. [Continue induction for 60 seconds.]

"I'd like you to stay with that situation and that feeling and focus carefully on any hot thoughts about that scene that come into your mind. When such a thought occurs, say to yourself, 'My mind is having a thought that . . . ' and state what the thought is (e.g., "I'm overloaded with things to do"). Don't judge the thought. Instead, tell yourself that it is 'just a thought.' Do that with each thought that comes into your mind." [Continue for 60 seconds.]

Instruct clients to return to imagining the scene and do a brief IA to increase arousal so that the letting-go-of-thoughts strategies can be experienced in the presence of a thought that is likely to be affect-laden. Continue for 2 minutes.

"Now, imagine that stressful scene once again and let that feeling grow. As a thought appears, imagine you're sitting on the bank of a beautiful mountain stream. To your right is a bend in the stream. When a thought arrives, imagine that it is a leaf that slowly floats down and lands in the stream. The leaf is caught by the current and is swept away around the bend in the stream, where it disappears from view.

"As the next thought appears, say, 'My mind is saying that . . . ' Then see the thought appear as print on a helium balloon and release the string so that the balloon floats away into the sky. Do that with each thought that comes to mind. [Continue for 60 seconds.]

"Focus again on that feeling and let it grow, stronger and stronger. . . . The next time a thought appears, see it attach itself to a billboard that you are approaching as you drive down the highway. Watch it pass out of sight as you drive past the billboard. [Continue for 60 seconds.]

"Now, turn your hand so that your palm is facing upward. Once again, as you imagine that stressful situation and a hot thought appears, let it fall down into your hand, then turn your palm downward or open your fingers and watch it drop out of your hand and out of sight. [Continue for 60 seconds.]

"Now, letting that feeling remain and letting the associated thoughts float into your conscious mind, use whichever technique you like best to release it." [Continue for 60 seconds.]

Discussion of Acceptance Rehearsal

"What was that like for you? Were you able to get into a feeling? Were you able to experience the thoughts associated with that situation and feeling? Did any of the distancing techniques work for you? My goal here was simply to try to give you an experience of using the acceptance techniques with some emotional arousal present to demonstrate this acceptance and mindfulness approach to dealing with stressful thoughts. These techniques are also in the handout I gave you last week, so you can practice them on your own.

"The techniques themselves are not very complicated, but because this way of dealing with thoughts and feelings is so different from the integrated coping response approach, it can take some time to master. But, as I said earlier, there's much research evidence that this approach works. It may be particularly useful if you encounter a situation in which your stress-reducing self-statements don't do the job. Some of our clients like the acceptance approach to coping so much that they make it their preferred coping skill."

As noted earlier, the acceptance/defusion techniques derived from ACT have been added recently as additional coping strategies. Postintervention feedback from our clients has been quite positive. However, we have no dismantling studies to assess the incremental benefits of adding these techniques.

Distraction: The 5-4-3-2-1 Technique

"So far, you've learned two different sets of stress management approaches. The first set involves active control, as in the integrated coping response. The other set includes mindfulness- and acceptance-based techniques that allow you to distance yourself from the thoughts. There is yet another approach that is useful under high-stress conditions, and that is distraction. It's based on the simple principle that we can't attend to more than one thing at a time (although we can switch our attention rapidly from one thing to another). If your attention is directed to something going on inside you, you're not attending to what's outside yourself. If I ask you what you're thinking right now and what sensations you can feel in your stomach, you'll direct attention there. If I ask you what color the wall is and what I'm wearing today, you'll direct your attention toward me, and you'll stop attending to what's inside.

"Research has shown that when people are stressed, their attention turns to negative thoughts and the internal physical sensations they are having. You've probably had this experience many times. People can become so focused on their internal thoughts and feelings that they don't process other information very well. That's one reason people with high levels of test anxiety perform poorly on tests. They often make mistakes because they don't process the test questions well or remember information they actually do know. The same thing happens with athletes who have high performance anxiety. Still another example involves getting angry: People who get very angry can lose the ability to process social cues that would keep them from acting in a hostile manner. When we're faced with a really disturbing situation, a good strategy can be to get out of our heads and our gut reactions by redirecting our attention elsewhere.

"Today I want to show you a simple strategy that directs your attention away from distressing thoughts and feelings and also creates a more relaxed state. It's called the 5-4-3-2-1 technique, and it involves directing your attention to things you see, hear, and feel in other (nonemotional) parts of your body. Breathe into your stomach, and with each breath, focus on something you see. Say to yourself in a slow, gentle rhythm with each breath, one at a time, five things you see, then five things you hear, then five things you feel in parts of your body that are not emotionally aroused, such as your feet. You can stop here or go on to say to yourself four things you see, four things you hear, four things you feel. Next, say three things you see, three things you hear, three things you feel in other parts of your body. Then two of each, and finally one of each. You'll find yourself repeating a lot, and that's fine. You can do this while sitting or in any other situation, such as while walking or waiting for a bus. Let me demonstrate for you. [Sit in a chair, adjust your posture, take a deep breath, fix your gaze, and begin, focusing on whatever might be present in your setting. The following is an example.]

"I see the picture on the wall, I see the trees out the window, I see the chairs in the room, I see the lamp in the corner, I see the white ceiling overhead. I hear the sound of my own voice, I hear the traffic outside, I hear the hum of the building's air conditioner, I hear the sound in the hallway outside the room, I hear the sound of an airplane flying over. I feel the chair supporting me, I feel my feet on the floor, I feel my watchband on my wrist, I feel my glasses on my nose. I feel the coolness of the air. I've now done five of each sense—vision, hearing, and touch stimuli. Now, let's return to the exercise and do four of each, then three, then two, then one. Or, I can just go along noticing what I'm noticing, and continue to relax and breathe deeply and evenly without the exercise.

"Like all the techniques we've learned, distraction has its place in some situations and not in others. For example, distraction should not be used in situations where you have to attend closely to the task at hand or have to process incoming information. In such situations, distraction could impair your performance."

Caution: Avoidance and Suppression as Maladaptive Coping Strategies

Given the empirical evidence concerning the undesirable consequences of habitual experiential avoidance and emotional suppression (as reviewed in Chapter 3), it is important to encourage clients to use the active coping skills they have learned in the CASMT program together with the acceptance-based methods as alternatives to avoidance.

"Today I want to talk about some other things that have implications for how we handle stress. One is the topic of avoidance. [If the Stress and Coping Diary was used, mention here that avoidance is one of the coping strategies that clients have been tracking on it.] We all tend to avoid things that we find unpleasant. Sometimes, avoidance is a perfectly fine strategy. For example, you might decide to simply avoid interacting with an obnoxious person, or you may decide to avoid an activity that you do not enjoy. That's okay as long as avoidance doesn't have other costs for you.

"A major principle in psychology is that behavior is affected by its consequences. If we are successful in avoiding something unpleasant, we get an immediate feeling of relief. This relief strengthens the avoidance response, leading you to avoid the unpleasant person or situation even more in the future. So when you avoid X, your difficulty in confronting and dealing with X becomes even stronger.

"Now, it is reasonable to avoid certain things that you fear. For example, I've avoided sky diving because jumping out of a plane would be very anxiety-provoking for me, but avoidance of sky diving is no big deal because passing on it has no negative effects on my life. But avoiding social situations or avoiding driving a car because of fear would negatively affect my life. It would not be in my best interest. You have to decide if what you are avoiding is negatively affecting your life. Is it really in your best interest to continue to avoid this X? If you make yourself face feared situations, especially if you do so in gradual steps, your fear will decrease. I'll show you a way to do that a bit later today.

"Another costly coping strategy is that of blocking or suppressing your emotions. There a time and place where that might be helpful, as in an emergency when you have to keep your head and focus on the task at hand. But habitual emotional suppression has negative effects on both physical and emotional well-being, and it has social costs as well. It keeps you from being genuine in your relationships and gets in the way of acknowledging and solving problems. The stored-up feelings boil beneath the surface and are associated with both medical and psychological problems.

"This is where your new coping skills can help you. They make it easier to face the things you might be inclined to avoid or the feelings that you would otherwise suppress. You do have to face problems in order to overcome them. Hopefully, in this program, you've developed some coping skills that can make these situations easier to deal with."

In this final session, we also provide guidelines for several other coping strategies that many of our clients report finding helpful in our post-training follow-up contacts.

Self-Desensitization and Mental Rehearsal

"I want to tell you about another technique that's proven successful in reducing the stressfulness of situations. It's a procedure called *desensitization*. Desensitization means that we strip a troublesome situation of its capacity to be stressful, sort of like an allergy shot desensitizes us to an allergen.

"Desensitization procedures have been used very successfully to help people get over phobias involving such things as heights, airplane travel, snakes, water, and so on. In addition to fear and anxiety, it's also been used to help people reduce anger. A nice feature of this treatment is that people can do it successfully on their own, without professional assistance, using the very coping skills you've already developed. I'm going to give you a handout with some examples to take with you, but let me briefly describe how it's done.

"One way to get yourself to face feared things more easily is to start by vividly imagining yourself approaching the stressful situation in gradual steps while you practice your coping response. This is called *self-desensitization*. Here's how you do it:

"First, select situations in your life that are challenging, particularly those that you have to encounter repeatedly. These can be situations that produce anxiety, anger, or other emotions. From your out-of-session assignments (Stress and Coping Diary or Analyzing Thoughts and Feelings form), you've learned about the situations that push your buttons.

"Let's say that there's a situation in your life that tends to elicit anger or anxiety in you. Create some scenes involving that type of situation that elicit varying degrees of anger or anxiety. Make a list of those scenes, ordering them from the least (bottom) to the most (top) stressful. This list is called a *situation hierarchy*. Here are some examples of anxiety-arousing and anger-inducing hierarchies that come from the handout I'm going to give you today. [Display hierarchies in Appendix B, Table B-2, by PowerPoint or hard copy.] Notice how they are arranged from the least difficult situation on the bottom to the most difficult one at the top.

"Always start with the least-arousing event. Imagine it while also focusing on signs of distress in your body and on any stress-inducing self-statements that might apply. When you've gotten into the feeling, apply an integrated coping response to it with a stress-reducing statement on inhalation, and relaxation on exhalation. See yourself doing the integrated coping response in the situation.

"When the feeling has been reduced, then imagine yourself behaving effectively in the situation—for example, speaking calmly rather than becoming angry, or acting effectively in a situation that causes you anxiety. You can observe yourself handling the situation from the outside, as if you were someone else. For example, see yourself responding calmly in a job interview and saying just what you'd like to say to the interviewer in order to get the job. Then imagine that the interviewer hires you. This combination of mental rehearsal techniques allows you to reduce the emotional arousal and rehearse an effective way of handling the situation at the same time. When you feel comfortable with this first imagined situation, you can proceed to the next scene in the hierarchy, and so on up to the top. This can be done in multiple sessions; you need not do the whole hierarchy at one sitting. If you find it too difficult to move up to a new hierarchy scene, insert an intermediate scene between them that you can handle.

"Self-desensitization is even more effective if you include some real-life practice after you have done the imagined practice. By putting yourself in relevant real-life situations and applying your coping responses, these situations lose their power to create uncontrollable negative feelings. Create a gradual hierarchy of actual situations, and then use your stress and coping skills at every step. For example, one college student who had severe social anxiety created a series of real-life situations that started with simply making eye contact with another passing student on campus while remaining relaxed, then saying hello to someone she passed while going to class (guaranteeing that she wouldn't have to converse), then saying hello to a person in her class, and then initiating a conversation about a class assignment with a fellow student. She chose controllable situations and used her favorite integrated coping response, in which she said to herself, 'I'm in control . . . so . . . relax.' She had used this coping response before, while imagining each of the real-life situations. Through this careful process, she gradually worked her way up the hierarchy and became less socially anxious."

Relapse Prevention

"At the start of our work together, I told you that you were going to become more effective in managing life stress, but that you were never going to be stress-free. I've also emphasized that managing stress is a complex thing and that what works in one situation may not work in another. Sometimes the best approach is to do something to change the situation and solve the problem. Other times, we can't control the situation, but we can change our reactions to it if we can manage our thoughts and physiological responses. Then there are times when the best bet may be to simply accept and tolerate our thoughts and feelings, but get some psychological distance from them with techniques like mindful acceptance. That's why we want you to have a flexible set of strategies at your disposal and the ability to apply them effectively.

"When people try to make changes in their lives, they can become discouraged if they sometimes falter. They can lose confidence in their ability to change and abandon their efforts to change. Scientists who study people who abuse substances call this the *abstinence violation effect*. It's when a lapse (a one-time misstep like returning to drinking and getting intoxicated on one occasion) becomes a full-blown relapse back into the original problem, such as uncontrolled drinking. Relapse prevention is a key goal in this treatment and in virtually every area of behavior change. A lapse back into anxiety and stress is simply that. It doesn't mean the treatment doesn't work or can't work, or that you are a hopeless failure. Instead, a lapse is an opportunity to learn how to more effectively deal with problem situations. It gives you the information you need to make adjustments. Research shows that if people can view a lapse in that way, they can avoid a full-blown relapse and reduce the likelihood of future lapses. When you learn from experience, you increase your self-control. The lapse becomes a blessing in disguise rather than something that triggers complete relapse.

"In this regard, I'd like to quote from John Wooden (Wooden & Jamison, 2010), the most successful college basketball coach of all time. Wooden coached his UCLA team to 10 national championships in 12 years, a record that still stands. Two aspects of his philosophy are especially noteworthy. First, he said, 'Success is peace of mind, a peace that comes from knowing that you've done your best to become the best that you are capable of becoming. No one can do more' [p. 33]. Wooden said that he never mentioned winning games, only giving maximum effort.

"Second, he told his players not to fear making mistakes. He said, 'Mistakes are the stepping stones to achievement, for they give us the feedback we need to improve performance' [p. 41]. He also said, 'The only true failure is the failure to learn from our mistakes' [p. 41]."

Final Comments

"We've come to the end of our final session, but I want to invite you to ask any questions you have or make any comments on your experience. We've covered a lot of ground and introduced you to many different coping skills, some of which may have been more useful for some folks than for others. I'd be interested in what you think worked well or didn't work as well for you. Also, I'd appreciate any suggestions you might have for how the program could have been more valuable for you.

[Following any discussion that ensues, distribute the handouts.] "I hope that you'll use the handouts I've given you in the future. Many people have reported that doing so helps them continue to develop their skills and perhaps to remind them of something they had not yet tried out in their lives.

"It is my hope that the skills you've learned in this program will help you deal more effectively with the challenges that arise in your life, and that these life skills will help you to become the best that you're capable of becoming. It's been a privilege to share this part of your journey with you."

Distribute the handout on Self-Desensitization and Mental Rehearsal (Handout A-6). It can also be helpful to clients to provide a nicely bound copy of all of the handouts so that they have a compendium of all resource materials to refer to or make copies from in the future.

If you plan to offer booster sessions, provide the required information and invite the participants to sign up. A follow-up letter or e-mail invitation in advance of the booster session(s) would be highly appropriate.

INDIVIDUAL ADMINISTRATION

There is only a limited opportunity to practice defusion in the group administration, and this kind of IA application might best be done in an individual administration that goes beyond six sessions. At this point, we have no research that has integrated IA into a mindfulness framework, but we expect, on theoretical grounds, that the technique could be useful in practicing mindfulness and acceptance skills under conditions of actual arousal. We regard this possibility as a topic worthy of future empirical attention.

In individual administration, clients can be assisted with the self-desensitization process introduced in Session 6, particularly with hierarchy construction, and they can be given introductory experiences in the process to supplement the Session 4 out-of-session homework in applying the integrated coping response using imaginal exposure to stressful events.

POTENTIAL TREATMENT ISSUES

Are Six Sessions Enough?

All interventions include an important issue regarding the dose–response relationship—that is, the question of how many sessions are needed to activate the mechanisms of change and thereby achieve a desired outcome. This issue has been the topic of much research, originally inspired by the work of Howard, Kopta, Krause, and Orlinsky (1986), who reported a negatively accelerating function in which about half of clients improve markedly with roughly eight sessions, with smaller improvements occurring thereafter to about 26 sessions. Subsequent analyses of dose–response relationships across a variety of therapies have indicated that substantial effects occur within a relatively small number of sessions, especially in mildly stressed individuals. Hansen, Lambert, and Forman (2002) analyzed a sample of randomized clinical trials ranging from three to around 25 sessions, and found that between 58 and 67% of patients improved within an average of 12.7 treatment sessions. Mildly dysphoric clients improved as much in eight sessions of CBT as in 16. Finally, in a large-scale analysis of results in a university counseling center sample of 4,676 clients, seen by 204 therapists, 100% of improvement in Outcome Questionnaire–45 scores occurred within the first 10 sessions, and 95% within the first six sessions (Baldwin, Berkeljon, Atkins, Olsen, & Nielsen, 2009). Newman, Kenardy, Herman, and Taylor (1997) found four sessions of CBT, supplemented by the use of palmtop computers for self-assessment and practicing therapy techniques, to be a close match for a longer 12-session therapy protocol in the treatment of panic disorder. Other examples of brief and efficacious interventions focused on specific disorders are a one-session exposure treatment for specific phobias (Ollendick & Davis, 2013; Öst, 1989) and a five-session treatment for panic disorder (Otto et al., 2012).

The dose–response question is an important one for us as treatment developers, and one for which we have no empirical data. In working with individual clients, we often extend the number of sessions to ensure that each leaves at the end of the treatment with a sufficient mastery of the program's coping skills. In addition to a more extensive application of cognitive restructuring, the recent addition of a mindfulness and acceptance component may very well warrant such an extension if the therapist wishes to place greater emphasis on those components. As noted earlier, the "six-session" format presented in Chapters 4 through 9 can also be seen as a flexible "six-phase" intervention. Finally, we should note that although CASMT is designed for one session per week, successful outcomes have been achieved with two sessions per week over a three-week period (Chen, 2015; Smith & Nye, 1989). However, the weekly format obviously creates more time and opportunity to develop and practice coping skills.

Promoting Posttreatment Gains and Generalization

The CASMT program focuses on the acquisition and rehearsal of coping skills. In order for the intervention to achieve its intended effects, the acquired skills must generalize beyond the treatment context to the real world. It is therefore important to emphasize to clients the importance of continuing to practice their skills in their daily lives so that they do not regress into ineffective past habits as their skills fall into disuse. In a sense, all treatments can be seen as attempts to "jump-start" more adaptive modes of responding that will be reinforced and strengthened as response-contingent positive consequences occur outside of therapy.

In the final phase of treatment, reviewing with clients the process of training, what they have learned, and the successes they have reported can contextualize not only what has occurred, but can also help enhance their coping self-efficacy—a major predictor of future effective behavior (Bandura, 1997).

When the intervention proper is ended, the therapist can continue to serve as a resource for the client. In both the group and individual format, booster sessions can be arranged, and even are advised. For groups, 1, 3, and 6 months are appropriate intervals for booster sessions. These sessions often reveal that the stressors clients are facing have changed, sometimes as a result of their own improved coping strategies. For example, a client whose social anxiety has improved may have been able to initiate a romantic relationship in which interpersonal difficulties have now arisen. Booster sessions can (1) provide useful reviews of the concepts and coping methods covered in previous training, (2) provide feedback regarding clients' posttreatment progress in refining coping skills, and (3) allow for troubleshooting ways of confronting new challenges. These sessions also offer opportunities to reinforce clients for their successes, ensure that they make internal attributions for their progress, and increase feelings of competence and self-efficacy. Discouraged clients can again be reminded that coping skills, like physical skills, often reach plateaus in which no further progress seems to be occurring, followed by subsequent gains as further practice occurs.

In booster sessions for groups, those who report success also serve as coping models for other members. However, trainers should discourage negative social comparison with others by emphasizing that everyone is different and has a specific set of life circumstances with which to deal. Although clients have learned some valuable coping skills, they are, and will continue to be, works in progress.

A booster session arranged in advance with an individual client allows the client to maintain a connection with the therapist as a source of professional and social support. Therapists may also have an open-door policy that invites clients to contact them if needed, as in other forms of treatment.

Motivational Factors, Attributions of Change, and Relapse Prevention

Many factors affect the maintenance of gains in behavior change interventions. Even when treatments are initially successful, posttreatment changes may not persist because clients do not continue to utilize the adaptive behaviors they have acquired in the intervention (Antony, Ledley, & Heimberg, 2005). This lack of longer-term utilization can occur for a number of reasons. Sometimes naturalistic environmental contingencies are not strong enough to maintain changes. For example, a client's new ability to control anger responses may upset the relational equilibrium in a relationship or family system characterized by mutually hostile interchanges, prompting more intense provocations.

Another factor involves the client's motivation for change. In Chapter 6, we described the transtheoretical model advanced by Prochaska and DiClemente (1984) and its relevance to the ability of clients to profit from a program that requires out-of-session assignments, such as CASMT. Clients at the contemplation stage, though participating in a program such as CASMT, may fail to commit themselves to homework assignments, or they may show uneven compliance with the program. In the action stage, clients are committed and actively involved in behavior change efforts both within and outside of the treatment context. The maintenance stage requires continued compliance with the program to improve and solidify the newly acquired coping skills as clients proceed toward the final stage of termination. At this point, the skills have (ideally) become ingrained and are under sufficient personal control that stress management is both improved and permanent.

Most clients who seek out stress management training are at least at the precontemplation stage, acknowledging that stress is having negative impacts on their lives and that it is worth looking into a program. From the first session on, we make it very clear that in order for the program to be helpful to them, clients will need to take personal responsibility for doing what is required to learn the coping skills we teach. The initial goal is to move such clients from precontemplation and preparation into the action stage, where they are committing themselves to attending sessions and doing the out-of-session training assignments. Early failures to comply with homework assignments should be explored and addressed promptly and assertively by the therapist, for they are an opportunity to move pre-action-phase clients into the action stage where they can help themselves develop stress resilience. Likewise, the importance of continually emphasizing and reinforcing self-attributed gains cannot be overemphasized. To the extent that clients attribute positive behavioral changes to their own efforts and skills, rather than to external factors (including what the therapist "did to them"), they increase the likelihood that the changes will be maintained (Bandura, 1997).

No matter how well stress management skills have been learned, clients are certain to encounter new situations in which their attempts at emotion regulation are unsuccessful, either because the situation is too demanding or because there is a mismatch between the demands and the coping strategy that is applied. It is essential to emphasize frequently to clients that these failed attempts can be anticipated and should not be an occasion for attributions of personal inadequacy or hopelessness. Rather, each failed attempt provides an opportunity to learn more about the features of high-risk situations and the development of action plans to deal with such situations in the future. Emphasize the importance of flexibility in selecting and applying coping strategies so that clients can minimize such mismatches. Properly appraised, lapse experiences can be a source of resilience as clients learn that by persisting in their coping strategies, they can bounce back from setbacks. Interventions like CASMT are not designed to make people "stress proof." As emphasized both in the CASMT sessions and in the resource materials, the goal is not to eliminate stress from clients' lives, but to increase their personal resourcefulness and resilience in the face of the inevitable demands of living.

APPENDIX A

Handouts and Forms for Clients

There are numerous sources of stress in modern life. Occupational demands, time pressures, and stresses in our personal lives all contribute to what has come to be called the "Age of Anxiety." There is mounting evidence that life stress has a strong negative impact on physical and psychological well-being. Many illnesses have been linked to stress, including high blood pressure, stroke, asthma, heart attacks, and ulcers. People who suffer from stress perform less efficiently on their jobs and at school, are more accident-prone, and are more likely to suffer from physical ailments. Although few of us can totally avoid stressful circumstances, we can learn to cope more effectively with them.

This Stress Management Training Program trains people to cope more effectively with stress. In this educational program, people learn both mental and physical coping skills to use in stressful situations. In this way, people gain increased control over their emotional responses and an increased ability to adapt to the demands of their daily lives.

Stress responses have both mental and physical elements. The mental elements include what people tell themselves about the stressful situation and their plans to cope with it. In important ways, these mental responses determine how stressful the situation will be for the person. People also react physically to stressful situations. Reactions include increased heart rate, blood pressure, muscle tension, and respiration. Stress hormones pour into the bloodstream and produce a state of physiological arousal. The body mobilizes its resources to cope with the stressor, which in turn places an increased demand on the body.

The above description of stress suggests that people can learn to cope with stress at both the mental and the physical levels. In the Stress Management Training Program you will learn both types of coping skills. First you will learn how to prevent or reduce the body's stress response by using deep muscle relaxation. You will be trained to detect tension in your body as soon as it begins to develop and to relax your muscles as a way to counteract the tension. On a mental level, you will learn to identify stress-producing statements you tell yourself and to replace them with stress-reducing statements. You will practice using these coping skills to control stress by imagining and reexperiencing stressful situations. You will find that such practice will help you cope more effectively with stress in real-life situations. You will also be taught two easily learned meditation techniques you can use daily to create a tranquil mental state as well as bodily changes that reduce stress and promote physical well-being.

(continued)

The Stress Management Training Program consists of six sessions, each lasting approximately an hour. You will also receive take-home materials that allow you to learn and practice the stress management coping skills. Doing the out-of-session assignments is essential to your success in the program.

Schedule of Training Sessions*

- *Session 1.* Orientation and muscle relaxation training. The nature of emotion and stress is discussed, as is the nature of coping with stress. Training is begun in deep muscular relaxation, which serves as a physical coping response.

- *Session 2.* Continuation of muscle relaxation training and discussion of the relationship between thoughts and feelings. Implications for coping with stress.

- *Session 3.* Practice in muscle relaxation and stress-reducing self-statements. These are used to control emotions induced during the session through the imagining of stressful situations. Continued development of mental coping skills.

- *Session 4.* Practice in muscle relaxation and stress-reducing self-statements to control emotions induced through imagination. Introduction to mindfulness meditation.

- *Session 5.* Continued practice of muscle relaxation with mental coping skills. Emphasis on application to actual life situations. Instruction in mindfulness stress reduction exercises.

- *Session 6.* Rehearsal of coping skills, summary of main principles, and description of procedures that can be used to build on the stress management program, including self-administered exercises.

---

*Take-home materials for coping skills practice and out-of-session training assignments will be provided for each session.

We respond to stressful events mentally, physically, and behaviorally. Physically, we are wired by nature to have a "fight or flight" response. It mobilizes our body to act in emergencies. The state of physical arousal that results is familiar to all of us. It involves increases in heart rate, respiration, and muscle tension. In an actual emergency, this physical arousal would help us flee or fight, but most of the stressors we experience are psychological, not physical. Thus, this response of arousal is not helpful, in addition to being unpleasant, and it can negatively affect our health and ability to act effectively.

You can learn to counter the physical aspects of stress in two important ways. The first is by learning to regulate your breathing. The second is by learning to relax your muscles to counteract tension. In both procedures, we ask you to choose and say a cue word, such as *relax* or *calm*, as you breathe and relax. With enough practice, this word will become a way to quickly relax. Because you can't be tense and relaxed at the same time, muscle relaxation becomes a powerful method for controlling the stress response.

Breath Training

Breathing comes naturally, so it may surprise you to learn that it plays such an important role in stress control. There are two breathing patterns that have very different effects. One involves breathing into the chest (often shallowly and rapidly). This is technically called *thoracic breathing*, and it is part of the stress response. The most extreme example occurs in hyperventilation, when rapid thoracic breathing decreases levels of body-calming carbon dioxide and increases muscle tension in the chest, shoulders, and neck regions. It can also produce feelings of lightheadedness, weakness, and anxiety.

The other form of breathing is called *abdominal breathing*, where the breath is taken into the stomach instead of the chest. This type of breathing occurs when someone is relaxed or asleep (and it is how babies naturally breathe). It has a calming influence on the body. This type of breathing is easy to learn and apply.

To experience the difference between chest and abdominal breathing, try the following: Place one hand over the center of your chest and the other over your navel. First, inhale in such a way that the top hand moves as you inhale, whereas the bottom one does not. Do this five times. Then reverse the procedure. Imagine that there's a

(continued)

bright red balloon in your stomach. Breathe in slowly; see and feel the balloon fill. Then slowly let the air out as you exhale; see and feel the balloon deflate.

Notice the sensations that accompany the two types of breathing—they are quite different. If you want to feel the difference even more clearly, try the exercise while lying on your back.

How to Practice Abdominal Breathing

For the first week, practice the following exercise at least twice a day for 5–10 minutes:

1. Find a quiet, comfortable place where you will not be disturbed. After you begin to master abdominal breathing, you'll be able to do the exercise anywhere at any time. As you begin breath training, you can use the two-handed placements to make sure only the bottom hand is moving in and out.

2. Take a slow, natural breath into your stomach, directing the air toward your belly button. Breathe at your natural depth and keep your breathing smooth; don't gulp in a big breath and let it out all at once. Instead, let the air flow out from your nose equally over the whole time you're exhaling.

3. Each time you inhale, focus on the air expanding your belly. Each time you exhale, stretch out the exhalation for at least 5 seconds as well as the word *relax* (or any other word that is meaningful for you, such as *calm, peace*, etc.) Pair this word with the natural relaxation produced by the exhalation phase of abdominal breathing. Do this every time you practice, as often as possible, so that the word itself becomes a trigger for relaxation.

4. Try to focus only on the breathing and the word. If thoughts begin to intrude, don't worry about them, don't try to suppress them, and don't get upset. Simply think "Oh, well" and turn your attention back to your breathing.

5. During the day, practice the abdominal breathing paired with the word *relax*. The greater the number of pairings, the stronger the link will become between the word *relax* and the relaxed state. You'll be surprised at how quickly you'll be able to relax yourself in this manner.

6. If you find yourself in a stressful situation and experience shallow chest breathing, try to counteract that response with abdominal breathing. There is nothing like practicing in actual stressful situations.

(continued)

Muscle Relaxation Training*

This procedure, known as *progressive muscle relaxation training*, is one of our most powerful anti-stress measures. As with the breathing program, we are going to pair the cue word (such as *relax*) with physical relaxation of your muscles. In as little as a week of serious practice, you can arm yourself with a powerful anti-stress weapon.

Progressive relaxation training involves tensing, then relaxing the muscles while focusing closely on the resulting sensations. This procedure can make you more sensitive to what's going on in your body. With practice, you should be able to detect low levels of tension and use your breathing and relaxation skills before high tension levels make things more difficult. It's easier to put out a campfire than a forest fire.

Get as comfortable as possible. We recommend doing this procedure while sitting in a recliner, a comfortable chair, a sofa, or while sitting propped up in bed. Tight clothing should be loosened and your legs should not be crossed. Take a deep breath, let it out slowly, and become as relaxed as possible.

We are going to divide the body's muscles into three groups: (1) feet, legs, and buttocks; (2) hands, arms, shoulders, chest, and abs; and (3) back, neck, jaw, and face.

In each case, you are going to tense the muscles, slowly release the tension, and think *relax* as you exhale and relax the muscles. When you tense, do not do so with such vigor that you risk pulling a muscle; a mild degree of tension is sufficient.

1. Feet, Legs, and Buttocks

Curl your toes, bend your feet downward to tense the calves, straighten the thighs to tense the muscles, and bunch up your buttocks, all at the same time. Hold that tension for 5 seconds, then *slowly* release the tension, thinking *relax* as you do so. Focus carefully on the sensations and note the many degrees of tension your muscles go through, from bunching up and stretching to letting go. After the tension is released, focus on relaxing the muscles. Imagine a wave of relaxation (in whatever form, or color, denotes relaxation to you) flowing down from your waist through all of those muscles, relaxing them as it moves slowly downward. Pair the wave and its sensations with the word *relax*. Keep doing so until your entire lower body is relaxed and without tension. Contrast those sensations with the tension you felt earlier. Breathe into your stomach and think *relax* as you exhale and let the relaxation deepen. When you inhale, you draw the tension out of the muscles, and when you exhale, you breathe the tension away.

(continued)

*An audio recording of this exercise is available to purchasers of this book for personal use or use with individual clients (see the box at the end of the table of contents).

2. Hands, Arms, Shoulders, Chest, and Abs

Make fists with both hands, bend your hands downward to tense your forearms, and tense your upper arms (biceps and triceps). Then press your arms in against your body, tensing your shoulders, chest, and crunching up your abdominal muscles. Hold for 5 seconds, then slowly let the tension out until the muscles are relaxed. Picture in your mind the wave of relaxation moving slowly through those muscles and seeing them let go from being bunched and tight to being loose, limp, and relaxed. Breathe into your stomach, and as you exhale, think *relax* to yourself. When you inhale, you draw the tension out of the muscles, and when you exhale, you breathe the tension away.

3. Back, Neck, Jaw, and Face

Push your shoulders back to tense your back muscles while thrusting your jaw outward, tensing your neck muscles, and scrunching your forehead and facial muscles. Focus on the sensations for 5 seconds, then slowly let the tension out, as before. Imagine the wave of relaxation flowing from the top of your head down through your face and jaw. Let your jaw and facial muscles comfortably release and let the wave move down to your neck and back. Let your head rest comfortably where you're seated so your neck muscles can relax. Breathe into your stomach and as you exhale, think *relax* to yourself.

4. Yoga Breath Exercise

Finish off your relaxation session with the following yoga exercise, which tends to produce a quick relaxation response. While sitting in a totally relaxed position, take a series of short inhalations, about 1 per second into your chest, until your chest is filled and tense. Hold this for about 5 seconds, then exhale slowly for at least 5 seconds while silently saying your cue word to yourself (e.g., *relax*) throughout the exhalation. Most people can produce a deeply relaxed state by doing this. Repeat this exercise three times.

We recommend that you repeat the above four-step sequence three to five times per session. Doing so should take less than 10 minutes. Like the breathing exercise, practice muscle relaxation twice a day for the first week. The more practice you can do early on, the more potent a relaxation response you will develop.

Thoughts and feelings are closely connected to one another. When we experience stress and other unpleasant emotions, we usually view these reactions as being directly triggered by disturbing situations. However, a careful analysis of what has taken place would disclose that when the upsetting event occurs, we tell ourselves something about it (e.g., "This is awful!"; "They're screwing things up for me!"), and it is this self-statement that triggers the emotion. This sequence of events can be represented as:

$$\text{Situation (A)} \rightarrow \text{Self-Statement (B)} \rightarrow \text{Emotion (C)}$$

In this model, *A* stands for the activating event, *C* stands for your emotional consequence, and *B* stands for your belief, in the form of a self-statement, concerning the situation. The A–B–C concept of emotion helps us understand why two different people can respond to the same situation with far different emotional reactions. It also suggests that by changing our internal self-statements at B, we can change our emotional responses at C.

The good news is that we can indeed change our internal self-talk. This change can be accomplished by noticing what we are telling ourselves at B, challenging these "hot thoughts" that are creating needless stress, and replacing them with more realistic statements that decrease or prevent the emotional response. This process adds a new element to the A–B–C model: *D*, for *dispute*). One goal of the Stress Management Training Program is to help you learn to use the A–B–C–D approach to cope with stress. Your task will be, first, to identify specifically what you say to yourself that makes you upset. Second, you will develop a set of alternative statements that you can use to cope with stressful situations. Thus, by the end of the program you will have a set of physical (relaxation) and mental (adaptive statements) tools at the ready to cope with stress. The goal is not to get rid of all unpleasant emotions; that would be impossible. Rather, it is to reduce the frequency and intensity of needlessly distressing reactions to situations.

How We Distress Ourselves

What kinds of automatic thoughts are involved when you experience stress, anger, and other negative emotions? One way to find out is to stop whenever you find yourself getting upset and ask yourself what you are silently thinking that is causing the distress. You will find that in most instances, the sentences take a form such as "Isn't it

(continued)

awful that . . . ?" or "Wouldn't it be *terrible* if . . . ?" or "What an (awful) (lousy) (rotten) thing for (me) (him) (her) (them) to do." In most cases you are either telling yourself that it is awful that things are not the way you are demanding that they be, or you are condemning yourself or something else because your demands are not being met. These automatic, emotion-triggering "hot thoughts" are often extreme and out of proportion to the actual state of affairs. They turn up the volume, "awfulizing" events and producing inappropriately strong emotional reactions. Automatic thoughts can tell us that a mildly threatening event is dangerous, has dire consequences, and that we are powerless to deal with it. We can therefore react to a minor stressor as if it were a catastrophe.

We use the term "catastrophizing" to describe the kind of thinking that leads to much stress and emotional disturbance. Catastrophizing means that relatively minor frustrations, inconveniences, and concerns are mentally blown up so that they become, for the moment, catastrophes to which we then reacted emotionally.

Much of our distress-producing thinking takes the form "I don't like this situation!"; "This is **terrible!** I can't **stand** it!"; "It's driving me **crazy!**"; "It **shouldn't** be this way!"; "It's simply **got to** change or I can't **possibly** be happy!"

The eminent psychologist Albert Ellis maintained that almost all of these stress-producing hot thoughts flow from one underlying toxic idea:

It's terrible, awful, and catastrophic when things (life, other people, the past, or me) are not (or are certain not to be) the way that I demand that they be, and I can't stand it when things are that way.

Several irrational elements can be found in this statement:

1. Most of the events that we upset ourselves about are not truly terrible, awful, and catastrophic. They are more likely to be unpleasant, annoying, or inconvenient. The same is true when we or others fail to measure up to the "musts" contained in irrational demands that we and others be perfect in all respects and that other people and life in general should always treat us fairly.

2. It is far more rational to think in terms of *preferences* than to *demand* that we, others, or the world conform to our wishes. God is not a special agent of ours.

3. We can almost always "stand" things that occur to us. People tolerate and survive things that are much more traumatic than the day-to-day stresses most of us have.

(continued)

The good news is that by systematically tuning in to your own internal self-talk about troublesome situations, you will find that you can pretty quickly pin down the thoughts that are producing your distress. If you stop and ask yourself "How is it *terrible* that . . . ?" or "Why would it actually be *awful* if . . . ?" or "Who am I to demand that things be exactly the way I'd like them to be?" you will often quickly get over being upset because you can readily see the irrational aspects of what you are telling yourself. Here are some ways to discover and replace such ideas.

Stress-Busters: Stress-Reducing Thoughts

A key to mentally coping with stress is to acknowledge the role that your own thoughts play in generating distress. Whenever you feel yourself becoming upset, the first thing you should tell yourself is this: "*I* am creating this feeling by the way I'm thinking. How can I stop myself from being upset?" This statement, or one like it, immediately alerts you that it is time to put things in perspective and to use the physical relaxation and mental coping techniques that are the focus of the Stress Management Training Program. If you are completing the Stress and Coping Diary (Form A-1) or the Analyzing Thoughts and Feelings form (Form A-2) that accompany the program, you have already been identifying stress-producing automatic thoughts and generating stress-reducing ones.

The idea that things *should* or *must* be the way we want/like/need them to be is an idea that we can focus on in developing stress-reducing thoughts. Here are some examples of "stress busters" that can be used to stop this irrational idea from triggering stress:

- "I don't like this situation, but I certainly can live with it. No sense getting strung out."
- "It's not that big a thing."
- "There's no reason why the world should revolve around my needs."
- "Unfortunately, people don't always behave like I want them to. That's the way it goes—no use getting upset."
- "Other people's needs are as important to them as mine are to me."
- "I don't have to be perfect. I can make mistakes, too. I don't have to please everyone."
- "I don't need to upset myself. *I* control how I feel."
- "In the end, how important is this, really?"
- "Okay, so I don't like this. It's not the end of the world."
- "Don't catastrophize now. Put this in perspective."

(continued)

- "It would be nice if everything always went perfectly, but that's not the way life is."
- "If I catastrophize about *this*, I deserve to be upset."
- "If I can change this situation, I should do so. Thinking about what I can do about this situation is better than getting upset."
- "I may not like this, but I can definitely stand it."
- "Keep cool. Take a slow breath and say, 'Relax.'"
- "Life is too short to let things like this make me miserable."
- "Is this really the worst that can happen? Put it in perspective."
- "Getting upset does me no good at all. No sense overreacting."

These examples should help you to develop your own set of self-statements for coping with difficult situations. You will find that you can almost always short-circuit unpleasant emotions by placing things in a noncatastrophizing perspective.

Logically Evaluating the Evidence

Another way to counter stress-producing hot thoughts is to challenge them on the basis of factual evidence. You can use the form Challenging and Replacing Stress-Producing Thoughts: Where's the Evidence? (Form A-3) for this purpose.

To use this form, list a stressful situation you've experienced and describe it in detail in the first column. This is the Activating Event (A). In the next column, name the Emotional Response (C) you experienced and rate how much discomfort you felt from 1 (complete calm) to 100 (unbearable) on the Units of Discomfort scale at the top of the form. In the third column, try to identify the hot thought(s) that created the feeling. (This is the same as *B* in the A-B-C-D sequence.)

Then, in fourth column, list any past or present facts, including experiences that support the thought (no impressions, beliefs, or assumptions allowed!). Here you take on the role of a prosecuting attorney. This list is the "evidence to convict." In the fifth column, you play the role of a defense attorney, marshaling as much factual evidence as you can think of that would render the hot thought invalid. A useful approach is to look for facts that counterbalance each item listed in the "evidence for" column. Here are some questions that can guide you:

- "What is the most probable outcome of this situation and how probable (from 0 to 100%) is it that the worst possible consequence will occur?"
- "I'm focusing on the bad aspects of the situation. Are there any good aspects that I'm ignoring?"

(continued)

- "Does it truly have catastrophic implications for who I am as a person, or for who someone else is?"
- "Is it true that I absolutely *can't* stand it?"
- "Have I had a similar experience in the past? Did I get through it without severe damage? What did I learn that could help me weather this storm?"
- "Is there an alternative interpretation of the situation besides the one in the hot thought?"
- "Have I had any past experiences that are inconsistent with the hot thought?"
- "Are there circumstances for which this thought is not true?"
- "What would I tell my best friend if he/she had this same hot thought?"
- "What might my best friend tell me about my thought?"
- "How much will this bother me tomorrow? Next week? Next month? Looking back, will I view the event the same way?"

Now it is time to move to the D (Dispute) stage, evaluate the evidence for and against the hot thought, and arrive at a balanced reappraisal of the Activating Event. The goal is to evaluate the evidence *for* and *against* the thought and see if a more balanced and realistic appraisal of the event emerges that reduces the stress response. Write a stress-reducing alternative thought in the next to last column.

Finally, imagine yourself back in the stressful situation, say the alternative thought to yourself, and rate the intensity of your emotional response using the 0-to-100 Discomfort scale. Record the rating in the last column. Does the new way of appraising the situation reduce your distress?

Self-Instructions: Performance-Enhancing Thoughts

Intense emotion often has a disruptive effect on performance. We can become so upset or angry that it is hard to function effectively. For example, some students become so anxious and fearful during tests that they cannot answer test questions. One reason why intense emotions can disrupt performance is that we become so bound up in self-defeating thoughts about how terrible the situation is that we cannot devote full attention to coping with it. Psychologist Donald Meichenbaum developed a technique called *self-instructional training* to teach people to talk to themselves more adaptively before, during, and after stressful situations. Here are some self-instructional self-statements that people have used to help them reduce stress and keep their minds on the task at hand:

(continued)

Preparing for a Stressful Event:

- "You can develop a plan to deal with this."
- "Run it through your mind and visualize how you want to respond."
- "Concentrate on keeping your cool. You can handle this."

Confronting the Stressful Event:

- "Don't think about being upset; just focus on what you have to do."
- "Don't get all bent out of shape; just do what has to be done."
- "Relax and slow things down. You're in control. Take a deep breath."
- "This upset is a signal for you to use your coping skills. Relax and think rationally."
- "Don't try to eliminate stress. Just keep it manageable and focus on the present."
- "Don't react now when you're angry. Take some time to cool down, then think about how to handle things in a better way."
- "You never got into trouble by keeping your mouth shut."

We all know that behaviors that lead to positive outcomes become stronger and more efficient. One important source of reward for saying adaptive things to yourself is that they work and help you control your level of stress. Used in conjunction with your relaxation coping response, these kinds of adaptive, performance-enhancing self-statements give you powerful weapons against negative emotions. You can help this strengthening process along by internally rewarding yourself immediately after you use them effectively. When you feel yourself handling stress effectively, reward yourself; you're winning out over your deadliest enemy. Here are some examples of self-rewarding self-statements:

Following the Stressful Event:

- "Way to go! You're in control."
- "Good—you're handling the stress."
- "Beautiful—you did it!"

If you're not satisfied with the outcome of your coping attempt, use it as a learning opportunity.

(continued)

- "How can you handle it better next time? You can visualize and mentally rehearse exactly what you'd do and say."

Coping more effectively with life stressors increases self-confidence and resiliency. By developing your coping abilities, you can gain increasing control over your emotional life.

Anti-Stress Log and Coping Cards

As you learn to analyze and change your stress-producing thoughts through the various exercises in this program, the end product will be an Anti-Stress Log (Form A-4), consisting of stress-producing thoughts in one column and stress-reducing ones in the other. Most people find that their lists are not very long because most of us have a limited number of "hot button" themes that pop up frequently in our lives. As these coping statements develop, transfer them to *coping cards*, 3" × 5" index cards that contain the A, B, and C elements on one side and the corresponding D statement on the other. You can keep these coping cards with you and commit the alternative statements to memory so that you can practice anywhere, anytime, either in your imagination or in actual situations. This repeated practice helps increase the strength of these stress-reducing thoughts until they eventually replace the old stress-producing automatic thoughts as you develop new habits of thinking and responding.

A Final Word

We hope that this handout and the exercises and forms associated with it will help you to develop new stress-reducing ways of thinking. We end with five key ideas:

1. You, not situations, cause your emotions.

2. You feel the way you think.

3. Things are rarely as catastrophic as they may seem in the moment.

4. You can stand anything.

5. You can control your emotions by controlling your thinking.

In this handout, we describe a meditation technique developed at Harvard Medical School for the treatment of stress and medical problems such as pain and hypertension. The technique developed by Herbert Benson is a general body–mind relaxation technique. It produces a biological relaxation response that counteracts the typical fight-or-flight response to the stresses of everyday living. Research has shown that the relaxation response can be learned quickly and that it lowers oxygen consumption, heart rate, respiration, and stress hormones, thereby producing a restful state. Clear health benefits have been documented in medical research and are described in the book *Relaxation Revolution.*

The Benson technique is a generalized version of a variety of Eastern and Western religious and lay meditation practices. It has four basic components that are common to many other techniques, such as yoga and transcendental meditation. These components are:

1. **A quiet environment**: A quiet, calm environment with as few distractions as possible is needed for this technique.

2. **A mental device**: A sound, word, or phrase is repeated silently or aloud, or fixed gazing at an object is used to focus attention.

3. **A passive attitude**: Thoughts and feelings are allowed to come and go without any attempt to actively suppress them, act on them, or hold on to them.

4. **A comfortable position**: A comfortable, relaxed posture is recommended so that there is no undue muscular tension. (There is a tendency to fall asleep if lying down.)

The subjective feelings that accompany the relaxation response vary among individuals. Most people feel a sense of calm and deep relaxation. Other descriptions involve feelings of pleasure, refreshment, well-being, renewal and energy after meditating. Still others report little change on the subjective level. Regardless of the subjective experience, however, there is objective evidence of the positive physiological changes that accompany a restful state in which bodily processes slow down.

(continued)

---

*Benson, Herbert, and Proctor, William. (2010). *Relaxation revolution: Enhancing your health through the science and genetics of mind–body healing*. Fort Worth, TX: Scribner.

Instructions for the Benson Technique

1. Sit quietly in a comfortable position.

2. Close your eyes.

3. Deeply relax all your muscles, beginning at your face and progressing down to your feet, using the cued relaxation technique you've already learned.

4. Breathe in through your nose and into your stomach. Concentrate on your breathing. As you breathe out, say the word, "one" (or a focus word of your choosing) silently to yourself (e.g., "calm," "peace"). For example, breathe in . . . out, while silently saying "one"; in . . . out, while silently saying "one"; and so on. Breathe easily and naturally.

5. When distracting thoughts occur, as they surely will, simply return to your breathing and the repetition of the focus word. Adopt a passive attitude. Simply say, "Oh, well" to yourself. Distracting thoughts and mind wandering do not mean you are performing the technique incorrectly. They are to be expected because our minds are always active. Do not worry about whether you are successful in achieving a deep level of relaxation. *Do not worry about how well you are performing the technique*, because this may prevent the relaxation response from occurring.

6. Continue for 12–15 minutes. You can open your eyes to check the time, but do not use a loud alarm that might startle you. There are smartphone apps available that make a gentle sound. When you finish, sit quietly for several minutes, at first with your eyes closed and later with your eyes open. In an optional second phase of the technique, you can visualize the most relaxing scene you can think of (e.g., sitting in a warm spa or in warm sand on a beautiful beach) for additional minutes before returning your attention to your surroundings, stretching, and then rising.

Mindfulness

Mindfulness is a state in which you observe your present-moment experiences in an accepting and nonjudgmental manner. Mindfulness leads to the realization that all thoughts, emotions, and physical sensations are transitory events that come and go on the stream of consciousness, independent of the "you" who observes their passage. This ability to detach from these experiences creates an awareness that has beneficial effects. Rather than being swept up into distressing automatic thoughts, we can calmly observe them as simply thoughts—that is, as transitory events in the mind—and so gain psychological distance from them. Mindfulness is also about having compassion and adopting a nonjudgmental stance, as best we can, toward whatever arises in our awareness. It is noticing with curiosity rather than evaluation. Mindfulness helps us recognize that we can experience and accept thoughts and emotions fully without a need to suppress them; they can be tolerated as temporary events that come and go, just as clouds in the sky come and go.

Regular practice of mindfulness has been shown to have positive effects on anxiety, depression, physical pain, substance abuse, and other physical and psychological problems. It is increasingly being incorporated into psychological treatments for a variety of problems. Studies of brain function during mindfulness practices reveal decreased activity in the parts of the brain that are involved in evaluation and emotion.

A good introduction to this mental state is through mindfulness meditation. In mindfulness meditation, you focus on your breathing, as in the Benson technique, but there is no focus word like "one" involved. Instead, when you become aware of any thoughts, sensations, or images, you just observe them nonjudgmentally. Here is how mindfulness meditation is done:

1. Sit in a comfortable position on a chair or in a cross-legged or lotus/half-lotus position on the floor.

2. Close your eyes and focus your attention on your breathing as you slowly inhale and exhale. Feel the coolness of the air as it enters your nose, and the sensations of your lungs expanding and contracting.

3. When thoughts, physical feelings, emotions, or external sounds come into your awareness, simply accept them, letting them come and go without getting

(continued)

involved with them. Regard them as events that "just are." Be an observer, not a reactor. No matter how often these experiences occur, just keep bringing your attention back to your breathing. This practice of "switching" gives you greater control over your mental and emotional experience.

4. Do this meditation exercise for 15 minutes each day for a week to see how it feels to incorporate it into your life. You may elect to do the Benson technique, mindfulness meditation, or both, depending on your own preferences.

Defusion

When we take negative thoughts literally and regard them as truth, we can suffer unnecessarily. A thought such as "I am a failure" means that you are, in reality, a failure. In fact, thoughts have *no reality* at all other than as events in our minds. Mindfulness is a way to achieve this distance from negative thoughts without changing them. We can learn to regard negative whisperings of the mind as what they are, "just thoughts" that come and go, and not as reflections of reality. When feelings are too intense to control, we can accept the sensory, "gut" aspects of them without getting swept away with thoughts and meanings. This distancing from the content of thoughts is technically called *defusion*. Defusion does not involve confronting, disputing, or ultimately changing the thought. Nor does it mean avoiding or suppressing the thought—which, by the way, doesn't work very well. Defusion simply changes your relationship to your thoughts: You can detach from them and see them as what they are—temporary mental events that will soon move on. You can tolerate them in the same manner that people who live with chronic pain learn to tolerate their painful sensations by stepping back and accepting them.

Defusion involves recognizing that you are not your thoughts and that the content of a thought is not the reality it seems to represent. Instead of "fusing" with painful thoughts, accepting them as truths and letting them trigger a vicious cycle of increasing misery, we can "*de*-fuse"—distance ourselves from their content—and let go of them. This handout is designed to build on the experiences you've had in the last session and help you learn this valuable skill.

Try these defusion exercises. They each begin by using the mindfulness meditation technique described above. Sit up straight in a chair, close your eyes, get comfortable, and relax. Focus on your breathing as you breathe into your stomach, effortlessly. Feel the sensations of the cool air passing into your nostrils and down your throat and the warmth of the air that you exhale. Each time you exhale, let yourself relax more deeply.

(continued)

Watching and Labeling Thoughts

As you've discovered in your previous meditation, thoughts and images are certain to enter your mind from time to time. Concentrate on your breathing, but when a thought appears, briefly note whether the thought is positive, neutral, or negative. That's all; do not get caught up in the thought's content. Then say to yourself, "Now my mind is having a positive thought," or "Now my mind is having a neutral thought," or "Now my mind is having a negative thought." Then return to concentrating on your breathing until the next thought appears.

White-Room Meditation

Picture your mind as an all-white room with nothing in it. You are wherever you want to be in the room—on the side or even on the ceiling—so you can observe what's going on. The room has two open doors, one to the left and one to the right. Imagine your thoughts are like misty clouds floating in from the door to your left and exiting through the door to your right. Allow each thought that comes into your mind to have a brief moment in your awareness as it passes through the room and disappears through the door before the next one floats in. You're only role is to observe how thoughts come and go.

Letting Go of Thoughts

You've now seen how you can be a passive, accepting observer of your thoughts with no need to respond to them as they come and go by themselves. However, there are also some ways of letting go of thoughts and gaining some distance from them so that they have less believability and less power to affect you.

LEAVES ON A STREAM

As you continue to meditate, imagine you're sitting on the bank of a beautiful mountain stream with crystal-clear water that is flowing through the forest. A canopy of fall trees reaches out across the stream. To your right is a bend in the stream. When a thought arrives, imagine that it is a leaf that slowly floats down from the trees above and lightly lands in the stream. The leaf is caught by the current and is swept away around the bend in the stream, where it disappears from view. As each thought arrives, let this process repeat itself.

(continued)

BILLBOARDS

Imagine you're driving down a long stretch of highway. At various points there are billboards to your right. When a thought occurs, imagine that it attaches itself to a billboard that soon disappears from sight as you pass it. As the next thought appears, let a new billboard pop up and the thought attach to it, so that each thought becomes a message on a billboard that you pass by.

HELIUM BALLOONS

Imagine you are holding a big collection of round helium balloons. As each thought occurs, it appears on the back side of a balloon that turns in the wind to face you. Say to yourself, "My mind put a thought on the balloon." Then let the string slip through your fingers and watch that balloon float away on the breeze into the sky until it disappears. Repeat with each new thought.

PHYSICALLY LETTING GO OF THOUGHTS

Here's a distancing technique that involves your body. This one has a physical component. Continue your meditation with your breath, and now hold your hand with the palm facing upward. When a thought comes into your mind, imagine that it floats down into the palm of your hand. Feel the texture, weight, and temperature of the thought as it settles into your hand. Then slowly rotate your hand so that the thought drops out of it and out of sight. Return your palm upward to receive the next thought. Alternatively, you can hold the thought in your hand with the fingers bent slightly to contain it, then let your fingers open slowly and jiggle them when you wish to release the thought. That's far less conspicuous. Many people report that letting thoughts go physically in this fashion makes the process seem more real and believable.

Mindfulness, acceptance, and defusion differ fundamentally from some other mental coping skills, such as reappraisal. They are not about disputing your thoughts, but about accepting them in a nonjudgmental manner that gives you some distance from their content. This can be especially useful when you are too highly stressed to use the integrated coping response you've learned in the program. Some people even find mindfulness and acceptance as a preferred way of managing their emotions and dealing with stressful life events.

You have already learned some mental and physical coping skills that can increase your personal resourcefulness and resilience in the face of stress. You've also learned how to create a mind–body integrated coping response. You are therefore able to use an additional stress-reduction technique known as *desensitization*. Desensitization means that we reduce the ability of a troublesome situation to evoke a stress response, much like an allergy shot desensitizes us to an allergen. Desensitization procedures have been used very successfully to help people get over phobias involving such things as heights, airplane travel, snakes, water, and so on. In addition to fear and anxiety, desensitization procedures have been used to help people reduce anger responses. And a great feature is that people like you, who have already mastered stress-reducing coping skills like relaxation, can do it successfully on your own—hence the term, "self-desensitization."

Situations in your life that are challenging and arouse unwanted emotional responses, particularly those encountered repeatedly, are suitable targets for self-applied desensitization. These can be situations that produce anxiety, anger, or other unwanted emotions. From your "personal scientist" homework assignments, you've learned more about the aspects of situations that push your buttons. Desensitization can involve two kinds of controlled exposure to the stressor. The first involves imagining relevant scenes, as we've done in the Stress Management Training Program, and the second involves gradual exposure to real-life situations. Often, the imaginal step is sufficient, especially if you don't have control over the situation (such as the level of misbehavior of another person). If you do have control, such as how closely you can approach a feared situation or interact with a troublesome relative, then you can use real-life exposure as well.

The first step is to create a hierarchy of scenes, from least negative to most negative, involving the person or situation that elicits varying degrees of anger or anxiety. The hierarchy is like a ladder whose bottom rungs are less emotionally arousing than the top ones. The desensitization process involves climbing the ladder and mastering each rung. The table illustrates some sample hierarchies used to deal with a phobia, anxiety, and anger

Start with the least-arousing event at the bottom of the hierarchy and imagine it while focusing on signs of distress in your body and on any stress-inducing self-statements that might come to mind. When you've gotten into the feeling, apply an integrated coping response to it, with a stress-reducing self-statement upon

(continued)

Anxiety and Anger Hierarchies for Self-Desensitization

Fear of Heights (fear reduction)	Test Anxiety (anxiety reduction)	Obnoxious Mother-in-Law (anger control)
Looking down from the edge of the Grand Canyon	Looking at a test question you cannot answer with confidence	Clara tells you your spouse should have married someone else
Looking over the edge of a high bridge at the ground below	Sitting in your seat as the test is passed out	Clara points out "mistakes" in your child-rearing practices
Standing at the railing of a 12th-floor open balcony	Arriving at the scene of the test	Clara makes a snide remark about your income or job
Looking out of a 12th-floor closed window	Getting up on the morning of the test and thinking about it	Clara ignores you during dinner at her house
Walking over an open 2nd-floor skyway and looking down	Studying a large amount of material the night before the test	Clara looking at you in a dismissing fashion when you express an opinion
Walking on a high, narrow trail in the mountains	Discussing difficulty of the material to be covered on the test with classmates	Clara describes successful past boyfriends of your spouse in glowing terms
Riding on a glass-walled elevator to the next level in a shopping center	Being reminded that the test will occur in 3 days	Clara criticizes your spouse's choice of carpeting
Watching a graphic film about skydivers	Finding that you will have another test on the same day	Clara complaining about not having a "loving family"
Standing 10 steps up on a ladder	Instructor announces a test in 2 weeks	Image of Clara's scowling face

inhalation and relaxation on exhalation. For each scene, prepare an integrated coping response consisting of a rational stress-reducing self-statement from your Anti-Stress Log. Apply the integrated coping response until the feeling has been reduced. Then imagine it again and see if you can arouse the feeling. If so, reduce it again using your coping skills. If you have trouble proceeding up the hierarchy at a particular point, the "rungs" might be too far apart. Insert one or more intermediate scenes that are easier to handle.

Next, you can combine another proven behavior change technique with the self-desensitization emotion control procedure—namely, mental rehearsal. After you have

(continued)

toned down the emotional arousal using your integrated coping response, imagine yourself coping with the situation behaviorally in an effective manner—for example, speaking calmly rather than becoming angry, or walking across a high bridge with less fear. There is much scientific evidence that mental rehearsal of desired behaviors translates into better performance in sports, work, and social behavior, so use this tool to your benefit. By mentally rehearsing behaving as you'd like to, you will be programming yourself to respond more effectively in the future.

The combination of self-desensitization and mental rehearsal allows you to cope with and reduce the emotional arousal and also to rehearse an effective way of handling the situation behaviorally. When you feel comfortable with each situation, you can proceed to the next-highest scene in the hierarchy, and so on up to the top. This trip up the hierarchy ladder is best done over multiple sessions; you should not try to traverse the whole hierarchy of scenes at one sitting.

Self-desensitization can be even more effective if you include some real-life exposure and coping after you have done the imagined practice. By exposing yourself to relevant real-life situations and applying your coping responses, these situations lose their power to create uncontrollable negative feelings. Again, use a gradual hierarchy of actual situations, and use your stress coping skills at every step. For example, one college student who had severe social anxiety created a series of real-life situations that started with simply making eye contact with another passing student on campus while remaining relaxed . . . then saying hello to someone she passed while going to class (guaranteeing that she wouldn't have to converse) . . . then saying hello to a person in her class . . . then initiating a conversation about the class assignment with a fellow student . . . and so on, proceeding eventually to more general conversations and social contact. By choosing controllable situations (and applying her favorite integrated coping response that said, "I'm in control . . . so . . . relax") that she had used beforehand while imagining the future real-life situation, she gradually worked her way up the hierarchy and became less socially anxious.

| **Stress and Coping Diary**

1. **Please respond to the following question based on how you have been feeling since your last diary entry.**

	Not at all stressful		Somewhat stressful		Extremely stressful	
In general, how stressful have your life circumstances been since your last diary entry?	O	O	O	O	O	O	O

2. **To what extent do these terms describe how you have been feeling since your last diary entry?**

	Not at all	A little	Some- what	Moder- ately	A fair amount	Quite a bit	Extremely
Optimistic	O	O	O	O	O	O	O
Irritable	O	O	O	O	O	O	O
Tense	O	O	O	O	O	O	O
Unhappy	O	O	O	O	O	O	O
Relaxed	O	O	O	O	O	O	O
Angry	O	O	O	O	O	O	O
Anxious	O	O	O	O	O	O	O
Enthusiastic	O	O	O	O	O	O	O
Discouraged	O	O	O	O	O	O	O
Resentful	O	O	O	O	O	O	O
Contented	O	O	O	O	O	O	O
Afraid	O	O	O	O	O	O	O
Depressed	O	O	O	O	O	O	O
Energetic	O	O	O	O	O	O	O

3. **Please describe a stressful event you experienced since your last diary entry.**
   In the box below, please indicate what happened. Please describe the event in enough detail so that when you read it later, you'll be able to reexperience the event. Please do the best you can to describe what made this event stressful to you.

(continued)

4. Please respond to the following questions based on the situation you just described.

	Not at all		Somewhat			Extremely
To what extent did you **feel incompetent** in this situation?	O	O	O	O	O	O	O
To what extent did you **feel exhausted** in this situation?	O	O	O	O	O	O	O
To what extent did you **feel excluded** in this situation?	O	O	O	O	O	O	O
To what extent did you **feel helpless** in this situation?	O	O	O	O	O	O	O
To what extent did you **feel irritated** in this situation?	O	O	O	O	O	O	O
To what extent did you **feel confused** in this situation?	O	O	O	O	O	O	O
To what extent did you **feel rushed** in this situation?	O	O	O	O	O	O	O
To what extent did you **feel as though your time was wasted** in this situation?	O	O	O	O	O	O	O
To what extent did you **feel betrayed** in this situation?	O	O	O	O	O	O	O
To what extent did you **feel bored** in this situation?	O	O	O	O	O	O	O
To what extent did you **feel as though your expectations were not met** in this situation?	O	O	O	O	O	O	O
To what extent did you **feel as though your goals were blocked** in this situation?	O	O	O	O	O	O	O
To what extent were you **afraid of letting others down** in this situation?	O	O	O	O	O	O	O

(continued)

5. How stressed did you feel?

	Not at all intense		Somewhat intense		Extremely intense	
How intense was your emotional reaction to this stressful event?	○	○	○	○	○	○	○

6. Please respond to the following questions based on the stressful event you described at the beginning of this diary entry.

	I felt I had little or no personal control		I felt I had some personal control		I felt I had a great deal of personal control	
To what extent did you feel you had **personal control** over this situation?	○	○	○	○	○	○	○
To what extent did you feel you were able to **control your emotional reaction** to this event?	○	○	○	○	○	○	○

7. We tend to have thoughts or perceptions that occur more or less automatically when we encounter certain situations. The following two questions ask you to describe what you may have mentally "said to yourself" about the stressful event.

A. In the box below, please indicate what you may have automatically "told yourself" about the event that could have contributed to your emotional reaction.

B. Instead of what you told yourself about the **event**, what could you have told yourself instead to prevent or reduce your emotional reaction?

(continued)

297

8. The following questions ask you to indicate what you did in response to the event you described at the beginning of this diary entry.

	Not at all		Somewhat			A great deal

Rethinking the situation involves reevaluating the situation and its meaning in ways that counteract stress-producing thoughts and thereby reduce the stress response. To what extent did you engage in rethinking the situation?

◯ ◯ ◯ ◯ ◯ ◯ ◯

If you engaged in **rethinking the situation,** to what extent did it help you reduce your stress response?

◯ ◯ ◯ ◯ ◯ ◯ ◯

Relaxation techniques involve attempts to reduce emotional arousal using muscle relaxation, meditation, or breathing techniques. To what extent did you engage in relaxation techniques in this situation?

◯ ◯ ◯ ◯ ◯ ◯ ◯

If you engaged in **relaxation techniques,** to what extent did they help you reduce your stress response?

◯ ◯ ◯ ◯ ◯ ◯ ◯

Seeking social support involves seeking or finding emotional support or advice from loved ones, friends, or professionals. To what extent did you seek social support in this situation?

◯ ◯ ◯ ◯ ◯ ◯ ◯

If you engaged in **seeking social support**, to what extent did it help you reduce your stress response?

◯ ◯ ◯ ◯ ◯ ◯ ◯

Direct problem solving involves thinking about solutions to the problem, gathering information about the problem, or actually doing something about the problem. To what extent did you engage in direct problem solving in this situation?

◯ ◯ ◯ ◯ ◯ ◯ ◯

If you engaged in **direct problem solving,** to what extent did it help you reduce your stress response?

◯ ◯ ◯ ◯ ◯ ◯ ◯

Blaming yourself involves being critical of yourself for the problem. To what extent did you blame yourself in this situation?

◯ ◯ ◯ ◯ ◯ ◯ ◯

(continued)

	Not at all		Somewhat			A great deal	
If you engaged in **blaming yourself**, to what extent did it help you reduce your stress response?	O	O	O	O	O	O	O
Blaming others involves criticizing and/or getting angry with the people you view as most responsible for the situation. To what extent did you blame others in this situation?	O	O	O	O	O	O	O
If you engaged in **blaming others**, to what extent did it help you reduce your stress response?	O	O	O	O	O	O	O
Wishful thinking involves daydreaming, fantasizing, or just **hoping** that things would be better or that the event will turn out differently. To what extent did you engage in wishful thinking in this situation?	O	O	O	O	O	O	O
If you engaged in **wishful thinking**, to what extent did it help you reduce your stress response?	O	O	O	O	O	O	O
Distraction involves diverting your attention from stressful thoughts and feelings by thinking about or imagining more pleasant things. To what extent did you engage in distraction in this situation?	O	O	O	O	O	O	O
If you engaged in **distraction**, to what extent did it help you reduce your stress response?	O	O	O	O	O	O	O
Avoidance involves doing things to sidestep confronting the problem or thinking about it, doing things to evade experiencing negative emotions, or not letting others know what is happening or how you are feeling. To what extent did you engage in avoidance in this situation?	O	O	O	O	O	O	O
If you engaged in **avoidance**, to what extent did it help you reduce your stress response?	O	O	O	O	O	O	O
Counting your blessings involves focusing on the good things in your life or reminding yourself that, no matter how difficult things might be, you are still better off than many people. To what extent did you count your blessings in this situation?	O	O	O	O	O	O	O

(continued)

	Not at all		Somewhat			A great deal
If you engaged in **counting your blessings**, to what extent did it help you reduce your stress response?	O	O	O	O	O	O O
Physical activity includes any form of exercise (e.g., jogging, swimming). To what extent did you engage in physical activity in this situation?	O	O	O	O	O	O O
If you engaged in **physical activity**, to what extent did it help you reduce your stress response?	O	O	O	O	O	O O
Acceptance involves simply allowing the presence of stressful thoughts and feelings and waiting for them to pass away rather than trying to control them. To what extent did you engage in acceptance in this situation?	O	O	O	O	O	O O
If you engaged in **acceptance**, to what extent did it help you reduce your stress response?	O	O	O	O	O	O O

9. **Please respond to the following questions based on the stressful event you described at the beginning of this diary entry.**

	Not at all stressful			Somewhat stressful			Extremely stressful
How stressful was the event **at the time you experienced it?**	O	O	O	O	O	O	O
How stressful was the event **after engaging in coping behaviors?**	O	O	O	O	O	O	O

10. **Current life satisfaction**

	Most unhappy									Most happy
Overall, how would you rate your general life satisfaction at this time?	O	O	O	O	O	O	O	O	O	O O

Thank you for completing today's entry.

Form A-2	Analyzing Thoughts and Feelings

This exercise helps you gain greater awareness of your stress-producing automatic thoughts and develop stress-reducing alternatives to replace them. It uses the A-B-C-D (**A**ctivating event; **B**elief or appraisal of the event; emotional **C**onsequence; **D**isputing thought) model of emotion and emotional change discussed in your session on thoughts and feelings. This form should be completed for each stressful event you encounter. Briefly answer the following questions about a recent event you found disturbing.

A. What happened? Briefly describe the event. _____

_____

_____

_____

B. How did you feel when (A) occurred? What was your emotional reaction to (A)?

_____

_____

_____

C. What must you have told yourself about (A) in order to produce (C)? _____

_____

_____

_____

D. Instead of (B), what could you have told yourself about (A) that might have prevented (C)? _____

_____

_____

_____

From *Promoting Emotional Resilience: Cognitive–Affective Stress Management Training* by Ronald E. Smith and James C. Ascough. Copyright © 2016 The Guilford Press. Permission to photocopy this material is granted to purchasers of this book for personal use or use with individual clients (see copyright page for details). Purchasers can download enlarged versions of this material (see the box at the end of the table of contents).

We tend to accept many of our "hot" automatic thoughts as "reality." This exercise helps you question the evidence for and against these hot thoughts. Upon reflection, we can often uncover evidence that calls the hot thoughts into question and use this evidence to adopt a more balanced or rational way of thinking about the situation prompted by the thought, thereby reducing our emotional response. In the worksheet that follows, imagine the situation at (A), the event, and then apply both the (B) and (D) thoughts. Use the "Units of Discomfort" scale when rating the emotional intensity resulting from the hot and alternative thoughts.

Units of Discomfort

0	10	20	30	40	50	60	70	80	90	100
None: calm, relaxed		Slight discom- fort	Mild: able to cope		Moderate discom- fort; hard to control		Severe discom- fort: nearly uncon- trollable		Intense and uncon- trollable	Unbear- able; worst imagin- able

Activating Event (A)	Your Emotional Response (C)	Stress- Producing Thought (B)	Factual Evi- dence That Supports (B)	Factual Evidence That Does Not Support (B)	Stress- Reducing Alternative Thought (D)	Your Emotional Response with (D)
Describe stressful situation in detail	*Rate intensity from 0 to 100*	*What were you thinking?*	(list below)	(list below)	(from #3, below)	*Rate intensity from 0 to 100*

1. List the evidence that **supports** B (include only objective facts, past experiences, etc.):

_____

_____

_____

(continued)

2. List any evidence **against** B, using questions like the following:

   • Is B an overreaction or an overgeneralization? Are there ever times when B is not true?

   _____

   • Is there an alternative interpretation of what happened?

   _____

   • Are there objective facts or past experiences that would contradict B?

   _____

   • What is the likelihood that any consequences you fear will actually occur? If they did, would they be true catastrophes, or could you tolerate them?

   _____

   • Do you have the skills needed to handle the situation or reduce its stressfulness? What could you do?

   _____

3. In light of the evidence you listed under #2, can you come up with a rational alternative thought (D) that would prevent or reduce the emotional impact of Situation A? If so, write it below and use it as you re-imagine Situation A. Then reevaluate your emotional response (E) using the Units of Discomfort scale.

   _____

   _____

   _____

   _____

   _____

What we say to ourselves about stressful situations shapes our emotions. Based on what you've learned in the stress management sessions, the handouts, and your homework exercises, you are ready to develop a list of stress-reducing self-statements that are specific to you and the situations you confront. By now, you should have a good idea of the specific things you tend to say to yourself that produce needless stress, and what you could say to yourself instead that would short-circuit the stress response or help you deal with it productively (e.g., telling yourself to focus on what you need to do in the situation).

Directions: In the left-hand column of the Anti-Stress Log, list the stress-producing self-statements you tend to say to yourself when you encounter demanding situations. Next to each one, in the right-hand column, list a rational anti-stress alternative that would reduce your emotion. Also list in the right-hand column any self-instructions that would help you deal with impending stress or with the situation as it happens. See Handout A-3, Mental Control of Emotions and Stress, for examples of helpful self-instructions.

As a result of this exercise, you will have the elements needed to reprogram your thinking and direct your behavior more effectively in stressful situations. With practice, these new ways of thinking will become habitual or automatic, just as the stress-producing "hot" thoughts are at this point.

It is recommended that you transfer these thoughts to your coping cards to remain mindful of them.

(continued)

My Anti-Stress Log

Stress–producing self–statements	Stress–reducing self–statements

APPENDIX B

Materials for Therapists/Trainers

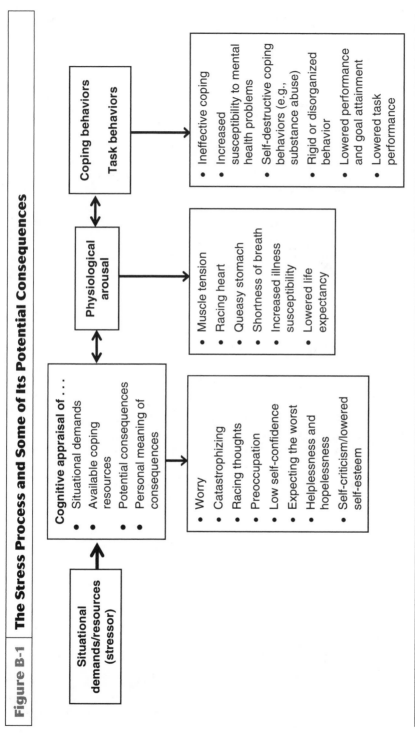

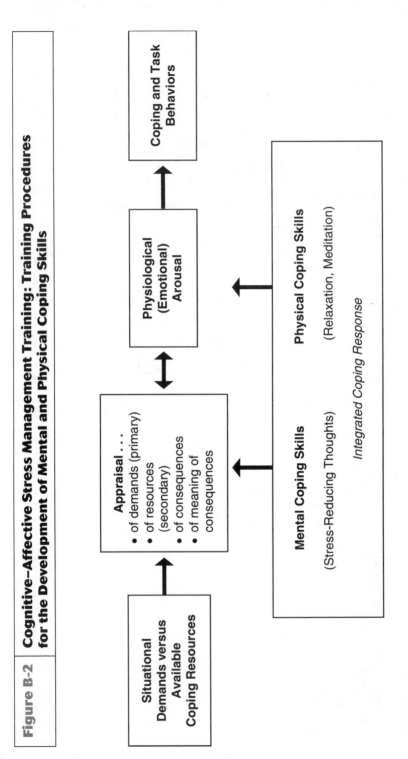

Figure B-2 | Cognitive–Affective Stress Management Training: Training Procedures for the Development of Mental and Physical Coping Skills

Situational Demands versus Available Coping Resources

Appraisal . . .
- of demands (primary)
- of resources (secondary)
- of consequences
- of meaning of consequences

Physiological (Emotional) Arousal

Coping and Task Behaviors

Mental Coping Skills

(Stress-Reducing Thoughts)

Physical Coping Skills

(Relaxation, Meditation)

Integrated Coping Response

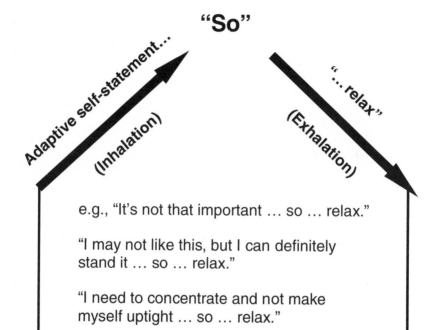

"So"

Adaptive self-statement... (Inhalation)

"...relax" (Exhalation)

e.g., "It's not that important ... so ... relax."

"I may not like this, but I can definitely stand it ... so ... relax."

"I need to concentrate and not make myself uptight ... so ... relax."

"I'm in control ... so ... relax."

Figure B-4 | Subjective Units of Discomfort Scale (SUDS)

Units of Discomfort

0	10	20	30	40	50	60	70	80	90	100
None; calm, relaxed		Slight discomfort	Mild; able to cope		Moderate discomfort; hard to control		Severe discomfort; nearly uncontrollable		Intense and uncontrollable	Unbearable; worst imaginable

Table B-1	Some Core Beliefs That Cause Needless Emotional Distress

- "To feel worthwhile, I must have the love and approval of virtually everyone."

  (Underlies excessive fear of disapproval or rejection.)

- "If I am not perfectly adequate, achieving, and competent in all possible respects, I can't feel good about myself."

  (Underlies distress-causing perfectionism and fear of failure.)

- "People who do not behave as they should deserve my wrath and should be punished for their misdeeds."

  (Underlies anger and hostility any time others violate our "shoulds.")

- "Unhappiness is caused by external and past circumstances, so there is nothing I can do about my distress."

  (Underlies feelings of helplessness, passivity, and inability to take positive steps to reduce distress.)

- "Dangerous or fearful things are causes for great concern, and their possibility of occurrence should be dwelt upon."

  (Underlies feelings of personal vulnerability, fear, and needless worry.)

- "I must have someone stronger upon whom to rely for support and guidance."

  (Underlies feelings of personal inadequacy and fosters excessive dependency.)

Table B-2	Samples of Anxiety and Anger Hierarchies for Self-Desensitization

Fear of Heights (fear reduction)	Test Anxiety (anxiety reduction)	Obnoxious Mother-in-Law (anger control)
Looking down from the edge of the Grand Canyon	Looking at a test question you cannot answer with confidence	Clara tells you your spouse should have married someone else
Looking over the edge of a high bridge at the ground below	Sitting in your seat as the test is passed out	Clara points out "mistakes" in your child-rearing practices
Standing at the railing of a 12th-floor open balcony	Arriving at the scene of the test	Clara makes a snide remark about your income or job
Looking out of a 12th-floor closed window	Getting up on the morning of the test and thinking about it	Clara ignores you during dinner at her house
Walking over an open 2nd-floor skyway and looking down	Studying a large amount of material the night before the test	Clara looking at you in a dismissing fashion when you express an opinion
Walking on a high, narrow trail in the mountains	Discussing difficulty of the material to be covered on the test with classmates	Clara describes successful past boyfriends of your spouse in glowing terms
Riding on a glass-walled elevator to the next level in a shopping center	Being reminded that the test will occur in 3 days	Clara criticizes your spouse's choice of carpeting
Watching a graphic film about skydivers	Finding that you will have another test on the same day	Clara complaining about not having a "loving family"
Standing 10 steps up on a ladder	Instructor announces a test in 2 weeks	Image of Clara's scowling face

From *Promoting Emotional Resilience: Cognitive–Affective Stress Management Training* by Ronald E. Smith and James C. Ascough. Copyright © 2016 The Guilford Press. Permission to photocopy this material is granted to purchasers of this book for personal use or use with individual clients (see copyright page for details). Purchasers can download enlarged versions of this material (see the box at the end of the table of contents).

References

Ackerman, S. J., Hilsenroth, M. J., Baity, M. R., & Blagys, M. D. (2000). Interaction of therapeutic process and alliance during psychological assessment. *Journal of Personality Assessment, 75,* 82–109.

Addis, M. E., & Jacobson, N. S. (2000). A closer look at the treatment rationale and homework compliance in cognitive-behavioral therapy for depression. *Cognitive Therapy and Research, 24,* 313–326.

Aldao, A., & Nolen-Hoeksema, S. (2012). When are adaptive strategies most predictive of psychopathology? *Journal of Abnormal Psychology, 121,* 276–281.

Aldao, A., Nolen-Hoeksema, S., & Schweizer, S. (2010). Emotion-regulation strategies across psychopathology: A meta-analytic review. *Clinical Psychology Review, 30,* 217–237.

Aldwin, C. M. (2007). *Stress, coping, and development: An integrative perspective* (2nd ed.). New York: Guilford Press.

Alidina, S. (2015). *The mindful way through stress: The proven 8-week path to health, happiness, and well-being.* New York: Guilford Press.

American Psychiatric Association. (2013). *Diagnostic and statistical manual of mental disorders* (5th ed.). Arlington, VA: Author.

American Psychological Association. (2013). Stress in America: Missing the health care connection. Retrieved from *www.apa.org/news/press/releases/2013/02/stress-management.aspx.*

Antony, M. M., Ledley, D. R., & Heimberg, R. G. (2005). *Improving outcomes and preventing relapse in cognitive-behavioral therapy.* New York: Guilford Press.

Antony, M. M., & Roemer, L. (2014). Behavior therapy process. In G. R. VandenBos, E. Meidenbauer, & J. Frank-McNeil (Eds.), *Psychotherapy theories and techniques* (pp. 29–34). Washington, DC: American Psychological Association.

Arnold, M. B. (1960). *Emotion and personality.* New York: Columbia University Press.

Arnold, M. B. (1970). *Feelings and emotion.* New York: Academic Press.

Ascough, J. C. (1975). *Manual for induced affect.* Unpublished document, Purdue University, West Lafayette, IN.

Ascough, J. C. (Ed.). (1981). *Case studies and research in induced affect.* Delphi, IN: Center for Induced Affect.

Ascough, J. C., Moore, C. H., & Sipprelle, C. N. (1981). *Induced anxiety: A method for research and behavior change.* Delphi, IN: Center for Induced Affect.

Ascough, J. C., & Sipprelle, C. N. (1968). Operant verbal conditioning of autonomic responses. *Behaviour Research and Therapy, 6,* 363–370.

Atkinson, J. W. (1964). *An introduction to motivation.* Princeton, NJ: Van Nostrand.

Auerbach, S. M. (1989). Stress management and coping research in the health care setting: An overview and methodological commentary. *Journal of Consulting and Clinical Psychology, 57,* 388–395.

Averill, J. A. (1980). A constructivist view of emotion. In R. Plutchik & H. Kellerman (Eds.), *Emotion: Theory, research and experience* (Vol. 1, pp. 127–158). New York: Academic Press.

Baldwin, M. W. (1999). Relational schemas: Research into social-cognitive aspects of interpersonal experience. In D. Cervone & Y. Shoda (Eds.), *The coherence of personality: Social-cognitive bases of consistency, variability, and organization* (pp. 127–154). New York: Guilford Press.

Baldwin, S. A., Berkeljon, A., Atkins, D. C., & Nielsen, S. L. (2009). Rates of change in naturalistic psychotherapy: Contrasting dose–effect and good-enough level models of change. *Journal of Consulting and Clinical Psychology, 77,* 201–211.

Bandura, A. (1986). *Social foundations of thought and action: A social-cognitive theory.* Englewood Cliffs, NJ: Prentice Hall.

Bandura, A. (1997). *Self-efficacy: The exercise of control.* New York: Freeman.

Bandura, A., Blanchard, E. B., & Ritter, B. (1969). The relative efficacy of desensitization and modeling approaches for inducing behavioral, affective, and attitudinal changes. *Journal of Personality and Social Psychology, 13,* 173–199.

Barlow, D. H. (2004). *Anxiety and its disorders: The nature and treatment of anxiety and panic* (2nd ed.). New York: Guilford Press.

Barlow, D. H., Allen, L. B., & Choate, M. L. (2004). Toward a unified treatment for emotional disorders. *Behavior Therapy, 35,* 205–230.

Barlow, D. H., Farchione, T. J., Fairholme, C. P., Ellard, K. K., Boisseau, C. L., Allen, L. B., et al. (2011). *Unified protocol for transdiagnostic treatment of emotional disorders: Therapist guide.* New York: Oxford University Press.

Barlow, D. H., Sauer-Savala, S., Carl, J. R., Bullis, J. R., & Ellard, K. K. (2014). The nature, diagnosis, and treatment of neuroticism: Back to the future. *Clinical Psychological Science, 2,* 344–365.

Beck, A. T. (1976). *Cognitive therapy and the emotional disorders.* New York: International Universities Press.

Beck, J. S. (2011). *Cognitive behavior therapy: Basics and beyond* (2nd ed.). New York: Guilford Press.

Benson, H., & Klipper, M. (1976). *The relaxation response.* New York: Morrow.

Benson, H., & Proctor, W. (2010). *Relaxation revolution: Enhancing your health through the science and genetics of mind–body healing.* Fort Worth, TX: Scribner.

Bereika, G. M. (1976). *The effects of induced affect on selected characteristics of drug-dependent patients.* Unpublished doctoral dissertation, Purdue University, West Lafayette, IN.

Berg, K. C., Peterson, C. B., Crosby, R. D., Cao, L., Crow, S. J., Engel, S. G., et al. (2014). The relation between daily affect and overeating-only, loss of control eating-only, and binge eating episodes in obese adults. *Psychiatry Research, 215,* 185–191.

Berking, M., & Schwarz, J. (2014). Affect regulation training. In J. J. Gross (Ed.), *Handbook of emotion regulation* (2nd ed., pp. 529–547). New York: Guilford Press.

Boer, A. P. (1970). *Toward preventative psychotherapy: Experimental reduction of psychophysiological stress through prior behavior therapy training.* Unpublished doctoral dissertation, University of South Dakota, Vermillion.

Boer, A. P., & Sipprelle, C. R. (1969). Induced anxiety in the treatment for LSD effects. *Psychotherapy and Psychosomatics, 17,* 108–113.

Boersma, K., MacDonald, S., & Linton, S. J. (2012). Longitudinal relationships between pain and stress problems in the general population: Predicting trajectories from cognitive behavioral variables. *Journal of Applied Biobehavioral Research, 17,* 229–248.

Bonanno, G. A., & Keltner, D. (1997). Facial expressions of emotion and the course of conjugal bereavement. *Journal of Abnormal Psychology, 106,* 126–137.

Bonanno, G. A., & Mancini, A. (2012). Beyond resilience and PTSD: Mapping the heterogeneity of responses to potential trauma. *Psychological Trauma: Theory, Research, Practice, and Policy, 4,* 74–83.

Bonanno, G. A., Papa, A., Lalande, K., & Coifman, K. (2004). The importance of being flexible. *Psychological Science, 15,* 482–487.

Borckardt, J. J., Nash, M. R., Murphy, M. D., Moore, M., Shaw, D., & O'Neil, P. (2008). Clinical practice as a natural laboratory for psychotherapy research: A guide to case-based time-series analysis. *American Psychologist, 63,* 77–95.

Borkovec, T. D., Alcaine, O., & Behar, E. (2004). Avoidance theory of worry and generalized anxiety disorder. In R. G. Heimberg, C. L. Turk, & D. S. Mennin (Eds.), *Generalized anxiety disorder: Advances in research and practice* (pp. 77–108). New York: Guilford Press.

Bornstein, P. H., & Sipprelle, C. N. (1973a). Induced anxiety in the treatment of obesity: A preliminary case report. *Behavior Therapy, 4,* 141–143.

Bornstein, P. H., & Sipprelle, C. N. (1973b). Group treatment of obesity by induced anxiety. *Behaviour Research and Therapy, 11,* 339–341.

Bornstein, P. H., & Sipprelle, C. N. (1981). Clinical applications of induced anxiety in the treatment of obesity. In J. C. Ascough (Ed.), *Case studies and research in induced affect* (pp. 29–34). Delphi, IN: Center for Induced Affect.

Boswell, J. F. (2013). Intervention strategies and clinical process in transdiagnostic cognitive-behavioral therapy. *Psychotherapy, 50,* 381–386.

Boswell, J. F., Anderson, L. M., & Barlow, D. H. (2014). An idiographic analysis of change processes in the unified transdiagnostic treatment of depression. *Journal of Consulting and Clinical Psychology, 82,* 1060–1071.

Bower, G. H. (1981). Mood and memory. *American Psychologist, 36,* 129–148.

Buske-Kirschbaum, A., Geiben, A., & Hellhammer, D. (2001). Psychobiological aspects of atopic dermatitis: An overview. *Psychotherapy and Psychosomatics, 70,* 6–16.

Campbell-Sills, L., Ellard, K. K., & Barlow, D. H. (2014). Emotion regulation in anxiety disorders. In J. J. Gross (Ed.), *Handbook of emotion regulation* (2nd ed., pp. 393–412). New York: Guilford Press.

Cannon, W. B. (1932). *The wisdom of the body.* New York: Norton.

Carroll, K. M. (1998). *Therapy manuals for drug addictions: A cognitive-behavioral approach.* Bethesda, MD: National Institute on Drug Abuse.

Carver, C. S., Scheier, M. F., & Weintraub, J. K. (1989). Assessing coping strategies: A theoretically based approach. *Journal of Personality and Social Psychology, 56,* 267–283.

Cattell, R. B. (1965). *The scientific analysis of personality.* Chicago: Aldine.

Cervone, D., Shadel, W. G., Smith, R. E., & Fiori, M. (2006). Self-regulation: Reminders and suggestions from personality science. *Applied Psychology: An International Review, 55,* 333–385.

Charles, S. T., Piazza, J. R., Mogle, J. S., Sliwinski, M. J., & Almeida, D. M. (2013).

The wear and tear of daily stressors on mental health. *Psychological Science, 24,* 733–741.

Chen, J. A. (2015). *The effects of systematic self-monitoring, feedback, and collaborative assessment on stress reduction.* Unpublished doctoral dissertation, University of Washington, Seattle.

Chen, J. A., Gilmore, A. K., Wilson, N. L., Smith, R. E., Shoda, Y., Quinn, K., et al. (in press). Enhancing stress management coping skills using induced affect and collaborative daily assessment. *Cognitive and Behavioral Practice.*

Chiesa, A., & Serretti, A. (2009). Mindfulness-based stress reduction for stress management in healthy people: A review and meta-analysis. *Journal of Alternative and Complementary Medicine, 15,* 593–600.

Childers, J. (1981). Induced anxiety as a function of massed versus spaced practice. In J. C. Ascough, C. H. Moore, & C. N. Sipprelle (Eds.), *Induced anxiety: A method for research and behavior change* (pp. 23–26). Delphi, IN: Center for Induced Affect.

Clark, L. A., & Watson, D. (1991). Tripartite model of anxiety and depression: Psychometric evidence and taxonomic implications. *Journal of Abnormal Psychology, 100,* 316–336.

Clum, G. A., & Watkins, P. (2008). Self-help therapies: Retrospect and prospects. In P. Watkins & G. A. Clum (Eds.), *Handbook of self-help therapies* (pp. 419–436). New York: Routledge.

Cockshott, J. B., & Ascough, J. C. (1981). An evaluation of the efficacy of induced anxiety for treatment of schizophrenia. In J. C. Ascough (Ed.), *Case studies and research in induced affect* (pp. 81–88). Delphi, IN: Center for Induced Affect.

Cohen, S., Kamarck, T., & Mermelstein, R. (1983). A global measure of perceived stress. *Journal of Health and Social Behavior, 24,* 385–396.

Cook, T. D., & Campbell, D. T. (1979). *Quasi-experimentation: Design and analysis issues for field settings.* Chicago: Rand-McNally.

Craske, M. G., & Barlow, D. H. (2014). Panic disorder and agoraphobia. In D. H. Barlow (Ed.), *Clinical handbook of psychological disorders* (5th ed., pp. 1–61). New York: Guilford Press.

Craske, M. G., Kircanski, K., Mystkowski, J., Chowdhury, N., & Baker, A. (2008). Optimizing inhibitory learning during exposure therapy. *Behaviour Research and Therapy, 46,* 5–27.

Crocker, P. R. E. (1989). A follow-up of cognitive–affective stress management training. *Journal of Sport and Exercise Psychology, 11,* 236–242.

Crocker, P. R. E., Alderman, R. B., & Smith, F. M. R. (1988). Cognitive–affective stress management training with high performance youth volleyball players: Effects on affect, cognition, and performance. *Journal of Sport and Exercise Psychology, 10,* 448–460.

Cromer, T. D. (2013). Integrative techniques related to positive processes in psychotherapy. *Psychotherapy, 50,* 307–311.

Culver, N. C., Stoyanova, M., & Craske, M. G. (2012). Emotional variability and sustained arousal during exposure. *Journal of Behavior Therapy and Experimental Psychiatry, 43,* 787–793.

Davidson, R. J., & Schwartz, G. E. (1976). The psychobiology of relaxation and related states: A multi-process theory. In D. I. Mostofsky (Ed.), *Behavioral control and the modification of physiological activity* (pp. 129–146). Englewood Cliffs, NJ: Prentice Hall.

Deffenbacher, J. K. (2013). Cognitive-behavioral therapy for angry drivers. In E. Fernandez (Ed.), *Treatments for anger in specific populations: Theory, application, and outcome* (pp. 15–32). New York: Oxford University Press.

Diener, E., & Larson, R. J. (1993). The subjective experience of emotional well-being. In M. Lewis & J. M. Haviland (Eds.), *Handbook of emotions* (pp. 405–415). New York: Guilford Press.

Dollard, J., & Miller, N. E. (1950). *Personality and psychotherapy*. New York: McGraw-Hill.

Dusek, J. A., Otu, H. H., Wohlheuter, A. L., Bhasin, L. F., Zerbini, L. F., Joseph, M. G., et al. (2008). Genomic counter-stress changes induced by the relaxation response. *PLoS ONE, 3*(7), e2576.

D'Zurilla, T. J., & Nezu, A. M. (2007). *Problem-solving therapy: A social competence approach to clinical intervention* (3rd ed.). New York: Springer.

Easterbrook, J. A. (1959). The effect of emotion on cue utilization and the organization of behavior. *Psychological Review, 66,* 183–201.

Edenfield, T. M., & Saeed, S. A. (2012). An update on mindfulness meditation as a self-help treatment for anxiety and depression. *Psychology Research and Behavior Management, 5,* 131–141.

Ehde, D. M., Dillworth, T. M., & Turner, J. A. (2014). Cognitive-behavioral therapy for individuals with chronic pain: Efficacy, innovations, and directions for research. *American Psychologist, 69,* 153–166.

Elliot, R., Watson, J. C., Goldman, R. N., & Greenberg, L. S. (2004). *Learning emotion-focused therapy*. Washington, DC: American Psychological Association.

Ellis, A. (1962). *Reason and emotion in psychotherapy*. New York: Lyle Stuart.

English, T., John, O. P., & Gross, J. J. (2013). Emotion regulation in close relationships. In J. A. Simpson & L. Campbell (Eds.), *The Oxford handbook of close relationships* (pp. 500–513). New York: Oxford University Press.

Eysenck, H. J. (1947). *Dimensions of personality*. Oxford, UK: Routledge & Kegan Paul.

Eysenck, H. J. (1994). Cancer, personality, and stress: Prediction and prevention. *Advances in Behaviour Research and Therapy, 16,* 167–215.

Eysenck, H. J., & Grossarth-Marticek, R. (1991). Creative novation behavior therapy as a prophylactic treatment for cancer and coronary heart disease: Part II—effects of treatment. *Behaviour Research and Therapy, 29,* 17–31.

Farb, N. A. S., Anderson, A. S., Irving, J. A., & Segal, Z. V. (2014). Mindfulness interventions and emotion regulation. In J. J. Gross (Ed.), *Handbook of emotion regulation* (2nd ed., pp. 548–570). New York: Guilford Press.

Farb, N. A. S., Segal, Z. V., & Anderson, A. K. (2013). Mindfulness meditation training alters cortical representations of interoceptive attention. *Social Cognitive and Affective Neuroscience, 8,* 15–26.

Fergusson, D. M., Woodward, L. J., & Horwood, L. J. (2000). Risk factors and life processes associated with the onset of suicidal behaviour during adolescence and early adulthood. *Psychological Medicine, 30,* 23–39.

Fiedler, F. E. (1995). Cognitive resources and leadership performance. *Applied Psychology: An International Journal, 44,* 5–28.

Fischer, C. T., & Finn, S. E. (2008). Developing life meaning of psychological test data: Collaborative and therapeutic approaches. In R. P. Archer & S. R. Smith (Eds.), *Personality assessment* (pp. 379–404). New York: Routledge.

Foa, E. B., & Jaycox, L. H. (1999). Cognitive-behavioral treatment of post-traumatic stress disorder. In D. Spiegel (Ed.), *Efficacy and cost-effectiveness of psychotherapy* (pp. 23–61). Washington, DC: American Psychiatric Press.

Folkman, S. (2011). *The Oxford handbook of stress, health, and coping*. New York: Oxford University Press.

Fredrickson, B. L. (1998). What good are positive emotions? *Review of General Psychology, 2,* 300–319.

Freitas, A. L., & Downey, G. (1998). Resilience: A dynamic perspective. *International Journal of Behavioral Development, 22,* 263–285.

Friedberg, F. T. (1969, April). *The effects of induced anxiety under verbal and nonverbal conditions in chronic hospitalized schizophrenics.* Paper presented at the meeting of the Southeastern Psychological Association, New Orleans, LA.

Frijda, N. H. (1986). *The emotions.* Cambridge, UK: Cambridge University Press.

Furmark, T., Carlbring, P., Hedman, E., Sonnenstein, A., Cleuberger, P., Bohman, B., et al. (2009). Guided and unguided self-help for social anxiety disorder: Randomised controlled trial. *British Journal of Psychiatry, 195,* 440–447.

Garnefski, N., Legerstee, J., Kraaij, V., van den Kommer, T., & Teerds, J. (2002). Cognitive coping strategies and symptoms of depression and anxiety: A comparison between adolescents and adults. *Journal of Adolescence, 25,* 603–611.

Gianini, L. M., White, M. A., & Masheb, R. M. (2013). Eating pathology, emotion regulation, and emotional overeating in obese adults with binge eating disorder. *Eating Behaviors, 14,* 309–313.

Goldfried, M. R. (1971). Systematic desensitization as training in self-control. *Journal of Consulting and Clinical Psychology, 37,* 228–234.

Goldfried, M. R. (2013). Evidence-based treatment and cognitive–affective–relational behavior therapy. *Psychotherapy, 50,* 376–380.

Goldin, P. R., McRae, K., Ramel, W., & Gross, J. J. (2007). The neural bases of emotion regulation: Reappraisal and suppression of negative emotion. *Biological Psychiatry, 63,* 577–586.

Goldin, P. R., Ziv, M., Jazaieri, H., Werner, K., Kraemer, H., Heimberg, R. G., et al. (2012). Cognitive reappraisal self-efficacy mediates the effects of individual cognitive-behavioral therapy for social anxiety disorder. *Journal of Consulting and Clinical Psychology, 80,* 1034–1040.

Gray, J. A. (1991). Neural systems, emotions, and personality. In J. Madden, IV (Ed.), *Neurobiology of learning, emotion, and affect* (pp. 171–223). New York: Raven Press.

Gregory, R. J., Schwer Canning, S., Lee, T., & Wise, J. (2004). Cognitive bibliotherapy for depression: A meta-analysis. *Professional Psychology: Research and Practice, 35,* 275–280.

Gross, J. J. (1998) Antecedent- and response-focused emotion regulation: Divergent consequences for experience, expression, and physiology. *Journal of Personality and Social Psychology, 74,* 224–237.

Gross, J. J. (Ed.). (2014a). *Handbook of emotion regulation* (2nd ed.). New York: Guilford Press.

Gross, J. J. (2014b). Emotion regulation: Conceptual and empirical foundations. In J. J. Gross (Ed.), *Handbook of emotion regulation* (2nd ed., pp. 3–22). New York: Guilford Press.

Hansen, N. B., Lambert, M. J., & Forman, E. M. (2002). The psychotherapy dose–response effect and its implications for treatment delivery services. *Clinical Psychology: Science and Practice, 9,* 329–343.

Harmon-Jones, E. (2003). Anger and the behavioral approach system. *Personality and Individual Differences, 35,* 995–1005.

Hayes, S. C., Strosahl, K., & Wilson, K. G. (2012). *Acceptance and commitment therapy: An experiential approach to behavior change* (2nd ed.). New York: Guilford Press.

Higher Education Research Institute. (2015). *The American freshman: National norms Fall, 2014.* Los Angeles: UCLA Cooperative Institutional Research Program.

Hoffman, H. G., Patterson, D. R., Canougher, G. J., & Sharar, S. R. (2001). Effectiveness of virtual reality-based pain control with multiple treatments. *Clinical Journal of Pain, 17,* 229–235.

Hoffman, S. G., Heering, S., Sawyer, A. T., & Asnaani, A. (2009). How to handle anxiety: The effects of reappraisal, acceptance, and suppression strategies on anxious arousal. *Behaviour Research and Therapy, 47*, 389–394.

Holahan, C. J., & Moos, R. H. (1986). Personality, coping, and family resources in stress resistance: A longitudinal analysis. *Journal of Personality and Social Psychology, 51*, 389–395.

Hollon, S. D., Thase, M. E., & Markowitz, J. C. (2002). Treatment and prevention of depression. *Psychological Science in the Public Interest, 3*, 39–77.

Holmes, G. D. (1981). Modeling, induced anxiety, and test-taking anxiety. In J. C. Ascough, C. H. Moore, & C. N. Sipprelle (Eds.), *Induced anxiety: A method for research and behavior change* (pp. 57–60). Delphi, IN: Center for Induced Affect.

Holmes, T. S., & Rahe, R. H. (1967). The Social Readjustment Rating Scale. *Journal of Psychosomatic Research, 11*, 213–218.

Holtzworth-Munroe, A., Munroe, M. S., & Smith, R. E. (1985). Effects of a stress management training program on first- and second-year medical students. *Journal of Medical Education, 60*, 417–419.

Hope, D. A., Heimberg, R. G., & Turk, C. L. (2006). *Managing social anxiety: A cognitive-behavioral therapy approach.* New York: Oxford University Press.

Howard, K. I., Kopta, S. M., Krause, M. S., & Orlinsky, D. E. (1986). The dose–response relationship in psychotherapy. *American Psychologist, 41*, 159–164.

Hoyle, R. H., Fejfar, M. C., & Miller, J. D. (2000). Personality and sexual risk taking: A quantitative review. *Journal of Personality, 68*, 1203–1231.

Huovinen, E., Kaprio, J., & Koskenvuo, M. (2001). Asthma in relation to personality traits, life satisfaction, and stress: A prospective study among 11,000 adults. *Allergy, 56*, 971–977.

Huprich, S. K., & Bornstein, R. F. (2007). An overview of issues related to categorical and dimensional models of personality disorder assessment. *Journal of Personality Assessment, 89*, 3–15.

Ingram, J. A. (1981). Induced anxiety as a therapeutic technique for the reduction of public speaking anxiety. In J. C. Ascough, C. H. Moore, & C. N. Sipprelle (Eds.), *Induced anxiety: A method for research and behavior change* (pp. 43–48). Delphi, IN: Center for Induced Affect.

Ingram, R. E., & Hollon, S. D. (1986). Cognitive therapy of depression from an information processing perspective. In R. E. Ingram (Ed.), *Information processing approaches to clinical psychology* (pp. 261–284). Orlando, FL: Academic Press.

Insel, T. R. (2012). Next-generation treatments for mental disorders. *Science and Translational Medicine, 4*, 1–9.

Insel, T. R., & Cuthbert, B. N. (2013). Toward precision medicine in psychiatry: The NIMH research domain criteria project. In D. S. Charney, J. D. Buxbaum, P. Skylar, & E. J. Nestler (Eds.), *Neurobiology of mental illness* (4th ed., pp. 1076–1088). New York: Oxford University Press.

Jacobs, R. S., Smith, R. E., Fiedler, F. E., & Link, T. G. (2013). Using stress management training to enhance leader performance and the utilization of intellectual abilities during stressful military training: An application of cognitive resource theory. In J. D. VanVactor (Ed.), *The psychology of leadership* (pp. 61–79). New York: Nova Science.

Jacobson, E. (1938). *Progressive relaxation.* Chicago: University of Chicago Press.

John, O. P., & Eng, J. (2014). Three approaches to individual differences in emotion regulation: Conceptualizations, measures, and findings. In J. J. Gross (Ed.), *Handbook of emotion regulation* (2nd ed., pp. 321–345). New York: Guilford Press.

Johnstone, B. M., Garrity, T. F., & Straus, R. (1997). The relationship between alcohol and life stress. In T. W. Miller (Ed.), *Clinical disorders and stressful life events* (pp. 247–279). Madison, NJ: International Universities Press.

Jones, R. G. (1968). *A factored measure of Ellis' irrational belief system, with personality and maladjustment correlates.* Unpublished doctoral dissertation, Texas Technical University, Lubbock, TX.

Joorman, J., & Siemer, M. (2014). Emotion regulation in mood disorders. In J. J. Gross (Ed.), *Handbook of emotion regulation* (2nd ed., pp. 413–427). New York: Guilford Press.

Jordan, C. S., & Sipprelle, C. N. (1972). Physiological correlates of induced anxiety in normal subjects. *Psychotherapy: Theory, Research, and Practice, 9,* 18–21.

Judge, T. A., Colbert, A. E., & Illies, R. (2004). Intelligence and leadership: A quantitative review and test of theoretical propositions. *Journal of Applied Psychology, 89,* 542–552.

Kabat-Zinn, J. (1982). An outpatient program in behavioral medicine for chronic pain patients based on the practice of mindfulness meditation: Theoretical considerations and preliminary results. *General Hospital Psychiatry, 4,* 33–47.

Kabat-Zinn, J. (1990). *Full catastrophe living: Using the wisdom of your body and mind to face stress, pain, and illness.* New York: Dell.

Kalisch, R., & Gerlicher, A. M. V. (2014). Making a mountain out of a molehill: On the role of the rostral dorsal anterior cingulate and dorsomedial prefrontal cortex in conscious threat appraisal, catastrophizing, and worrying. *Neuroscience and Biobehavioral Reviews, 42,* 1–8.

Kazdin, A. E. (2008). Evidence-based treatment and practice: New opportunities to bridge clinical research and practice, enhance the knowledge base, and improve patient care. *American Psychologist, 63,* 146–159.

Kazdin, A. E., & Blase, S. L. (2011). Rebooting psychotherapy research to reduce the burden of mental illness. *Perspectives on Psychological Science, 6,* 21–37.

Kendler, K. S., Gatz, M., Gardner, C. O., & Pederse, N. L. (2006). Personality and major depression. *Archives of General Psychiatry, 63,* 1113–1120.

Kessler, R. C., Chiu, W. T., Demler, O., & Walters, E. E. (2005). Prevalence, severity, and comorbidity of 12-month DSM-IV disorders in the National Comorbidity Survey Replication. *Archives of General Psychiatry, 62,* 617–627.

Kiesler, D. J. (1966). Some myths of psychotherapy research and the search for a paradigm. *Psychological Bulletin, 65,* 110–136.

Kihlstrom, J. F. (2008). The psychological unconscious. In O. P. John, R. W. Robins, & L. A. Pervin (Eds.), *Handbook of personality: Theory and research* (3rd ed., pp. 234–258). New York: Guilford Press.

Kober, H. (2014). Emotion regulation in substance use disorders. In J. J. Gross (Ed.), *Handbook of emotion regulation* (2nd ed., pp. 428–446). New York: Guilford Press.

Korn, E. J., Ascough, J. C., & Kleemeier, R. B. (1972). The effects of induced anxiety on state–trait measures of anxiety in high, middle, and low trait-anxious individuals. *Behavior Therapy, 3,* 547–554.

Kring, A. M., & Sloan, D. S. (Eds.). (2010). *Emotion regulation and psychopathology: A transdiagnostic approach to etiology and treatment.* New York: Guilford Press.

Kross, E., & Ayduk, O. (2008). Facilitating adaptive emotional analysis: Distinguishing distanced-analysis of depressive experiences from immersed-analysis and distraction. *Personality and Social Psychology Bulletin, 34,* 924–938.

Lahey, B. B. (2009). Public health significance of neuroticism. *American Psychologist, 64,* 241–256.

Lang, P. J., & Lazovik, A. D. (1963). Experimental desensitization of a phobia. *Journal of Abnormal and Social Psychology, 66,* 519–525.

Lazarus, R. S. (1966). *Psychological stress and the coping process*. New York: McGraw-Hill.

Lazarus, R. S. (1991a). *Emotion and adaptation*. New York: Oxford University Press.

Lazarus, R. S. (1991b). Progress on a cognitive–motivational–relational theory of emotion. *American Psychologist, 46*, 819–834.

Lazarus, R. S. (1993). From psychological stress to the emotions: A history of changing outlooks. *Annual Review of Psychology, 44*, 1–21.

Lazarus, R. S., & Folkman, S. (1984). *Stress, appraisal, and coping*. New York: Springer.

Leahy, R. L., Tirch, D., & Napolitano, L. A. (2011). *Emotion regulation in psychotherapy*. New York: Guilford Press.

LeDoux, J. E. (2000). Emotion circuits in the brain. *Annual Review of Neuroscience, 23*, 155–184.

Levin, M. E., Hildebrandt, M. J., Lillis, J., & Hayes, S. C. (2012). The impact of treatment components suggested by the psychological flexibility model: A meta-analysis of laboratory-based component studies. *Behavior Therapy, 43*, 741–756.

Levis, D. J. (2009). The prolonged CS exposure techniques of implosive (flooding) therapy. In W. T. O'Donoghue & J. E. Fisher (Eds.), *General principles and empirically supported techniques of cognitive behavior therapy* (pp. 272–282). Hoboken, NJ: Wiley.

Linehan, M. M. (1993). *Cognitive-behavioral treatment of borderline personality disorder*. New York: Guilford Press.

Linehan, M. M. (2015). *DBT skills training manual* (2nd ed.). New York: Guilford Press.

Lorr, M., & Vestre, N. D. (1968). *Psychotic Inpatient Profile manual*. Beverly Hills, CA: Western Psychological Services.

MacLeod, C., & Grafton, B. (2014). Regulation of emotion through modification of attention. In J. J. Gross (Ed.), *Handbook of emotion regulation* (2nd ed., pp. 508–528). New York: Guilford Press.

Malouff, J. M., Thorsteinsson, E. B., & Schutte, N. S. (2006). The five-factor model of personality and smoking: A meta-analysis. *Journal of Drug Education, 36*, 47–58.

Marlatt, G. A., & Gordon, J. R. (Eds.). (1985). *Relapse prevention: Maintenance strategies in the treatment of addictive behaviors*. New York: Guilford Press.

Mathews, A., & MacLeod, C. (2005). Cognitive vulnerability in emotional disorders. *Annual Review of Clinical Psychology, 1*, 167–195.

Maxwell, W. A. (1981). Some relationships between induced anxiety and systematic desensitization. In J. C. Ascough (Ed.), *Case studies and research in induced affect* (pp. 69–74). Delphi, IN: Center for Induced Affect.

McCaul, K. D., & Mallott, J. J. (1984). Distraction and coping with pain. *Psychological Bulletin, 95*, 516–533.

McCracken, L. M., & Vowles, K. E. (2014). Acceptance and commitment therapy and mindfulness for chronic pain: Model, process, and progress. *American Psychologist, 69*, 178–187.

McCrae, R. R., & Costa, P. T. (2003). *Personality in adulthood: A five-factor theory perspective*. New York: Guilford Press.

McRae, K., Cielielski, B., & Gross, J. J. (2012). Unpacking cognitive reappraisal: Goals, tactics, and outcomes. *Emotion, 12*, 250–255.

Meichenbaum, D. (1974). Self-instructional methods. In F. H. Kanfer & A. P. Goldstein (Eds.), *Helping people change* (pp. 67–91). New York: Pergamon Press.

Meichenbaum, D. (1977). *Cognitive-behavior modification*. New York: Plenum Press.

Meichenbaum, D. (1985). *Stress inoculation training*. New York: Pergamon Press.

Melzack, R. (1973). *The puzzle of pain*. New York: Basic Books.

Mennin, D. S., & Fresco, D. M. (2010). Emotion regulation as an integrative framework for understanding and treating psychopathology. In A. M. Kring & D. M.

Sloan (Eds.), *Emotion regulation in psychopathology: A transdiagnostic approach to etiology and treatment* (pp. 356–379). New York: Guilford Press.

Mennin, D. S., & Fresco, D. M. (2014). Emotion regulation therapy. In J. J. Gross (Ed.), *Handbook of emotion regulation* (2nd ed., pp. 469–490). New York: Guilford Press.

Messer, S. B. (2013). Three mechanisms of change in psychodynamic therapy: Insight, affect, and alliance. *Psychotherapy, 50,* 408–412.

Meuret, A. E., Seidel, A., Rosenfield, B., Hofmann, S. G., & Rosenfield, D. (2012). Does fear reactivity during exposure predict panic symptom reduction? *Journal of Consulting and Clinical Psychology, 80,* 773–785.

Meuret, A. E., Wolitzky-Taylor, K. B., Twohig, M. P., & Craske, M. G. (2012). Coping skills and exposure therapy in panic disorder and agoraphobia: Latest advances and future directions. *Behavior Therapy, 43,* 271–284.

Meyer, T. D., & Baur, M. (2009). Positive and negative affect in individuals at high and low risk for bipolar disorders. *Journal of Individual Differences, 30,* 169–175.

Miller, W. R., & Rollnick, S. (2002). *Motivational interviewing: Preparing people for change.* New York: Guilford Press.

Mischel, W., & Shoda, Y. (1995). A cognitive–affective system theory of personality: Reconceptualizing situations, dispositions, dynamics, and invariance in personality structure. *Psychological Review, 102,* 246–268.

Moore, C. H. (1981). Induced anxiety as a therapy technique. In J. C. Ascough (Ed.), *Case studies and research in induced affect* (pp. 35–40). Delphi, IN: Center for Induced Affect.

Morrison, C., Bradley, R., & Westen, D. (2003). The external validity of efficacy trials for depression and anxiety: A naturalistic study. *Psychology and Psychotherapy: Theory, Research, and Practice, 76,* 109–132.

Mueser, K. T., Gottlieb, J. D., & Gingerich, S. (2014). Social skills and problem-solving therapy. In S. G. Hofmann, D. J. A. Dozois, W. Rief, & J. A. Smits (Eds.), *The Wiley handbook of behavior therapy* (pp. 243–271). Hoboken, NJ: Wiley-Blackwell.

Mumma, G. H. (2011). Validity issues in cognitive-behavioral case formulation. *European Journal of Psychological Assessment, 27,* 29–49.

Narrow, W. E., Rae, D. S., Robins, L. N., & Regier, D. A. (2002). Revised prevalence estimates of mental disorders in the United States: Using a clinical significance criterion to reconcile 2 surveys' estimates. *Archives of General Psychiatry, 59,* 115–123.

National Institute of Mental Health. (2008). *National Institute of Mental Health strategic plan* (NIH Publication No. 08-6388). Rockville, MD: Author.

Neacsiu, A. D., Bohus, M., & Linehan, M. M. (2014). Dialectical behavior therapy: An intervention for emotion regulation. In J. J. Gross (Ed.), *Handbook of emotion regulation* (2nd ed., pp. 491–507). New York: Guilford Press.

Newman, M. G., Kenardy, J., Herman, S., & Taylor, C. B. (1997). Comparison of palmtop-computer assisted brief cognitive-behavioral treatment to cognitive-behavioral treatment for panic disorder. *Journal of Consulting and Clinical Psychology, 65,* 178–183.

Newman, M. L., & Greenway, P. (1997). Therapeutic effects of providing MMPI-2 test feedback to clients at a university counseling service: A collaborative approach. *Psychological Assessment, 9,* 122–131.

Nideffer, R. M., & Sharpe, R. (1987). *A.C.T.: Attention control training.* New York: Wyden Books.

Ochsner, K. N., & Gross, J. J. (2014). The neural basis of emotion and emotion regulation: A valuation perspective. In J. J. Gross (Ed.), *Handbook of emotion regulation* (2nd ed., pp. 23–42). New York: Guilford Press.

O'Donohue, W. T., & Fisher, J. E. (Eds.). (2009). *General principles and empirically supported techniques of cognitive behavior therapy.* Hoboken, NJ: Wiley.

Ollendick, T. H., & Davis, T. E., III. (2013). One session treatment for specific phobias: A review of Ost's single-session exposure with children and adolescents. *Cognitive Behaviour Therapy, 42,* 275–283.

Onken, L. S., Carroll, K. M., Shoham, V., Cuthbert, B. N., & Riddle, M. (2014). Reenvisioning clinical science: Unifying the discipline to improve the public health. *Clinical Psychological Science, 2,* 22–34.

Öst, L.-G. (1989). One-session treatment for specific phobias. *Behaviour Research and Therapy, 27,* 1–7.

Otto, M. W., Tolin, D. F., Nations, K. R., Utschig, A. C., Rothbaum, B. O., Hofmann, S. G., et al. (2012). Five sessions and counting: Considering ultra-brief treatment for panic disorder. *Depression and Anxiety, 29,* 465–470.

Pagano, R. R., Rose, R. M., Stivers, R. M., & Warrenburg, S. (1976). Sleep during transcendental meditation. *Science, 191,* 308–310.

Paivio, S. C. (2013). Essential processes in emotion-focused psychotherapy. *Psychotherapy, 50,* 341–345.

Park, C. L., Armeli, S., & Tennen, H. (2004). Appraisal–coping goodness of fit: A daily Internet study. *Personality and Social Psychology Bulletin, 30,* 558–569.

Pascal, G. R. (1959). *Behavior change in the clinic.* New York: Grune & Stratton.

Pegg, P. O., Jr., Auerbach, S. M., Seel, R. T., Buenaver, L. F., Kiesler, D. J., & Plybon, L. E. (2005). The impact of patient-centered information on patients' treatment satisfaction and outcomes in traumatic brain injury rehabilitation. *Rehabilitation Psychology, 50,* 366–374.

Pennebaker, J. W. (1995). *Emotion, disclosure, and health.* Washington, DC: American Psychological Association.

Pennebaker, J. W. (1997). *Opening up: The healing power of expressing emotions.* New York: Guilford Press.

Perls, F. S. (1969). *Gestalt therapy verbatim.* Lafayette, CA: Real People Press.

Pollak, S. M., Pedulla, T., & Siegel, R. D. (2014). *Sitting together: Essential skills for mindfulness-based psychotherapy.* New York: Guilford Press.

Poston, J. M., & Hanson, W. E. (2010). Meta-analysis of psychological assessment as a therapeutic intervention. *Psychological Assessment, 22,* 203–212.

Powers, M. B., Halpern, J. M., Ferenschak, M. P., Gillihan, S. J., & Foa, E. B. (2010). A meta-analytic review of prolonged exposure for posttraumatic stress disorder. *Clinical Psychology Review, 30,* 635–641.

Powers, M. B., Zum Vorde Sive Vording, M. B., & Emmelkamp, P. (2009). Acceptance and commitment therapy: A meta-analytic review. *Psychotherapy and Psychosomatics, 78,* 73–80.

Prochaska, J., & DiClemente, C. (1984). *The transtheoretical approach: Crossing traditional boundaries of therapy.* Homewood, IL: Dow Jones-Irwin.

Ptacek, J. T., Smith, R. E., Raffety, B., & Lindgren, K. P. (2008). Coherence and transituational generality in coping: The unity and the diversity. *Anxiety, Stress, and Coping, 21,* 155–172.

Raine, A. (2008). From genes to brain to antisocial behavior. *Current Directions in Psychological Science, 17,* 323–328.

Renninger, S. M. (2013). Clinical application of meta-concepts that are essential to client change. *Psychotherapy, 50,* 302–306.

Rescorla, R. A., & Solomon, R. L. (1967). Two-process learning theory: Relationships between Pavlovian learning and operant conditioning. *Psychological Review, 74*, 151–182.

Rhadigan, C., & Huprich, S. K. (2012). The utility of the cognitive–affective processing system in the diagnosis of personality disorders: Some preliminary evidence. *Journal of Personality Disorders, 26*, 162–178.

Rimm, D. C., DeGroot, J. C., Boord, P, Heiman, J., & Dillow, P. V. (1971). Systematic desensitization of an anger response. *Behaviour Research and Therapy, 9*, 273–280).

Ro, E., & Clark, L. A. (2013). Interrelations between psychosocial functioning and adaptive- and maladaptive-range personality traits. *Journal of Abnormal Psychology, 122*, 822–835.

Rogers, M. E., Creed, P. A., & Searle, J. (2012). Person and environmental factors associated with well-being in medical students. *Personality and Individual Differences, 52*, 472–477.

Rohsenow, D. J., Smith, R. E., & Johnson, S. (1985). Stress management training as a prevention program for heavy social drinkers: Cognitions, affect, drinking, and individual differences. *Addictive Behaviors, 10*, 45–54.

Rose, R. D., Juckley, J. C., Zbozinek, T. D. Motivala, S. J., Glenn, D. E., Cartreine, J. A., et al. (2013). A randomized controlled trial of a self-guided, multimedia, stress management and resilience training program. *Behaviour Research and Therapy, 51*, 106–112.

Rosen, G. M., Glasgow, R. E., & Barrera, M. (1976). A controlled study to assess the clinical efficach of totally self-administered systematic desensitization. *Journal of Consulting and Clinical Psychology, 44*, 208–217.

Rotter, J. B. (1966). Generalized expectancies for internal versus external control of reinforcement. *Psychological Monographs, 80* (Whole No. 609).

Rumbold, J. L., Fletcher, D., & Daniels, K. (2012). A systematic review of stress management interventions with sport performers. *Sport, Exercise, and Performance Psychology, 1*, 173–193.

Rumelhart, D. E., & McClelland, J. L. (1986). *Parallel distributed processing: Explorations in the microstructure of cognition* (Vols. 1 and 2). Cambridge, MA: MIT Press.

Russell, J. A., & Carroll, J. M. (1999). The phoenix of bipolarity: Reply to Watson and Tellegen (1999). *Psychological Bulletin, 125*, 611–617.

Sarason, I. G. (1958). The effects of anxiety, reassurance, and meaningfulness of material to be learned on verbal learning. *Journal of Experimental Psychology, 56*, 472–477.

Sarason, I. G. (1975). Test anxiety and the self-disclosing coping model. *Journal of Consulting and Clinical Psychology, 43*, 148–153.

Sarason, I. G. (1984). Stress, anxiety, and cognitive interference: Reactions to tests. *Journal of Personality and Social Psychology, 46*, 929–938.

Sarason, I. G., Johnson, J. H., & Siegel, J. M. (1978). Assessing the impact of life changes: Development of the Life Experiences Survey. *Journal of Consulting and Clinical Psychology, 46*, 932–946.

Sareen, J., Cox, B. J., Clara, I., & Asmundson, G. J. G. (2005). The relationship between anxiety disorders and physical disorders in the U.S. National Comorbidity Survey. *Depression and Anxiety, 21*, 193–202.

Saulsman, L. M., & Page, A. C. (2004). The five-factor model and personality disorder empirical literature: A meta-analytic review. *Clinical Psychology Review, 23*, 1055–1085.

Schachter, S. (1966). The interaction of cognitive and physiological determinants of emotional state. In C. D. Spielberger (Ed.), *Anxiety and behavior* (pp. 193–244). New York: Academic Press.

Schelver, S. R., & Gutsch, K. U. (1983). The effects of self-administered cognitive therapy on social-evaluative anxiety. *Journal of Clinical Psychology, 39,* 658–666.

Scherer, K. R., Schorr, A., & Johnstone, T. (2001). *Appraisal processes in emotion: Theory, methods, research.* New York: Oxford University Press.

Segal, Z. V., Williams, J. M., & Teasdale, J. D. (2002). *Mindfulness-based cognitive therapy for depression: A new approach to preventing relapse.* New York: Guilford Press.

Selye, H. (1956). *The stress of life.* New York: McGraw-Hill.

Sheppes, G. (2014). Emotion regulation choice: Theory and findings. In J. J. Gross (Ed.), *Handbook of emotion regulation* (2nd ed., pp. 126–139). New York: Guilford Press.

Sherrington, C. S. (1906). *Integrative action of the nervous system.* New Haven, CT: Yale University Press.

Shoda, Y., & Smith, R. E. (2004). Conceptualizing personality as a cognitive–affective processing system: A framework for models of maladaptive behavior patterns and change. *Behavior Therapy, 35,* 147–165.

Shoda, Y., Wilson, N. L., Chen, J., Gilmore, A. K., & Smith, R. E. (2013). Cognitive-affective processing system analysis of intra-individual dynamics in collaborative therapeutic assessment: Translating basic theory and research into clinical applications. *Journal of Personality, 81,* 554–568.

Shoham, V., Rohrbaugh, M. J., Onken, L. S., Cuthbert, B. N., Beveridge, R. M., & Fowles, T. R. (2014). Redefining clinical science training: Purpose and products of the Delaware project. *Clinical Psychological Science, 2,* 8–21.

Sipprelle, C. N. (1967). Induced anxiety. *Psychotherapy: Theory, Research, and Practice, 4,* 36–40.

Sipprelle, C. N. (1981). Development and theory of induced anxiety. In J. C. Ascough, C. H. Moore, & C. N. Sipprelle (Eds.), *Induced affect: A method for research and behavior change* (pp. 1–8). West Lafayette, IN: Center for Induced Affect.

Sloan, D., & Marx, D. (2004). A closer examination of the structured written disclosure procedure. *Journal of Consulting and Clinical Psychology, 72,* 165–175.

Smith, R. E. (1980). Development of an integrated coping response through cognitive-affective stress management training. In I. G. Sarason & C. D. Spielberger (Eds.), *Stress and anxiety* (Vol. 7, pp. 265–280). Washington, DC: Hemisphere.

Smith, R. E. (1984). Theoretical and treatment approaches to anxiety reduction. In J. M. Silva & R. S. Weinberg (Eds.), *Psychological foundations of sport* (pp. 157–170). Champaign, IL: Human Kinetics.

Smith, R. E. (1993). *Psychology.* Minneapolis/St. Paul: West.

Smith, R. E., & Ascough, J. C. (1985). Induced affect in stress management training. In S. Burchfield (Ed.), *Stress: Psychological and physiological interactions* (pp. 359–378). New York: Hemisphere.

Smith, R. E., Fagan, C., Wilson, N. L., Chen, J., Corona, M., Nguyen, H., et al. (2011). Internet-based approaches to collaborative therapeutic assessment: New opportunities for professional psychologists. *Professional Psychology: Research and Practice, 42,* 494–504.

Smith, R. E., & Johnson, J. (1990). An organizational empowerment approach to consultation in professional baseball. *The Sport Psychologist, 4,* 347–357.

Smith, R. E., Leffingwell, T. R., & Ptacek, J. T. (1999). Can people remember how they coped?: Factors associated with discordance between same-day and retrospective reports. *Journal of Personality and Social Psychology, 76,* 1050–1061.

Smith, R. E., & Nye, S. L. (1989). A comparison of induced affect and covert rehearsal in the acquisition of stress-management coping skills. *Journal of Counseling Psychology, 36,* 17–23.

Smith, R. E., Smoll, F. L., Cumming, S. P., & Grossbard, J. R. (2006). Measurement of multidimensional sport performance anxiety in children and adults: The Sport Anxiety Scale–2. *Journal of Sport and Exercise Psychology, 28,* 479–501.

Smith, T. W., & MacKenzie, J. (2006). Personality and risk of physical illness. *Annual Review of Clinical Psychology, 2,* 435–467.

Smyth, J. M., Pennebaker, J. W., & Arigo, D. (2012). What are the health effects of disclosure? In A. Baum, T. A. Revenson, & J. Singer (Eds.), *Handbook of health psychology* (2nd ed., pp. 175–191). New York: Psychology Press.

Snyder, C. R. (Ed.). (2001). *Coping with stress: Effective people and processes.* New York: Oxford University Press.

Soto, J. A., Perez, C. R., Kim, Y.-H., Lee, E. A., & Minnick, M. R. (2011). Is expressive *supresión* always associated with poorer psychological functioning?: A cross-cultural comparison between European Americans and Hong Kong Chinese. *Emotion, 11,* 1450–1455.

Speisman, J. C., Lazarus, R. S., Mordoff, A. M., & Davison, L. A. (1964). The experimental reduction of threat based on ego-defense theory. *Journal of Abnormal and Social Psychology, 68,* 367–380.

Spiegler, M. D., & Guevremont, D. C. (2003). *Contemporary behavior therapy* (5th ed.). Belmont, CA: Wadsworth.

Spiller, R. C. (2007). Role of infection in irritable bowel syndrome. *Journal of Gastroenterology, 42,* S41–S47.

Strauman, T. J., Goetz, E. L., Detloff, A. M., MacDuffie, K. E., Zaunmuller, L., & Lutz, W. (2013). Self-regulation and mechanisms of action in psychotherapy: A theory-based translational perspective. *Journal of Personality, 81,* 542–553.

Suinn, R. M. (1990). *Anxiety management training: A behavior therapy.* New York: Springer.

Suinn, R. M., & Richardson, F. (1971). Anxiety management training: A nonspecific behavior therapy program for anxiety control. *Behavior Therapy, 2,* 498–510.

Suls, J., & Bunde, J. (2005). Anger, anxiety, and depression as risk factors for cardiovascular disease: The problems and implications of overlapping affective dispositions. *Psychological Bulletin, 131,* 260–300.

Szabo, M. (2011). The emotional experience associated with worrying: Anxiety, depression, or stress? *Anxiety, Stress, and Coping, 24,* 91–105.

Taylor, J. A. (1953). A personality scale of manifest anxiety. *Journal of Abnormal and Social Psychology, 48,* 285–290.

Taylor, S. E. (2014). *Health psychology* (8th ed.). New York: McGraw-Hill.

Teasdale, J. D., Segal, Z., & Williams, J. M. (1995). How does cognitive therapy prevent relapse and why should attentional control (mindfulness) training help? *Behavioural Therapy and Research, 33,* 25–39.

Tellegen, A., Watson, D., & Clark, L. A. (1999). On the dimensional and hierarchical nature of affect. *Psychological Science, 10,* 297–303.

Tichener, E. B. (1916). *A textbook of psychology.* New York: Macmillan.

Tugade, M. M. (2011). Positive emotions and coping: Examining dual-process models of resilience. In S. Folkman (Ed.), *The Oxford handbook of stress, health, and coping* (pp. 186–199). New York: Oxford University Press.

Turner, J., Holtzman, S., & Mancl, L. (2009). Mediators, moderators, and predictors of therapeutic change in cognitive-behavioral therapy for chronic pain. *Pain, 127,* 276–286.

van Dixhoorn, J., & White, A. (2005). Relaxation therapy for rehabilitation and prevention of ischemic heart disease: A systematic review and meta-analysis. *European Journal of Cardiovascular Prevention and Rehabilitation, 12*, 193–202.

van Os, J., & Jones, P. B. (2001). Neuroticism as a risk factor for schizophrenia. *Psychological Medicine, 31*, 1129–1134.

Vogeltanz, N. D., & Hecker, J. E. (1999). The roles of neuroticism and controllability/predictability in physiological response to aversive stimuli. *Personality and Individual Differences, 27*, 599–612.

Watson, D. (2000). *Mood and temperament.* New York: Guilford Press.

Watson, J. C. (1998). The effects of cognitive–affective stress management training on game-time stress reactivity in high school volleyball coaches. *Dissertation Abstracts International: Section B: The Sciences and Engineering, 59*(6-B), 3045.

Webb, T. L., Miles, E., & Sheeran, P. (2012). Dealing with feeling: A meta-analysis of the effectiveness of strategies derived from the process model of emotion regulation. *Psychological Bulletin, 138*, 775–808.

Weinstock, L. M., & Whisman, M. A. (2006). Neuroticism as a common feature of depressive and anxiety disorders: A test of the revised integrative hierarchical model in a national sample. *Journal of Abnormal Psychology, 115*, 68–74.

Weisz, J. R., Ng, M. Y, & Bearman, S. K. (2014). Odd couple?: Reenvisioning the relation between science and practice in the dissemination-implementation era. *Clinical Psychological Science, 2*, 58–74.

Westen, D., Novotny, C. M., & Thompson-Brenner, H. (2004). The empirical status of empirically supported psychotherapies: Assumptions, findings, and reporting in controlled clinical trials. *Psychological Bulletin, 130*, 631–663.

Williams, S. L., Kinney, P. J., Harap, S. T., & Liebmann, M. (1997). Thoughts of agoraphobic people during scary tasks. *Journal of Abnormal Psychology, 106*, 511–520.

Wolberg, L. R. (1967). *The technique of psychotherapy.* New York: Grune & Stratton.

Wolff, H. G. (1953). *Stress and disease.* Springfield, IL: Thomas.

Wolgast, M., Lundh, I. G., & Viborg, G. (2011). Cognitive reappraisal and acceptance: An experimental comparison of two emotion regulation strategies. *Behaviour Research and Therapy, 49*, 858–866.

Wolpe, J. (1958). *Psychotherapy by reciprocal inhibition.* Stanford, CA: Stanford University Press.

Wooden, J., & Jamison, J. (2010) *The wisdom of Wooden: My century on and off the court.* New York: McGraw-Hill Education.

Young, J. E., Klosko, J. S., & Weishaar, M. E. (2003). *Schema therapy: A practitioner's guide.* New York: Guilford Press.

Zautra, A. J. (2006). *Emotions, stress, and health.* New York: Oxford University Press.

Ziegler, S. G., Klinzing, J., & Williamson, K. (1982). The effects of two stress management training programs on cardiorespiratory efficiency. *Journal of Sport Psychology, 4*, 280–289.

Index